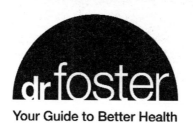

Your Guide to Better Health

# GOOD
# COMPLEMENTARY
# THERAPIST
# GUIDE

1   3   5   7   9   10   8   6   4   2

First published 2002 by Vermilion, an imprint of Ebury Press, Random House, 20 Vauxhall Bridge Road, London SW1V 2SA www.randomhouse.co.uk

Random House Australia (Pty) Limited 20 Alfred Street, Milsons Point, Sydney, New South Wales 2061, Australia

Random House New Zealand Limited 18 Poland Road, Glenfield, Auckland 10, New Zealand

Random House South Africa (Pty) Limited Endulini, 5a Jubilee Road, Parktown 2193, South Africa

The Random House Group Limited Reg. No. 954009

Papers used by Vermilion are natural, recyclable products made from wood grown in sustainable forests.

Printed and bound in Great Britain by Bookmarque Ltd,Croydon, Surrey

A CIP catalogue record for this book is available from the British Library.

ISBN 0091883784

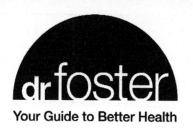

**Your Guide to Better Health**

# GOOD COMPLEMENTARY THERAPIST GUIDE

## Text and Data Compiled by Dr Foster

**LONDON**

# Acknowlegements

Dr Foster would like to thank the following for their time and help in compiling the information in this book. They are not, however, in any way responsible for anything included or omitted from the guide.

Gordon Brown

Mary Clarke

Christina Cunliffe

Michael Dixon

Liz Ellis

Edzard Ernst

Michael Fox

Andrew Gilmour

Torben Hersborg

Charles Hunt

Peter Jackson-Maine

Laurence Kirk

Nick Lampert

Michael McIntyre

Simon Mills

Renzo Molinari

NS Moorthy

Michael Murray

Trudy Norris

Mike O'Farrell

Sally Penrose

Margot Pinder

Persis Tamboly

Sue Wakefield

Lord Walton of Detchant

John Wheeler

Adrian White

Sarah Williams

Anne Woodham

# Contents

# Who is Dr Foster?

Dr Foster provides authoritative information on health services of all kinds in the UK. Our aim is to empower patients with information to help them access the best possible care. We are supervised by an independent Ethics committee that has legal powers to ensure that guides meet the highest standards and to investigate complaints.

The Ethics committee currently comprises the following membership:

**Dr Jack Tinker**, dean of the Royal Society of Medicine and chair of the committee
**Sir Donald Irvine**, former president, General Medical Council
**Dr Michael Dixon**, chair, NHS Alliance
**Peter Griffiths**, chief executive, Health Quality Service
**Dianne Hayter**, member of the board of the National Patient Safety Agency and the National Consumer Council
**Professor Alan Maynard**, director, Health Policy Unit, York University and chair, York Health Services NHS Trust
**Wilma MacPherson**, visiting professor at King's College London and a consultant in Health Services
**Bridget Gill**, chair of the Northern and Yorkshire Regional Council of the Institute of Healthcare Management
**Trevor Campbell Davis**, chief executive, Whittington Hospital
**Douglas Webb**, operations and development director, Friends of the Elderly
**Vanessa Bourne**, chair, Patients Association

**Dr Philip Davies**, medical director, Pontypridd and Rhondda NHS Trust
**Professor Nairn Wilson,** president of the General Dental Council.

---

## Dr Foster Help at Hand

Dr Foster collects data on local hospital, maternity and fertility services. It also has comprehensive information on hospital doctors and complementary therapists. Call the
**Help at Hand Service** on
**0906 190 0212**
to find the right solution to your health needs.
You can also visit
**www.drfoster.co.uk**
for information.

Calls cost £1.50 per minute; costs from mobile phones and some other networks may be more. Callers must be aged 18 or over. Lines are open Mon to Fri from 8.30am – 8pm, Sat 8.30am – 6pm.

Dr Foster Ltd.
Sir John Lyon House
5 High Timber Street
London EC4V 3NX

---

# Contributors

**Traditional Chinese Acupuncture**
John Wheeler holds a Licentiate in
Acupuncture from the College of
Traditional Acupuncture in
Leamington Spa. He is currently an
Executive Committee member,
Treasurer and Secretary of the
British Acupuncture Council. As
well as editing *Traditional
Acupuncture* Volumes 2 and 3 by
Professor JR Worsley, he has written
extensively within the profession
over the last decade and jointly
published occasional articles in peer
reviewed journals.

**Medical Acupuncture**
Dr Richard Halvorsen has worked as
a GP in central London for 13 years
and has studied traditional and
western acupuncture in the UK and
China. He is Chairman of a bi-
annual educational conference for
GPs and PR Officer for the BMAS.
He has published articles and
columns for a number of medical
magazines and papers, including a
regular column for The *Express*. He
has also talked about acupuncture
on TV and radio.

**Homeopathy**
The Faculty of Homeopathy, which
was incorporated by Act of
Parliament 1950, promotes the
academic and scientific
development of homeopathy. It
also regulates the education,
training and practice of
homeopathy by doctors, veterinary
surgeons, dentists, nurses,
midwives, pharmacists, podiatrists
and other statutorily registered
healthcare professionals. It
publishes the leading international
journal in the field, *Homeopathy*
(formerly the British Homeopathic
Journal) and is a founder member of
the European Committee for
Homeopathy.

The Faculty works closely with
the charity the British Homeopathic
Association and both organisations
aim to ensure that the benefits of
homeopathy are available to all.

**Chiropractic**
Dr Christina Cunliffe is a Fellow of
the College of Chiropractors and
currently holds the position of
Treasurer on the College Council.
She has been the Principal of the
McTimoney Chiropractic College
since 1998, and as well as
presenting extensively on the
McTimoney approach to
chiropractic around the world, is a
visiting lecturer at Oxford
University and Oxford Brookes
University.

**Chiropractic**
Manya McMahon BA (Hons),
MCIM, is a writer, editor and
chartered marketer with a special
interest in complementary health.
She has worked with the British
Chiropractic Association (BCA) for
over five years, producing a wide
range of information leaflets, web
pages and publicity material as well
as internal communications and

*Contact,* the BCA's quarterly members' journal. On this guide, she has worked closely with the BCA's Executive Director, Sue Wakefield, and Tim Hutchful, Chairman of their Marketing and PR Committee.

## Osteopathy

Andrew Gilmour is Senior Partner of one of the largest Osteopathic and Integrated Healthcare practices in the UK. He has been in full-time practice and at the forefront of the profession's development for more than 20 years. He has been a council member of The General Osteopathic Council with responsibilities for Education and Research, a board member of the British School of Osteopathy and is currently involved in a National Audit project.

## Western Herbalism

Charlotte Stedman is a member of the National Institute of Medical Herbalists (NIMH) and an ex-director of the NIMH Educational Foundation, which is responsible for the NIMH herbal medicine training clinics. Her publication, *Herbal Medicine – an information pack for health care professionals,* is available on the NIMH website. She is currently practising as a Medical Herbalist in an NHS Health Centre in North London.

## Chinese Herbalism

Jethro Rowland trained in Acupuncture and Traditional Chinese Medicine at the London School of Acupuncture and Traditional Chinese Medicine (LSATCM), and the London

Academy of Oriental Medicine. He has private practices in Hertfordshire, where he specialises in the treatment of people with drug problems, and he co-ordinates complementary therapies at the Chrysalis drug project in Hertford hospital.

## Ayurvedic medicine

Namasivayam Sathiyamoorthy has been practising Ayurvedic medicine and acupuncture in the UK since 1989 and is Director of the Eastern Clinic in South London. He is secretary of the Ayurvedic Medical Association and in 1991 helped in the founding of the World Ayurvedic Foundation. He appears twice a week on Sky's *Health Matters* programme, and has written for publications such as The *Daily Telegraph* and *Health and Fitness.*

## Methodology

Dr Adrian White worked for 5 years in general practice and 12 years in acupuncture practice, before joining the Department of Complementary Medicine in the University of Exeter in 1994, where he is now Senior Lecturer. Dr White has published widely on the subject of complementary medicine in general and acupuncture in particular, has edited 2 books on acupuncture, and is Editor of the journal *Complementary Therapies in Medicine.*

# Preface

In 2000, I was privileged to chair an inquiry launched by the House of Lords Select Committee on Science and Technology into complementary and alternative medicine (CAM). The report was published in March 2001 and subsequently debated in the House. My committee was aware that many individuals in the UK, and particularly those suffering from chronic and progressive conditions, were turning increasingly to complementary and alternative medicine in order to seek relief of their symptoms.

In my committee's enquiries, we were particularly concerned with issues such as definition, regulation, education, research and the availability of CAM in the NHS.

Two alternative disciplines, osteopathy and chiropractic, are now regulated by Acts of Parliament. People consulting these practitioners will know that if they are registered, they have achieved a high standard of education and training. Statutory regulation (regulation by law) may soon become possible in the case of western acupuncture, herbal medicine and homeopathy. Each of these professions has achieved satisfactory voluntary self-regulation (the achievement of uniformly high standards of education, training, and practice). While my committee recognised that Ayurvedic medicine and ancient Chinese medicine have been practised for many centuries, we were not convinced that the evidence supporting their respective philosophies was sound, but we fully recognised that many of the herbal preparations used by such practitioners contain effective herbal remedies which in due course we hope will be standardised so that they can be regulated by law in the same way as drugs used in conventional medicine are regulated at present. Increasing public interest, and indeed public demand, will undoubtedly result in the expansion of integrated medicine, and Dr Foster is to be congratulated. This guide will inform the British public about the present position with respect to many complementary and alternative disciplines available to the British public.

**Lord Walton of Detchant**, Kt, TD, MA, MD, DSc, FRCP, F MedSci
House of Lords Select Committee on Science and Technology

# Introduction

Whether you are new to complementary medicine or already visit an alternative practitioner, negotiating the bewildering mix of therapies available can be a daunting and perhaps even risky undertaking. How much do you know about your therapist's professional standards? How can you be sure that they are properly trained? Do they belong to a regulatory body should something go wrong? Although in Europe and the US it is very difficult to practice as an alternative therapist without state authorisation, most therapists in this country are unregulated: anybody can call themselves an acupuncturist, for example, with little or no training.

For the first time, *The Dr Foster Good Complementary Therapist Guide* has set out to measure and quantify certain standards to which we believe all complementary therapists should adhere. We have taken the 'big five' therapies – acupuncture, homoeopathy, osteopathy, chiropractic and herbal medicine – and asked some tough questions as to how they work and what, if any, are their benefits.

From now on, finding a good practitioner need not be such a lottery. With the help of the Department of Health, the Department of Complementary Medicine at the University of Exeter, The Foundation for Integrated Medicine, the NHS Alliance and leading practitioner bodies, we have formulated a series of benchmarks for best practice and questioned over 6000 practitioners as to whether they meet them. All those practitioners are listed in this guide. They are fully trained, belong to a professional regulating body, covered by insurance and follow a Code of Ethics. Whether you want to find out more about complementary medicine, or are simply looking to find a reliable practitioner in your area, this guide is an essential and unprecedented resource.

### How we produced this guide

We chose to look at the five therapies that were identified by the recent House of Lords Select Committee Report on CAM as being professionally organised with some scientific evidence of effectiveness and recognised systems of training.

Firstly we conducted consumer research to identify what information the public would most like to have when looking for a complementary therapist. We then teamed up with the Department of Complementary Medicine at the University of Exeter who assisted us in the development of a questionnaire which was sent to all practitioners of relevant bodies.

The questionnaires look at a range of issues that people said they wanted to know. For example, whether the therapist is a member of a properly regulated body, how much training they have, whether they are medically trained and the kind of environment they practise in.

We also asked the practitioners if they had communicated with a patient's GP regularly about diagnoses, should they feel this necessary. It does not mean a therapist is any worse at what they do if they rarely communicate with GPs – it may be more a reflection of the types of patients they treat rather than policy. However, we believe that complementary practitioners should always inform GPs about the treatments they provide, assuming that patients agree. There are rarely any great risks attached to seeing a complementary therapist, but problems have at times occurred when people with serious medical problems have visited a complementary practitioner who has failed to properly identify their illness. Keeping your GP informed is a good safety measure that can help prevent this.

This book also aims to answer other questions you may have about complementary therapists for example:

**Do I need a referral from my GP to visit a homeopath?**
Although you can refer yourself to any complementary practitioner, it is always a good idea to tell your GP what form of alternative treatment you are undertaking, and ask them to suggest a practitioner they know to be good. On p73 we tell you how to ask for homeopathy on the NHS and how your GP will decide to refer you to an appropriate practitioner.

**How do I know what will be in my herbal medicine?**
It is essential that you always visit a regulated practitioner who will tell you exactly what your medicine contains and how to take it. Herbal medicines can be harmful if not taken properly. Seeing a

properly regulated practitioner is also the only way you can be sure that your medicine does not contain harmful substances or steroids. On p129 of this guide, we tell you what to look out for when using herbal medicine.

**What are the risks associated with osteopathy?**
Osteopathy is safe and effective and serious side-effects are extremely rare. When they do occur, side-effects are usually due to poorly trained practitioners. On p94 of this guide, we explain how you can be sure your osteopath is properly trained.

**Where to find what you need**
This guide is unique. It falls into three sections, designed specifically to give you the information you need to decide whether a therapy is right for you and then how to find a professional, fully qualified practitioner in your area.

The first section explores the current issues surrounding complementary and alternative medicine (CAM). We look at how CAM works alongside orthodox medicine, discuss the importance of regulation, look into what research is being undertaken and what, if any, evidence there is as to CAM's efficacy. We also give general guidelines on how to find a reliable practitioner should you want to find a practitioner of a therapy not covered in this guide.

The second section explores the therapies themselves. We take you through them step by step and tell you whether your treatment is safe and what research has been done to qualify this, what your medicines will contain and how to make sure that your practitioner is properly trained and regulated.

The third section lists over 6000 practitioners by region and town, all of whom will be fully qualified and registered with an appropriate regulatory body. We tell you where they practise (whether privately or with the NHS), how much they cost (and if they offer reduced rates) and whether they meet our suggested benchmarks for best practice (for instance, how many hours training acupuncturists have taken and whether they will work alongside your GP as part of your treatment).

## What we tell you about the practitioners

Among other things (see p188 for more information), we tell you:

### Who regulates the practitioner

All practitioners in this guide are members of organisations that require proper training, professional indemnity insurance and which maintain adequate complaints and disciplinary procedures.

### Where and when they practise

Some therapists work from home, others work in clinics and some may work alongside practitioners of other therapies. It is up to you as to where you feel more comfortable visiting your practitioner. We tell you where they work, whether they work outside normal working hours and give you the contact details of their main practice.

### Their relationship with orthodox medicine

We believe that your practitioner should communicate with your GP and give them details of your treatment. We tell you which practitioners do this.

Your practitioner should never advise you to stop taking your conventional medication, although they may choose to work with you alongside your GP to help you find an alternative form of treatment for your condition.

We also tell you if a practitioner regularly takes referrals from the NHS as this suggests that they will have a good working relationship with your GP.

### Their fees

Fees vary geographically – practitioners in London are more expensive than those in other parts of the country. Also, the first consultation is often longer and so costs more. We also tell you which practitioners offer reduced fees.

Section One:

# An Introduction to Complementary and Alternative Medicine (CAM)

# Why is complementary medicine so popular?

A 1995 survey[1] found that many people turn to complementary medicine because they believe it to be more effective for their condition than conventional medicine. In a 1999 BBC survey, 25 per cent of respondents said they use CAM because it helps or relieves their condition; 21 per cent 'just like it', 19 per cent find it relaxing. Intriguingly, 11 per cent use CAM because they do not believe that conventional medicine works, the same percentage as those referred or recommended by conventional doctors. The question of expense was not included, but the fact of paying for treatment, in commitment as well as financially, could be seen as adding to its value.

An earlier American survey[2] concluded that people did not necessarily use CAM because they were dissatisfied with conventional care. As well as being better educated and in poorer overall health, most users choose CAM therapies because they find them to be 'more congruent with their own values, beliefs and philosophical orientations towards health and life'. Added to this is the fact that CAM patients prefer the overall experience that alternative therapies provide, not least the amount of time that practitioners can afford to give.

Many of us combine complementary and conventional medicine without even thinking. At the first sign of a cold, we'll dose ourselves with the herbal immunity-booster echinacea in the hope of staving off the worst, then turn to paracetamol to ease the symptoms. Someone on medication for high blood pressure may practise yoga to ease stress, or someone with migraine may see an acupuncturist as well as taking sumatriptan prescribed by the doctor.

A form of medicine that combines these two different approaches – though in a less pick and mix fashion – is seen by many experts as a

---

[1] *British Journal of Clinical Psychology,* 1995

[2] *Journal of the American Medical Association,* 1998

pattern for twenty-first-century healthcare. For one thing, orthodox medicine can no longer ignore the overwhelming popularity of complementary and alternative medicine. The 1999 BBC survey found that one in five people had used complementary therapy in the last 12 months, spending on average £14 per month in paying practitioners and buying products – about £1.6 billion a year. Industry sources estimate that the market for herbal and homeopathic medicines and aromatherapy essential oils was worth £109 million in 2000, and predict a rise to £126 million in 2002.

To coin a phrase, complementary medicine is in the pink of health. And the situation in the UK is reflected in other western countries. Surveys show that roughly half of all Americans and Australians use some form of CAM.

With all the sophisticated wizardry of modern medical science, why have complementary and alternative therapies gained such a following? The very success of conventional medicine in the twentieth century may itself be a factor. Medical and scientific breakthroughs – such as the discovery of antibiotics and other wonder drugs, dramatic open-heart operations, keyhole surgery, MRI scans and gene therapy – have combined with improved living standards and mass inoculation programmes to raise people's expectations of health and healthcare. The medical profession has found itself on a pedestal, an exalted position that many physicians have come to believe is their right.

When miracle drugs were found to have unpleasant and even fatal side-effects, and bacteria developed resistance to 'infallible' antibiotics, the public's faith was shaken. Progress in fighting cancer appears painstakingly slow and complicated. Pharmaceutical drugs and surgical procedures do not seem able to deliver trouble-free cures for chronic and uncomfortable conditions like back pain and arthritis. Many have begun to feel that conventional medicine no longer holds all the answers and could even be responsible for some of the problems.

A flight from science, fuelled by associated issues like environmental pollution and the power of multinational business corporations, is one element in the interest in complementary and alternative medicine. Disenchantment with the medical profession and its perceived authoritarian attitude is another. This is not the whole story, however. Easier access to information through mass media and the Internet has enabled lay people to become extraordinarily savvy about health and medicine. Add to this a government-backed health policy that encourages responsibility for our own wellbeing and a healthy lifestyle, and the resulting patient-power means that we want to be involved in discussions about treatment. This is not something that the average hard-pressed General Practitioner (GP) has the time or perhaps the inclination or training to provide.

Enter complementary medicine, in which the initial consultation is often an hour or more, with plenty of time to discuss symptoms, lifestyle, past experiences, and relationships. Practitioners follow a holistic approach in which all aspects of a person – emotional, mental, even spiritual as well as physical – are regarded as equally important in the restoration and maintenance of health.

## What is the medical support for CAM?

Patients' enthusiasm has led a number of doctors and nurses to investigate complementary medicine for themselves and medical attitudes have softened considerably since 1980, when the British Medical Association suggested chiropractic was no better than the 'examination of a bird's entrails'. Now nearly 40 per cent of general practices in England provide access to some form of complementary therapy for NHS patients, though not necessarily free of charge. Acupuncture is the most favoured. GPs are so impressed with acupuncture that almost half (47 per cent) now arrange treatment for their patients, 46 per cent would like training so they can practise it themselves, and 79 per cent want acupuncture available on the NHS[1]. In fact, 86 per cent of NHS pain clinics already offer it. And this is a therapy

---

[1] according to a *British Medical Association* report in 2000

that as recently as 1986 BMA doctors labelled ineffective and dangerous!

The terminology has changed too. Twenty years ago 'alternative' referred to any therapy that was not generally provided by or taught to orthodox health professionals such as doctors, dentists and nurses. Today it is reserved for treatments that are truly 'alternative', those therapies given in place of orthodox medical care as, for example, when cancer patients are urged to abandon chemotherapy and radiotherapy to follow extreme dietary regimes or take controversial supplements like laetrile or shark cartilage.

Gradually the word 'complementary' has come to describe treatments that could be used alongside conventional treatment – osteopathy, chiropractic and massage therapy, for instance. Or self-help measures like yoga or meditation. Far from having to choose one approach or the other, both patients and complementary therapists expect orthodox medication and procedures to continue. Complementary therapies have even found their way into hospices and NHS cancer units like the one at Charing Cross Hospital, London. Here, nurses and supervised practitioners use 'touch' therapies like aromatherapy and reflexology, or mind-body techniques such as relaxation, visualisation or hypnotherapy to relieve anxiety and help patients cope with intimidating procedures.

Alternative medicine is most popular for the treatment of chronic conditions like arthritis and back pain, or stubborn stress-related ailments that come and go like eczema, hay fever, irritable bowel syndrome and headaches. These are also the ones that doctors find the most difficult and frustrating to deal with and so might welcome another approach, especially if it is a therapy like massage or homoeopathy.

However, complementary medicine is still controversial among doctors. We asked two GPs – one in favour of CAM and the other opposed – to explain their views. Mike Dixon makes his case for increased availability of alternative medicine on the NHS on p8 while Lorna Gold explains why she is adamantly against it on p12.

## What is integrated medicine?

Medical practitioners who are persuaded of the benefits of complementary therapies now talk of 'integrated medicine' that combines the best of both fields. Rather than making your own 'ad hoc' choice of therapy, influenced perhaps by a magazine article, an advertisement or a friend's experience, you would visit your GP, who, while prescribing drugs or further tests if necessary, might refer you to one of the complementary therapists attached to the practice.

Integrated medicine focuses on health and healing rather than disease and treatment, say Professor Lesley Rees, director of education at the Royal College of Physicians, and Dr Andrew Weil, director of the integrative medicine programme at the University of Arizona[1]. 'It views patients as whole people with minds and spirits as well as bodies and includes these dimensions into diagnosis and treatment. It also involves patients and doctors working to maintain health by paying attention to lifestyle factors such as diet, exercise, quality of rest and sleep, and the nature of relationships.'

Strangely, things have come full circle. This holistic ethos is not only intrinsic to the ideology of health systems such as homeopathy, Chinese and Ayurvedic medicine, but was advocated over 2000 years ago by the Greek physician Hippocrates, the 'father' of modern medicine. The body is said to have a natural tendency towards equilibrium or 'homeostasis', and maintaining this internal balance and boosting the body's self-healing powers are crucial to long-term good health and wellbeing. Poor diet, lack of exercise and other lifestyle failings create a weakness in homeostasis that leaves the individual susceptible to disease, and balanced treatment will address these problems as well as specific symptoms. As Lorna Gold points out on p13, this kind of 'holistic' care is not confined only to complementary practitioners. To some extent, most good NHS doctors will take lifestyle factors into account. However, GPs are often pressed for time and

---

[1] *British Medical Journal*, January 2001

complementary practitioners believe that orthodox medicine often focuses too much on identifying a patient's illness rather than considering other aspects of their lives that may be relevant.

At present, apart from a handful of innovative general practices, there is not much in the way of genuinely integrated health care provision around. Marylebone Health Centre in London, which opened in 1987, was the first NHS practice to employ complementary therapists, and is the subject of a long-term research study into implementing integrated medicine. The team comprises three full-time and two part-time family doctors, an osteopath, homeopath, naturopath, acupuncturist, massage therapist and a counsellor. The GPs act as 'gatekeepers' and will refer a patient to a therapist if they think it appropriate, according to guidelines hammered out over hours of discussion and regular re-evaluation. Dr Sue Morrison, who is in charge of the practice, believes that complementary medicine has helped to cut referrals to specialists and led to a drug-prescribing rate that is half the national average.

Glastonbury Health Centre, Glastonbury, is another example of an integrated NHS practice that has supported its cost-effectiveness. Patients are offered acupuncture, herbal medicine, homeopathy, massage therapy and osteopathy in the same way that orthodox practices offer physiotherapy or medication. According to an evaluation study in the 1990s, 85 per cent of patients referred to complementary therapists reported some or much improvement. In two-thirds of patients, general vitality, social functioning, emotional and mental health improved significantly.

The Foundation of Integrated Medicine makes Awards for Good Practice in Integrated Healthcare. Short-listed projects for 2001 included a smoking cessation programme at the Clayton NHS Health Centre, Manchester, that integrates conventional treatments with hypnosis and acupuncture, and the Maternity Acupuncture Service at Derriford Hospital, Plymouth, which provides acupuncture for antenatal and postnatal problems and pain-relief during labour.

# A Doctor's view

Mike Dixon, GP

The introduction of complementary medicine to my own practice was patient rather than doctor led. Several of my patients were seeing local healers and saying that they were doing them more good than my medicine. I was intrigued and my purpose in asking a healer to come and work at College Surgery, Cullompton, in 1992 was largely to fuel my own curiosity. Now, in 2001, there are two healers working in my surgery and these are testimony to a service that both local GPs and patients value and wish to continue.

In those early days, our 'healing clinic' was financed by money provided by the previous government for 'health promotion clinics'. The definition of these clinics was hazy to say the least and provided an ideal opportunity for innovations of this sort. The healers saw all the kinds of patients with conditions that conventional medicine did not seem to help much – eg long-term skin conditions, ME, depression, stress, back pain, some forms of arthritis, etc. Patients seemed to get better but also to call upon conventional GP services less. These impressions were confirmed in a controlled trial that we eventually published in the *Journal of the Royal Society of Medicine.* This showed that our patients seeing a healer were significantly better 50 per cent of the time (having tried all other remedies previously), were able to do more and were generally happier and less anxious.

Funding the provision of complementary medicine within the NHS is always difficult – especially for services based at practice level. Health promotion clinics were a useful device for surgeries such as my own, while GP fundholders were also able to use money for the same purpose. Neither system currently exists and in our own surgery we have had to be inventive with the use of research money in order to provide an ongoing service to patients in the practice. Currently, this money has now run out and we are having to look at voluntary donations by patients. We see this as the only means of continuing a service that is free at the point of delivery and available to all. The alternative will be to invite private practitioners into the surgery and for them to charge patients who see them.

However we do it, I am sure the clinic will continue. There are too many benefits that come from orthodox and complementary practitioners working together. Orthodox practitioners would say that it is safer because patients are medically screened before referral. The good communication between orthodox and complementary practitioners ensures that patients get the best of both worlds and the exchange of ideas between orthodox and complementary practitioners leads to more patient-orientated attitudes. The benefit for doctors is that they end up with better, happier and frequently less demanding patients because the holistic nature of complementary medicine means that patient perception and attitude is affected by treatment as well as the bare symptoms. It also makes the best use of everyone's time. Though GPs in the partnership variously practice hypnosis and manipulation, for instance, it is more cost effective for the GP to use their time and skills on complex diagnosis and conventional treatment, while leaving the complementary therapist (where appropriate) to provide specialist treatment according to their own skills.

Many GPs are now happy to suggest complementary alternatives for their patients but seeing a private practitioner will remain the main means of access for the time being, while NHS resources are so scarce.

## The House of Lords Report

The widespread proliferation of complementary and alternative medicine led the House of Lords Select Committee on Science and Technology to make a 15-month study of CAM. Its report, published in November 2000, came to several blunt conclusions. Research into whether these therapies work is virtually non-existent. Training courses in complementary and alternative therapies vary unacceptably in content, depth and duration. And regulation of the multiplying number of different specialities is fragmented and inadequate.

'There is a clear need for more effective guidance for the public as to what does or does not work and what is or is not safe in CAM,' said the Select Committee report. Most therapies were considered relatively harmless in themselves, although acupuncture, osteopathy, chiropractic and herbal medicine were recognised as having the potential to cause damage in the hands of inadequately trained practitioners. But the main danger of CAM, the Committee felt, lay in the possibility that patients could miss a conventional medical diagnosis and treatment because they chose only to consult a CAM practitioner, who may not have the skills or experience to recognise serious symptoms.

It divided therapies into three groups, based on the claims they make, the supporting evidence they could produce, and the degree to which they are professionally organised.

In Group 1, which best fulfilled these criteria, were the 'big five': acupuncture, chiropractic, herbal medicine, homeopathy and osteopathy. Group 2 included therapies where supporting evidence was lacking but which could safely be used to complement – though not replace – conventional medicine: Alexander technique, aromatherapy, Bach and other flower remedies, bodywork therapies such as massage, counselling stress therapies, hypnotherapy, meditation, reflexology, shiatsu, healing, nutritional medicine and yoga. Into Group 3 were bundled alternative and diagnostic treatments that the Committee found scientifically unproven and unregulated: anthroposophical medicine, Ayurvedic medicine, traditional Chinese medicine, Eastern medicine (Tibb), naturopathy, crystal therapy, dowsing, iridology, kinesiology and radionics.

## Research

Demands on NHS funds are enormous and doctors and healthcare managers are understandably reluctant to fund treatments that lack a strong evidence base to show that they work. Although the 50,000 or so CAM therapists in the UK (who outnumber GPs by 10,000) might argue that only 20 per cent of modern medicine is evidence-based, this situation is rapidly being addressed and new drugs or procedures are backed by rigorous trials. By contrast, much complementary therapy is still taken largely on trust and high-quality research studies are few and far between.

There are a number of reasons for this. 'Gold standard' randomised clinical trials cost money and funding is difficult to find. Conventional medicine derives much of its research income from two sources: universities and hospitals who may hesitate to compromise their reputation by dabbling in unorthodox therapies; and pharmaceutical companies who are unlikely to invest in a therapy without the prospect of financially attractive patents. Most herbal remedies, for example, have been in use for centuries, and manufacturers of herbal and homeopathic remedies are usually relatively small companies who lack funds for large-scale trials.

What serious trials of complementary medicine have been carried out have been predominantly in the US or Europe. The US government's National Center for Complementary and Alternative Medicine (NCCAM) has a research budget of nearly $80 million to fund 11 research centres across the country which evaluate alternative treatment for chronic health conditions, such as asthma, arthritis and addictions. NCCAM also collaborates with other governmental bodies, as, for example, the US National Cancer Institutes.

The picture in the UK is very different. Although the Lords Report recommended that the NHS and the Medical Research Council siphon

# A Doctor's view

Lorna Gold, GP

I do not believe that mainstream medical practice should be making room for complementary therapy. I cannot understand how those doctors who recommend or even practise complementary therapies can reconcile the meaningless pseudoscience that underpins aromatherapy and flower remedies with their medical training and their conscience, and I regard the British Medical Association's recent decision to move towards working more closely with the complementary therapy industry as a betrayal.

What is a complementary therapy, after all? Acupuncture with its meridians, and homoeopathy with its serial dilutions, are based on theory which, although completely fictitious, is plausible enough to convince the scientifically naïve that there might be something in it. But what about iridology? Or crystal healing? Or the ludicrous LaStone therapy? How naked does an emperor have to be before his nakedness becomes obvious to everyone? Where does one draw the line between therapy and non-therapy – before or after feng shui?

What these products all have in common, in my view, is that there is no consistent hard evidence for their effectiveness. This situation has nothing to do with the oft-recited argument that therapeutic testing is funded by a pharmaceutical industry which has no interest in researching cheap traditional remedies. Nothing is cheaper or more traditional than aspirin, yet it has been extensively researched, and found to be of benefit in previously unsuspected treatment areas, in recent years. There is a simple explanation for the lack of evidence that alternative remedies have any medicinal value: they have nothing like the impact that orthodox medicines have – medicines which have been proven to cure infections, prevent heart attacks or save the lives of premature babies. There are no complementary therapies you could trust to have the same effect. No complementary therapy has ever been shown to cure an infection, prevent a single heart attack, or save the life of a premature baby. They are no more effective than placebo treatment even when tested using softer criteria such as making allergy symptoms a little bit better or easing pain. If a substance or intervention shows promise, it is quickly taken up, tested, and, if its effectiveness can be proven, it becomes conventional medicine.

Nor does the popularity of complementary therapy add to its credibility. Complementary therapy is the ultimate consumer product for this generation. It is overwhelmingly self-indulgent and its place in society is alongside lavishly packaged cosmetics and designer clothing.

Complementary therapy cannot claim to be holistic – treating people rather than symptoms. On the contrary, there is nothing at all holistic about answering an exhaustive list of leading questions which sound as if the practitioner is interested in you as an individual, but which is really designed to elicit a 'diagnosis' from a limited professional vocabulary.

Truly holistic healthcare is found where, according to the complementary therapy industry, you might least expect it – in the NHS. Your GP and the team with whom he or she works is likely to have known you and other members of your family for many years and to have learned a great deal about your cultural background, about the personal and family beliefs and attitudes which will influence your response to healthcare, about your own and your family's medical history which can help to predict – and prevent – the health problems to which you are particularly susceptible. An average consultation with your GP may last a meagre 8 minutes, but over the years they will get to know you pretty well.

I do not object to the existence of complementary therapy. On the whole, it is harmless. All I ask is that we recognise it for what it is – a sophisticated and heavily marketed lifestyle product – and stop trying to call it medicine.

more funding into CAM research, little has happened. Figures from the Department of Complementary Medicine at the University of Exeter show that 0.08 per cent of NHS funds for medical research was spent on complementary medicine. In 1998–99 the Medical Research Council spent nothing at all, and in 1999 only 0.05 per cent of the total research budget of UK charities went to this area. The Arthritis Research Campaign is one of the very few to allocate funds to study CAM, starting with a trial of acupuncture and knee osteoarthritis at Newcastle University and another of magnetic bracelets in Devon. But then, 66 per cent of arthritis patients are known to use alternative therapies already, and most say they prefer approaches that allow them to feel they are doing something for themselves, rather than drug-based treatments that may have severe side-effects.

Apart from the expense, the protocol involved in setting up clinical trials is exhaustive. The most convincing, and the most difficult, is the randomised placebo-controlled trial. To avoid any bias, patients are assigned at random to two or three groups: one that receives the treatment under investigation, one (the control) that receives nothing and/or another that receives a seemingly identical but inactive treatment (the placebo). The more subjects the better – a study of 200 or 2000 people has greater credibility than one of 20 – but large numbers of patients are usually only available through big organisations like the NHS or university hospitals. The ultimate challenge is the double-blind study, in which not even the practitioners know which patients are receiving the real treatment or the placebo, so that individual influences are ruled out.

A cheaper alternative is the systematic review or meta-analysis which evaluates the results of a number of trials. For most complementary therapies, however, not enough studies have been carried out to make this analysis worthwhile, although in the 1990s several reviews of this type did show that homeopathic treatments, acupuncture and chiropractic have clinical benefits.

Who carries out these studies? So far most research in complementary medicine has been done by doctors with an interest in the field. Few complementary therapists yet have the expertise to conduct a scientifically acceptable study; colleges that train practitioners have only recently begun to include research in the curriculum, and few are linked to universities or hospitals with research facilities. Exceptions are the Department of Complementary Medicine at the University of Exeter, and the University of Southampton, where academic researchers work with complementary practitioners in devising and conducting trials. Funding, however, is still a major hurdle.

And besides, many complementary therapists are wary of the constraints of scientific trials. How can you measure something as subtle as Qi, the 'vital force', or 'healing energy'? Is it possible to devise a trial that takes into account treatment that is tailored to individual patients, or rate a result that makes someone feel better, even if they are not cured or even physiologically improved?

Even so, growing consumer awareness and European Community regulations that demand proof for products making medicinal claims are driving greater research efforts. Good evidence already exists, published in top peer-reviewed medical journals, that some complementary treatments can help certain conditions. Studies[1] have shown that the herbal remedy St John's wort worked as well as tri-cyclic antidepressants for mild to moderate depression. A systematic review in the *Journal of the American Medical Association* in 1998 found that another herb, saw palmetto, could help relieve the symptoms of benign prostate problems. And in 2000, sufficient rigorous clinical trials showed that acupuncture was more effective than control procedures for back pain, nausea and vomiting, migraine and dental pain to persuade the British Medical Association to recommend it be made available on the NHS.

It helps if there is a possible scientific explanation. Increasing evidence shows that acupuncture, for instance, may influence the

---

[1] *British Medical Journal,* 1996 and *The Lancet,* 2000

nervous system, triggering the release of endorphins, the body's natural painkillers, mood-enhancing chemical messengers like serotonin and noradrenaline, and certain hormones such as oxytocin. It is also easy to understand how herbal medicine and manipulative therapies like osteopathy and chiropractic could work, but even non-sceptical medics stumble over homeopathy. The idea that minute quantities of a substance might affect physiology is just about acceptable, but that a substance becomes more powerful the more it is diluted, to the point where scarcely a molecule remains, defies current scientific knowledge. But we may yet find scientific support for homeopathic theories. A recent South Korean study has surprised chemists by appearing to show that some molecules can clump together as a solution is diluted. It may provide the first serious indication that homeopathic theory is on to something.

**Regulation**

In this guide we discuss in depth how each therapy is regulated. The main purpose of regulation for any health care profession is to protect the public from unqualified or inadequately trained practitioners. Without it, anyone can pass themselves off – as already happens – as an 'acupuncturist', with little or no training.

The House of Lords Committee was disturbed to discover that a number of therapists practised on the basis of 'seriously inadequate' home study courses. Within some therapies, various professional bodies with widely differing standards were often in active competition. 'It is very hard for the public to know where to look to find a "competent" therapist', said the Committee, strongly urging each complementary therapy to unite its practitioners under a single regulatory body that could promote itself to the public and supply information to doctors and other healthcare professionals.

In the case of therapies in Group 2 (Alexander technique, aromatherapy, Bach and other flower remedies, bodywork therapies such as massage, counselling stress therapies, hypnotherapy, meditation, reflexology, shiatsu, healing, nutritional medicine and yoga) whose potential to harm is minimal, voluntary self-regulation was considered sufficient. A regulatory body would:

- Maintain a register of individual members or member organisations
- Set educational standards and accredit training establishments
- Run a continuing professional development programme
- Provide codes of conduct, ethics and practice
- Organise a complaints mechanism and disciplinary procedure accessible to the public
- Require members to take out adequate professional indemnity insurance.

Such bodies, however, could not stop someone practising as, for example, an 'aromatherapist' or 'reflexologist', however inadequate their qualifications.

Those in Group 1 (acupuncture, homeopathy, osteopathy, chiropractic and herbal medicine) which have the potential in untrained hands to cause harm, should work towards statutory regulation, says the Report. This differs from voluntary regulation in being enforceable by law. Statutory regulation is achieved either by an Act of Parliament, as the osteopaths and chiropractors have already done, or through provisions in the Health Act 1999 which allow new professions to join the Health Professions Council and which create the possibility of new uni-professional statutory bodies.

Statutory regulation would undoubtedly facilitate a therapy's integration into the NHS. There are other advantages. Protection of title means that practitioners who are struck off a register for misconduct or malpractice cannot continue to practise as a member of that profession, and disciplinary procedures are underpinned by law. (For example, General Medical Council [GMC] registration is necessary in order to practise as a doctor in the UK.) A single register of practitioners is legally required, which makes it easy for the public to find out who is, and who is not, properly qualified. Specific advantages might also apply to herbal medicine. Anomalies in the Medicines Act 1968 currently permit unregulated practitioners to supply potentially harmful herbs, but these could become available only to herbalists on the statutory register.

Gaining statutory regulation has its pitfalls, as the osteopaths discovered after the Osteopathy Act was passed in 1993 (see p96). Among those already calling themselves osteopaths training ranged from four-year degree courses to as little as a handful of weekends, and there were nine different voluntary registers. The new regulatory body, the General Osteopathic Council, decided that all would-be members, no matter how many years in practice, must complete a professional portfolio and profile to demonstrate their competence. Inevitably there were some failures, which caused considerable discontent, but from the patient's point of view, a rigorous vetting procedure is reassuring. Like chiropractic, which went through a similar process after the Chiropractic Act of 1994, osteopathy involves manipulation that could be harmful in conditions like cancer or osteoporosis. It is vital that practitioners know their own limitations and know when to refer to a doctor.

Of the other 'big five', acupuncture and herbal medicine are actively moving towards statutory regulation. The European Herbal Practitioners Association (EPHA) (see p133), which represents the majority of UK herbalists, is following the Health Act route and seems set for success. Although the EHPA has had to contend recently with a rash of alarming stories about adverse reactions to Chinese herbs and public statements about the potential for harm in herbal medicines, it has argued with great clarity its members' conviction that statutory regulation is the single most effective way to bring the levels of safety and guarantees of standards which the public has a right to expect. This view is shared by the policy makers, and rapid progress towards statutory regulation will preserve the benefits to the public while reducing the risk.

## Complementary Therapies and Evidence

There is growing demand for hard statistical evidence that shows whether particular medical treatments work – both in conventional and complementary medicine.

The gold standard for testing a therapy is the double-blind randomised controlled trial. Patients are given either the treatment, or a fake treatment, known as a placebo. Double-blind means that neither the people receiving the treatment, nor the people managing the trial, know who is receiving the real treatment until after the trial is finished. This is important since, in trials that are not blind, the bias of the patients and those conducting the test will tend to influence the results.

Randomised trials were developed to test pharmaceuticals and are not always appropriate for complementary therapies where every patient is given an individualised treatment. Despite this, there have been many trials of complementary therapies. These trials compare therapies to sham therapies (eg acupuncture where needles are incorrectly placed). This is to discount the placebo effect where patients feel better simply because they are being treated – regardless of how they are treated.

Some are small or are poorly designed (for example they are not double-blind) and often a badly designed trial will suggest that the therapy works, when more stringent tests fail to find any effect.

Several organisations conduct systematic reviews of clinical trials which weigh up all the evidence for and against a particular treatment. Two well-regarded organisations that publish such reviews are the Cochrane Library (www.cochrane.org) and Bandolier (www.jr2.ox.ac.uk/bandolier/).

Systematic reviews often conclude that, although some trials support a particular therapy, overall there is insufficient evidence to recommend it. This may be because the therapy does not work, or it may just be that no no one has yet proved that it does. But treat with caution any claim that a therapy has been 'clinically proven' to work.

**Training**

The greatest hurdles in forming a single professional body are education and training criteria. In the relevant therapy sections of this guide, we explain your practitioner's training. The acupuncturists and homeopaths have some particularly thorny problems in this area. In both therapies, some practitioners are doctors while others are not. The problem is compounded for the acupuncturists by the range in levels of training required by the various providers of acupuncture, and the widely differing philosophies behind them (see p47). The British Medical Acupuncture Society, for example, has over 1700 members who can practise within the NHS. With anatomy and physiology already under their belts – so there's little risk of someone sticking a needle in a vital organ (rare but possible) – medics can gain the Society's certificate of basic competence in acupuncture after a couple of residential weekends. The diploma is more demanding, requiring half a dozen weekend courses and 100 case histories over a two-year period.

Many non-medical acupuncturists who practise Traditional Chinese Medicine (TCM), however, tend to dismiss the doctors' acupuncture training as a 'cop-out', arguing that a few weekends is not long enough to comprehend the ancient philosophy behind the procedure. The Lords Select Committee also pointed out that, even though medically qualified, doctors who practise a complementary therapy owe it to the public to be as competent in that therapy as any other practitioner of it.

The British Medical Acupuncture Society and the Acupuncture Association of Chartered Physiotherapists are working with the leading non-medical organisation, the British Acupuncture Council, to establish common ground. The Council's stringent three-year educational requirements, which include courses in conventional anatomy and physiology, are privately accepted by many doctors as more than satisfactory, and hopes are high that regulation can eventually be achieved.

Homeopathy is another story, however (see p70). On the one hand, the Faculty of Homeopathy regulates the practice of homeopathy by statutorily registered health professionals – doctors, dentists, nurses, vets and pharmacists. If, for instance, the GMC received a complaint about the practice of homeopathy by a doctor, it could call on the Faculty to advise on their competence.

Professional homeopaths, on the other hand, have neither conventional medical qualifications nor a single registering body. The largest self-regulatory organisation is the Society of Homeopaths, whose 800 members complete a testing six-month registration process over and above their training at Society-accredited colleges. While there are now several three-year full-time courses, including a BSc Hons in Homeopathy at Westminster University, that offer a grounding in medical sciences, other courses are by correspondence or involve only one weekend a month.

The various bodies representing professional homeopaths have set up the Council of Organisations Representing Homeopaths (CORH) to seek common ground to establish a register of non-medically qualified homeopaths, and recently there have been meetings with the Faculty. But education and training standards are likely to be major stumbling blocks. As Dr Bob Leckridge, president of the Faculty, has pointed out, 'We don't all start from the same place'.

Scientific evidence for homeopathy is contentious, although *The Lancet* has published well-devised trials by Dr David Reilly of Glasgow Homeopathic Hospital, that found homeopathic remedies relieved symptoms of hay fever, asthma and rhinitis. Nor does it carry inherent risks in practice, which would make statutory regulation advisable. But the Lords Select Committee believes that because some patients see homeopathy as a complete alternative to conventional medicine, homeopaths are in a position of great responsibility. 'It is imperative that there is a way of ensuring that this position is handled professionally, that all homeopaths are registered, that they know the limits of their competence, and there are disciplinary procedures with real teeth in place,' says the report. Statutory regulation for professional homeopaths might facilitate more co-operation and collaboration with the Faculty.

**You and your practitioner**

This guide is specifically designed to help you find a professional and fully trained practitioner in your area. As well as listing practitioners who will meet these standards, we also give you guidelines on what questions to ask before you visit them for each therapy we cover. Should things go wrong, we also tell you how to complain and who to. However, as a general rule, your should be aware of the following issues when visiting any alternative practitioner.

**Before the consultation**

Always ensure that a practitioner is adequately trained and insured, especially if the therapy involves either physical manipulation (osteopathy, chiropractic) or invasive techniques (ie swallowing herbal or any other medicine or having acupuncture needles inserted into you). The best way to ensure this is to check whether they are members of an appropriate professional body. Use the practitioners listed in this guide, or contact the relevant professional organisation for a list of practitioners in your area. You can also ask your GP as they may well have had good (or bad) experience of therapists from your area.

If a practitioner is recommended by another person or is listed in a directory or advertisement, ask if they are registered with a professional organisation and check that the organisation is represented in this guide.

**Ask the organisation**

- Does it publish a professional register?
- What sort of training is undertaken, for how long and whether there is continuing professional education?
- Does it publish a Code of Practice specifying the professional conduct required?
- Does the organisation have a complaints system and an effective disciplinary procedure and sanctions?

## Ask the practitioner

- Do they have professional indemnity insurance so that you could receive compensation if they were negligent?
- Can you claim for treatment through your private health insurance scheme, if you have one?

## At the consultation

Being able to trust your practitioner and feeling a sense of rapport with them is important to the therapeutic relationship that is part of the healing process. It can make a quantitative as well as a qualitative difference. According to Professor Herbert Benson of the Mind/Body Medical Institute, Harvard Medical School, the essence of healing depends on three elements

- The patient's belief or expectancy of a good outcome
- The caregiver's belief or expectancy of a good outcome
- A relationship between the patient and caregiver that generates positive belief and expectancies. This belief and expectation is thought to lie behind the 'placebo response', which often accounts for a substantial part of patients' improvement.

By the same token, avoid any practitioner with whom you feel uncomfortable. This is particularly relevant if the therapy involves removing clothes and being touched.

The practitioner should take a detailed medical history, particularly noting any current medication you are taking or medical procedures you are receiving.

## You should be told (and ask if you are not)

- What the treatment will involve
- How many sessions you are likely to need
- Any possible side-effects or risks it may have
- What the treatment can't be expected to do
- What other treatment options are

- How much the treatment will cost and how payment should be made

An acupuncturist should use single-use disposable needles that are all removed at the end of treatment. From a herbalist, expect to be given information on herbal medicines, any contraindications (eg alcohol or other medications), how and when to take them, what dosage and how often, and the expiry date.

The practitioner should note your GP's details and be prepared to communicate with your doctor about any diagnosis and treatment.

## After the consultation

Ask yourself

- Was the practitioner's conduct entirely professional?
- Did the practitioner answer your questions clearly and thoroughly?
- Were you given further information to study later?
- What was the practitioner's attitude towards any conventional medicine you were taking?
- Did any of the claims sound unrealistic?

## As treatment continues

- Is the practitioner prepared to refer you to another therapist if the treatment isn't working?
- Do they ask about any side-effects you are experiencing?
- Do they document what is happening?

Beware any therapist who claims miracle cures, charges exorbitant fees, stresses that you continue treatment despite a lack of success after several sessions, or suggests that you abandon conventional medicine without consulting your doctor. Report them to their professional regulatory organisation if they belong to one.

Should you be unhappy about any aspect of your treatment you should in the first instance approach your practitioner. This allows them the opportunity to clarify, explain or rectify the situation, as it may be that you are experiencing a temporary adverse reaction to treatment.

If you are not satisfied by the response from your practitioner, you may want to take the matter to the practitioner's professional or regulatory body, all of which have a Code of Practice and Ethics and a complaints procedure set in place. The association will usually involve the practitioner in trying to resolve the problem. In the event of malpractice a statutory regulatory body has the power to suspend registration or remove a practitioner from its register, which would deny him or her the right to practise legally in the UK.

If you see your practitioner through the NHS, for instance in a clinic or GP practice, these are required by law to have their own local complaints policy. Complaints about the practice of any doctor can be made directly to the General Medical Council. If your GP has referred you to a complementary practitioner with whom you are dissatisfied, you should firstly complain to the practitioner concerned, and then to your GP. GPs who 'refer' you to a complementary practitioner still remain responsible for your welfare during your treatment.

If you think you may have suffered injury or harm as a result of inappropriate care or poor treatment, or feel that your practitioner has misled you about their service, you will need to talk to an experienced personal injury lawyer. The Law Society may be able to give you contacts, or get in touch with Action for Victims of Medical Accidents, who are able to refer you to an expert solicitor.

If you feel that you have been assaulted or treated without your consent, your first course of action should be to call the police. You will still need advice from an expert solicitor, but only the police can start a prosecution for criminal assault.

# Section Two:
# **The Therapies**

# Acupuncture

## What is acupuncture?

Acupuncture is a system of healing which has been practised in China and other Far Eastern countries for thousands of years. It usually involves the insertion of very fine needles into specific points on the body to alleviate a variety of symptoms and restore overall health. It is often described as a means of pain relief, but in fact it is used to treat a wide range of illnesses. There are two main styles of acupuncture in use in the UK – Traditional Chinese Acupuncture and Western Medical Acupuncture.

## HISTORY

The earliest archaeological evidence of acupuncture dates back to the phenomenon of the Alpine 'ice man', who lived approximately 3000 years ago and was discovered to have acupuncture points tattooed on his body. In China, stone needles, dating back to before 1000BC have been found. In the next 2000 years the use of acupuncture spread through Japan, Korea and Vietnam, which developed traditions of their own, and into countries such as Tibet and India, which incorporated acupuncture into their systems of traditional healing. Acupuncture is now used extensively in China and the Far East in hospital-based systems for the treatment of both acute and chronic conditions. There were some practitioners of acupuncture in Europe as early as the nineteenth century, but it was not until the 1960s and early 1970s that the West began to take the therapy seriously.

Acupuncture demonstrated its greater acceptance by conventional medicine in the UK with the publication of a British Medical Association report in June 2000 which concluded that based on current evidence, acupuncture is effective in treating nausea, vomiting, back pain, dental pain and migraine. However, it found that for a wide range of conditions the evidence was inconclusive, and for smoking cessation and weight loss it was actually negative. The findings of the BMA's Board of Science and Education Committee represented a sea change in the BMA's attitude compared to its two previous reviews of complementary therapies in 1986 and 1993. The report also showed that acupuncture is the most popular complementary therapy amongst GPs; at least 47 per cent had arranged acupuncture treatment for their patients.

Although there are no precise figures for those in practice in the UK there are around 7000 acupuncturists who belong to the existing professional registers. There is no statutory regulation of acupuncture in the UK, although doctors and physiotherapists who practise acupuncture are statutorily regulated for the use of acupuncture as an adjunct to their primary skills. The Government has indicated that it wishes to see the statutory regulation of acupuncture as soon as is practicable.

The evidence base for acupuncture is increasing each year. As well as the conditions mentioned above, many others are being researched.

**How does acupuncture work?**

The two styles of acupuncture are based on different views of how the body works.

**Traditional Chinese Medicine (TCM)** believes that the flow of Qi (pronounced Chee) or energy in the body determines our physical and mental well-being. This flow is concentrated in clearly defined channels of energy or meridians both on the surface of and within the body. When there is insufficient or excess Qi in a meridian, or when the Qi is blocked or becomes stagnant, it can lead to illness. The flow of Qi can be disturbed by many factors. These can be physical, such as exposure to weather conditions, poor nutrition, poisons and trauma, or emotional and psychological, such as stress, anger, fear and anxiety. Hereditary factors can also play a major part in illness.

Each meridian is believed to be linked to the internal organs at specific locations on the body's surface known as 'acupuncture points'. By inserting fine needles into these energy channels the acupuncturist can affect the flow of energy, restore the natural balance of energy and promote a healing response in the body.

**Western Medical Acupuncture**  Within the context of western medicine, many physicians have discovered independently that pressing, stimulating or injecting various superficial body points may help to relieve pain, particularly muscular or rheumatic-like pains. These points are not necessarily at the site of pain, but often over distant areas known as 'referred pain'. These points have a variety of names, such as trigger points (for pain), or motor points. Western physicians have discovered that these trigger points by and large correlate with traditional acupuncture points.

Western medical acupuncture is based on a modern understanding of how acupuncture works involving the body's nervous system. Its use is premised on a western medical diagnosis made by a health professional such as a doctor or physiotherapist, and it is based on a more conventional western view of the structure and functions of the body and its internal organs. It is more commonly used as an adjunct to conventional treatment rather than as a primary treatment in itself.

**What conditions do acupuncturists treat?**
Both Traditional Acupuncturists and Medical Acupuncturists will treat a variety of conditions from anxiety states, arthritis and asthma, through to back pain, circulatory problems, depression and digestive problems. Acupuncture can also be used to treat fibrositis, high blood pressure, indeterminate aches and pains, infertility, menstrual problems, migraines, rheumatism, sciatica, skin conditions and ulcers. It is also commonly used in childbirth and to treat addictions.

Traditional Acupuncturists may also treat people who simply feel generally unwell without necessarily being 'ill' in the western sense, while others use traditional acupuncture as a preventative treatment to strengthen their constitution. Medical Acupuncturists more commonly focus on musculo-skeletal pain, pain management, sports injuries, and conditions where acupuncture's proven effect can enhance conventional treatment.

### Are there any conditions which an acupuncturist should not treat?

There is a comprehensive published list of notifiable diseases (which includes serious infectious diseases such as tuberculosis, typhoid, yellow fever, cholera, etc.) for which conventional treatment must be offered as a primary therapy, although acupuncture may be used as an adjunctive treatment to help with the symptoms and the side-effects of conventional treatment. The treatment of conditions such as cancer, Parkinson's disease and other chronic degenerative disorders should be discussed in great detail so you are very clear what purpose the treatment serves and what expectations you should have.

However, if you are on an anticoagulant medicine such as warfarin, you should not receive acupuncture without special precautions. If you have artificial or damaged heart valves, you should not be treated with the type of needles that remain in place for days or weeks before removal. Nor should electro-acupuncture be used on you if you have a pacemaker. Acupuncturists need to take extra precautions if you are on immuno-suppressant drugs and treatment should only be used with great caution if you have epilepsy or a tendency to bleed profusely or faint.

Many acupuncturists would not try to treat you for weight loss or giving up smoking, and some may not treat conditions where success of treatment is known to be limited, such as with tinnitus.

## Is acupuncture safe and are there any possible side-effects?

In two recent surveys, both of 34,000 treatments, adverse reactions were found in only 43 cases in each. These included symptoms such as mild headache or nausea. Inadequately trained practitioners pose the greatest risk but in the hands of a competent and properly trained practitioner, acupuncture is a comparatively safe medical intervention. However, occasional side-effects include a temporary increase in pain, bruising and dizziness. There have been no fatalities from acupuncture in the UK for the last twenty years although, rarely, a pneumothorax may result from poor technique and training.

## Is there research that shows acupuncture really works?

The British Medical Association has reviewed the evidence for acupuncture as a treatment for back and neck pain, osteoarthritis, recurrent headache, nausea and vomiting, smoking cessation, weight loss, stroke and dental pain. The report concludes that according to current evidence, acupuncture appears to be more effective than control interventions for nausea and vomiting (particularly for post-operative symptoms in adults), back pain, dental pain and migraine. Evidence is unclear about a specific response to acupuncture in osteoarthritis and neck pain cases. It considers that the jury is still out for its use in treating recovery from stroke, tension headache, fibromyalgia and certain joint dysfunctions. The report states: 'Acupuncture appears not to be superior to sham acupuncture (used as a control in research) for smoking cessation and weight loss.'

There are a number of Cochrane reviews of clinical trials of acupuncture. A review of 26 trials of acupuncture as a treatment for migraines and tension headaches found evidence that acupuncture was an effective treatment although it said more thorough testing was needed to confirm this. A systematic review of trials of acupuncture for tennis elbow found four small trials of reasonable quality which showed some reduction of pain in the short term but no evidence of longer-term improvement. Other reviews have looked at using acupuncture as a treatment for asthma (insufficient evidence to recommend acupuncture as an effective treatment); lower back pain (no evidence for acupuncture as an effective treatment); and smoking cessation (no clear evidence of efficacy).

## What happens on a first visit?

On a first visit the Traditional Acupuncturist will assess your general state of health, noting your current symptoms and any treatments you may have already had. They will take a detailed medical history and ask you questions about your diet, digestive system, sleeping patterns, emotional state and various other physical functions. The practitioner may also undertake a short physical examination, often checking posture and range of movement, and use a variety of pressure points to test any underlying pathology. The structure, colour and coating of the tongue are particularly important as a guide to overall health and the acupuncturist will pay great attention to the pulses in both your wrists. It is the rhythm, quality and strength of the pulses, together with the tongue diagnosis and the other details given by the patient which give the practitioner a comprehensive picture of the patient's energy flow and a good idea of what treatment to give.

The Medical Acupuncturist will take a different approach. Since they will often be working from your existing medical notes they may ask you further questions about the outcome of the various tests and treatments you have had as well as questions about your overall health. Physiotherapists who use acupuncture may also undertake a number of 'range of movement' tests. Both will gear their treatment to techniques and point selections indicated for the western diagnosis you already have.

# Case history

Sara Williams, TCM Acupuncturist

I arrive at 8:45am, confirm bookings and return an enquiry about acupuncture for infertility. For the rest of the day I will be seeing patients until 4pm when I prepare files for the following day. Among my cases today are four quite different complaints.

At 9am I welcome Mr Knight, a builder who has regular treatment for his arthritic knees. He has been doing roofing work, and this and the damp autumn weather have exacerbated his stiff, swollen knees. These symptoms fall under the category of 'Bi (or 'painful obstruction') syndromes', when pain, soreness or numbness of muscles, tendons and joints occur due to the obstruction of 'Qi' and blood in the body caused by external factors such as wind, cold and damp.

TCM acupunturists believe Qi is the life force or vital energy that flows throughout the body in the meridians that connect our internal organs and the surface of our body. When the Qi flows freely, there is inner harmony and balance and we feel healthy. Illness occurs when the flow of Qi is insufficient, unbalanced or interrupted. Acupuncture is one way of tapping into or manipulating this energy. By inserting needles into specific points where the energy is most accessible, we can balance, unblock or strengthen Qi.

I treat on acupuncture points around his knees and apply small cones of moxibustion to the needles. Moxa eliminates dampness and cold and also tonifies the Qi and blood. I use other body points to treat the underlying constitution.

At ten o'clock Julia arrives for her fourth session. She has noticed considerable changes to the intensity and duration of her cluster headaches over the past few weeks. She has been suffering from periods of one-sided headaches with sharp stabbing pain and tearing for thirty years. Scans and tests have revealed nothing.

The headaches no longer wake her at night, but she is still getting short attacks throughout the day. I use acupuncture points in the head, and along the stomach and gall bladder meridians to eliminate blood stagnation, the cause of the pain. Meridians are mapped channels through which energy flows in the body, and the acupuncture points are located along them. I use the appropriate acupuncture points to treat the root cause of the headaches, an underlying liver blood deficiency.

At 11am Simon arrives for treatment for hypertension. He is currently taking beta-blockers and diuretics but he and his GP want to look at alternative means of reducing his blood pressure. When he first came he felt constantly anxious and ill at ease. I have been treating him with a combination of body and ear acupuncture. His blood pressure has reduced and he has relaxed considerably. Today he is feeling quite anxious – he is moving house soon. I use a triangular needle to prick the pressure-lowering groove behind one ear, and perform body acupuncture to treat the root cause of his hypertension. Before he leaves, I insert press needles into the ear to sustain the treatment.

At 2pm Nick arrives – the pins and needles in both hands have improved, and the tingling after using power tools is gone. He is feeling more optimistic about being able to continue landscape gardening, but he has a sore throat and an impending cold, just when a big contract is about to start.

I do 20 minutes of cupping on lung points on his upper back to induce a mild sweat to eliminate the pathogen, and treat acupuncture points on the forearms and hands to support this treatment and treat the pins and needles in his hands. I then recommend he has a hot drink, keeps warm, and takes a Chinese herbal remedy to promote the sweating.

## What does the treatment involve?

Treatment usually involves the insertion of fine filiform (solid) needles into specific locations on the body ('points'). The needles, often as many as ten or more in a treatment session, are sometimes manipulated gently but may just be inserted and left in place for between 20 to 30 minutes.

## Does acupuncture hurt?

The needles used in acupuncture are so fine that there is usually very little sensation. Many are now inserted with the aid of a plastic 'guide tube' in which the needle is packed and which further reduces sensation. Once inserted, there is usually no further feeling until the needle reaches the required depth. Many people then experience a slight tingling, and often a dull ache. There may be a slight redness around the needle, which is believed to signify that the treatment is working.

## How big are the needles?

The most commonly used needles are between an inch and three inches long. The needles vary in diameter from around 0.16mm ('40-gauge') to around 0.30mm ('30-gauge'). All acupuncture needles are made from stainless steel and solid, unlike the hollow hypodermic needles with which most people are familiar.

## How deeply are they inserted?

Most needles are inserted no more than 3mm to 5mm beneath the skin. In fleshier areas, or in the treatment of the larger joints, the needles may be inserted more deeply. The appropriate depths of insertion for each point are well documented in the textbooks, as are specific instructions for techniques to maximise safety in areas of potential risk. Needles inserted in the upper torso, for example, will often be put in at a shallow angle to avoid accidental penetration of the lung.

### How long are the needles left in?

The length of time varies on the individual treatment – some needles are inserted and immediately withdrawn – the majority are left in place for up to 20 or 30 minutes, depending on the effect required.

### Does an acupuncture needle draw blood?

In general, the needles are too fine to cause bleeding. Bleeding may occur occasionally if you move while they are in place or if the needle penetrates a small blood vessel.

### How many treatments will I need?

Some people respond quickly while others may take longer. A responsible practitioner will review progress regularly and you would expect to see some improvement after about five treatments. If this is not the case, the practitioner may discuss with you whether or not to continue treatment. On each follow-up visit the practitioner will ask for detailed feedback on the effects of the treatment, whether there are any changes in your symptoms and other significant developments. If more treatment is needed, it will then be further refined to suit your individual needs.

### How often are treatments arranged?

At the beginning most acupuncturists see you once or twice a week and the interval between visits may increase as progress continues. If you have an acute condition, you may have to see your acupuncturist daily for a short while.

### How long does a treatment take?

First appointments can last anything from 30 minutes to two hours. Subsequent treatment times vary between 15 minutes and an hour.

# Case history

Richard Halvorsen, GP and medical acupuncturist

Like the majority of acupuncturists in the British Medical
Acupuncture Society, I am a GP who practices acupuncture
alongside other orthodox medical techniques. All medical
acupuncturists are either GPs or chartered physiotherapists. The
big advantage to medical acupuncture in my view is that a
patient is unlikely to be treated with acupuncture whatever the
diagnosis. It is offered as one of a range of options, or in
combination with other treatment. The important thing is to
establish when acupuncture is the most appropriate treatment.

I use acupuncture opportunistically, which means that it may
form part of a consultation, say for an acute muscle strain, and will
normally be very short, sometimes lasting only a few seconds.
Often when treating musculo-skeletal disorders, I will be needling
'trigger' points rather than specific traditional Chinese acupuncture
points, focusing on the tender areas where the muscle has knotted
up with pain. With acute problems I can get dramatic results;
sometimes only one or two treatments are required. With chronic
conditions, such as migraine or back pain, it may take longer. We
usually review the situation after about 4–6 sessions, to see if
acupuncture really is the most appropriate treatment.

When I give acupuncture, it is always after taking a detailed
history, as is my practice with all my patients. I will then come to
a western medical diagnosis, which is made in a completely
different language to that of Traditional Chinese Medicine. For
example, where a Chinese herbal medicine practitioner might
talk about 'rising liver fire', I might diagnose dyspepsia. I take a
number of factors into consideration before opting to use
acupuncture, not least the patient's own attitude to the
treatment. However, I will always recommend acupuncture over
another treatment if I think it appropriate. There is, for example,

good evidence to suggest that acupuncture helps reduce nausea during pregnancy, so in that evidence-based situation, I might urge the patient to consider it.

I recently treated a patient who installed central heating for a living with severe pain in his elbow. When I first saw him, he had been suffering constant acute pain in his right elbow for two weeks. I prescribed him anti-inflammatory painkillers and an X-ray. Two weeks later, the pain was still so bad he couldn't sleep. I referred him urgently to a consultant rheumatologist who was able to give him an appointment three days later. The consultant diagnosed a kind of tennis elbow injury, related to Repetitive Strain Injury, and gave the patient a steroid injection.

Three weeks later he was back to see me, the pain as bad as ever. At this point I suggested we try acupuncture, and he replied that I 'could hang him out of the window by his feet' as long as it helped the pain. So, I placed two needles in his arm, one in his hand, and one in his elbow near the site of the pain. I left them for ten minutes, during which time I also administered a brief periosteal pecking (a tapping of the bone around the area containing the needle). The results were dramatic. Before treatment, the patient had said his pain registered a ten on a possible scale of ten, afterwards he gave it a score of one. He described the pain as draining out of his arm like water from a sieve.

I saw him again two weeks later. He told me that he had been practically pain-free for three days after the treatment, although he had experienced some stiffness, and then some pain had returned. I have since given him a further three treatments, and he is now back at work.

**I've heard that my condition may get worse before it gets better. Is this true?**

Some conditions may respond in this way, although so much depends on the response of each individual that there are no general rules. Where the symptoms do occasionally become more intense they may soon pass and if this is a healing response (sometimes referred to as a 'healing crisis') you will quickly begin to feel much better. If the symptoms remain worse for a prolonged period you will need to discuss this with your practitioner.

**Are there any different acupuncture techniques?**

Traditional Acupuncturists may use a herb called moxa, which is allowed to smoulder directly on points or via special needles to warm and stimulate the flow of energy. Some practitioners also use a form of massage called 'tui na', or may tap points with a probe called a seven star hammer. These techniques are very useful for treating small children or people who are afraid of needles.

Medical Acupuncturists often use trigger point acupuncture. This technique is useful for treating painful muscular problems and involves inserting needles into tender areas of muscle known as 'trigger points'. Some Medical Acupuncturists employ a technique called periosteal acupuncture. This involves gently tapping areas of bone near the skin's surface and can be useful where a patient does not like needles. Segmental acupuncture can be used to treat an internal organ such as the stomach or bladder. Needles are inserted into areas of skin or muscle that share the same nerve supply originating from the same level of the spinal cord as the organ being treated.

Many practitioners of both styles also treat some conditions by inserting tiny needles into the ear and then stimulating them either manually or electrically. Electro-acupuncture, where electrodes are attached to the needles and create an electrical stimulation often experienced as a tingling or twitching, is becoming increasingly popular. Laser acupuncture, an experimental form of treatment used by a few practitioners, uses a laser beam to stimulate acupuncture points without piercing the skin.

### How do I know that the needles used are sterilised?

All practitioners should follow strict Codes of Safe Practice with stringent requirements for hygienic procedure. The Codes are regularly updated in consultation with health and safety experts as well as with the Department of Health. The majority of UK practitioners now use pre-sterilised disposable needles. Manufacturers are required to pass rigorous inspections before being granted the European-standard CE certificate, which appears on the needle boxes. Most importers carry out further safety checks of their own.

### How are used needles and clinical waste disposed of?

Each needle should be disposed of in a yellow Sharps Box. Once full, these are collected by registered clinical waste disposal agents and are taken away to be burned. All low-grade clinical waste, couch roll paper, tissues, etc, should be bagged in yellow bags and collected by a registered collection agent. Clinical waste should never be mixed with or disposed of as household waste.

### How much does a consultation cost?

Costs of treatment vary across the country. In London a first consultation may cost between £50 and £60 with subsequent visits costing between £30 and £45. In other parts of the country these figures can be £10 to £15 less.

### Can I have acupuncture at reduced rates?

Many practitioners will reduce their fees if you cannot afford the full rate. You will have to negotiate this directly with your practitioner, however, and your individual circumstances will be taken into account. Training schools sometimes offer sessions at reduced rates.

## Can I get my private health insurers to pay for my acupuncture treatment?

Many health insurance policies now cover acupuncture. If this is the case, the exact terms and conditions will be displayed in their policy literature, as well as the limits of cover provided. Some larger providers, however, still offer only very limited cover. Most are waiting for acupuncture to become statutorily regulated and for more research into its cost-effectiveness as an alternative to conventional treatments.

Some doctors and GPs offer acupuncture privately and some of these are recognised by BUPA, PPP and other health insurance companies. A GP is not allowed to charge his own NHS patients for providing acupuncture.

## Will my acupuncturist belong to a professional body?

The majority of acupuncture practitioners working in the UK belong to professional associations.

The largest group of Traditional Acupuncturists belong to the British Acupuncture Council (BAcC) which has published Codes of Ethics, Safe Practice and Professional Conduct and provides all of its members automatically with professional indemnity and public liability insurance.

The two largest groups of Medical Acupuncturists are the British Medical Acupuncture Society (BMAS) and the Acupuncture Association of Chartered Physiotherapists (AACP). Most of their members are doctors or physiotherapists, along with a few nurses who already have extensive medical training. They have then gone on to study acupuncture in order to use it alongside conventional western medicine. Many of the doctors are GPs but some are specialists such as rheumatologists or anaesthetists. Many work within the NHS and some work privately.

There are several smaller organisations representing both Traditional Acupuncturists and Medical Acupuncturists, all of which are usually happy to supply you with details of their membership and their professional codes.

## Where can I find a qualified acupuncturist?

The Traditional Chinese Acupuncturists listed in this guide are members of the BAcC and as such abide by a common code of practice and have over 1200 hours of training in acupuncture.

The Medical Acupuncturists listed in this guide will either be members of the BMAS or the AACP and as such will be trained to practice acupuncture within the bounds of their medical profession. Some may also be members of the BAcC.

The majority of referrals still come via word of mouth. Most acupuncturists who have practised in an area for several years will have cross-referred many patients to and from other health professionals, and it may be possible to get a referral from them. All practitioners should be able to offer the same basic professional service and many are happy to arrange short pre-treatment meetings to allow patients to meet them and discuss possible treatments.

The professional associations can also help you to find a suitable practitioner; The British Acupuncture Council, for example, publishes an annual register of members which also appears on its website. A member of the public can use the search facility on the website or call the BAcC directly to request a list of practitioners local to them. The British Medical Acupuncture Society and the Acupuncture Association of Chartered Physiotherapists also provide database searches and have websites from which you can identify practitioners near to where you live.

# Case history

Emily Childs, Acupuncture patient

Shortly before Christmas 2000, I was moving a bookcase when I felt something 'give' in my lower back. In considerable pain, I decided to see a chiropractor, but the day after treatment I could hardly walk. My bones felt as though they were grating together. The GP explained that my muscles had gone into spasm, and recommended physiotherapy. The physiotherapist, realising that I couldn't bear anyone to touch my back, suggested we try acupuncture.

In that first session she put the needles down the right-hand side of my lower spine, feeling for places where the muscles were in spasm. She also inserted them in and above my hip. In the early sessions, she used eight needles (this was later reduced to six), leaving them in for 20 minutes without touching them. In later sessions, she would come back two or three times to tweak the needles.

The change I felt after that first visit was immediate. When I arrived, I could barely walk and was in tears. After the treatment, I was still unable to walk far, but the pain was slightly easier, and I felt more comfortable. My recovery was also helped by the fact that my GP agreed to sign me off work for two weeks. I was initially worried that my complaint would flare up after treatment, as it had done with the chiropractic, but fortunately I carried on making gradual improvements. The sciatic pain that had been coursing down my legs gradually receded; and after about six sessions I was left with only a dull ache, which was due to an unrelated back problem caused by a hysterectomy some years before.

At the moment I am having acupuncture again, this time for a problem with my left elbow caused by a fracture I had as a child. The joint at the top of my elbow is now arthritic, and was operated on in March 2001. During the operation they moved a nerve to the inside of my arm. I knew that it would take some time for the pain to settle, but I was left with discomfort around my elbow joint and a tingling sensation in my left hand. I also developed a large triangular patch of sensitivity between my elbow joint and the wrist, and I couldn't bear anything to touch it or knock it. The tingling sensation made it uncomfortable to pick anything up, and my sensitivity to touch was affected. I felt as if I was wearing a rubber glove. I also had less strength in that hand.

My acupuncturist is currently working on my hand, inserting needles into various places, including between my thumb and forefinger and below the knuckle in my fingers. When she first put them in my hand I felt a kind of 'popping' sensation, and she told me that this was a sign that she had found the right 'meridian'. I also felt a peculiar referral of sensation; a needle inserted into my wrist, for example, could be felt in my middle finger. I feel sensations in different places in my elbow according to where the acupuncturist has put needles in my hand or wrist. This is also a good sign, and means that the needles are channelling the right places.

Immediately after the first session I felt a change of sensation in my elbow, and soon into the treatment the strange tingling and 'humming' in my hand disappeared. I have now had about six sessions, going twice a week, and am noticing steady improvements, including more feeling and strength coming back into my hand.

## What questions should I ask before making an appointment with an acupuncturist?

- Are they properly trained and a member of a recognised professional body?
- Do they have experience in treating similar health problems to yours?
- Are there any risks involved in treatment?
- Are there other treatment options available?
- How long is the treatment likely to last?
- Are they willing to discuss your condition with your GP if you request it?
- How much do they charge and do they offer concessionary rates?
- Do they have full professional indemnity and public liability insurance?

You should also make sure that on the first consultation a full case history is taken. The consultation should last at least 40 minutes. If your practitioner does not speak English, make sure that there is a translator present.

Perhaps the most important consideration is that you have a rapport with the practitioner and feel that you can communicate with them. You should feel comfortable asking questions about your problems and your practitioner should be forthcoming about what the treatment will involve, how much it will cost and how payment should be made. It may be helpful to visit the premises so try to book your first appointment in person.

## What training will my acupuncturist have?

The majority of Traditional Acupuncturists will have been trained in the UK. The British Acupuncture Accreditation Board (BAAB) was established in 1989 to set standards for all schools and colleges of acupuncture in the UK. There are currently seven accredited schools from which around 250 practitioners graduate each year.

Some universities now offer degree courses in acupuncture. Graduates of accredited schools have to complete a three-year part-time training equivalent to a two-year full-time degree course. That is set to rise to 3600 hours of training, the equivalent of a three-year full-time degree course.

Some Traditional Acupuncturists will have undertaken their original training in the Far East. Most have joined professional bodies in the UK and are individually interviewed and admitted only after showing they meet standards at least equivalent to those of a graduate from a UK college.

The largest provider of Medical Acupuncture training in the UK is the BMAS. As doctors, all members of the BMAS will already have completed a minimum of five years undergraduate training in medicine and usually many more years of postgraduate training. This education will already have provided them with a working knowledge of anatomy, physiology, hygiene, first aid, pathology and diagnosis. The requirements for acupuncture training for doctors are lower because of Medical Acupuncture's basis in western medicine – a minimum of 70 hours as an entry requirement for their professional associations. Other training courses in specialised techniques such as detoxification procedures or in basic acupuncture skills for GPs may be shorter still.

There are two levels of acupuncture training for BMAS members. The CoBC (Certificate of Basic Competence) means a doctor must have been practising acupuncture for at least three months and have submitted a logbook of 30 cases to the examiners, five of which should be considerably detailed. The CoA (Certificate of Accreditation) requires a further 100 hours minimum of training, a written logbook of 100 cases, 15 of which must be completed in detail, as well as a clinical interview and assessment of the applicant by two experienced trainers. The entry level qualification for this course is a Diploma in Medical Acupuncture, which means a doctor must have completed intermediate level training and also updated their training every five years with postgraduate courses examined by independent assessors.

Many physiotherapists will have been trained by the AACP, which offers its own introductory course containing elements of both Western and Chinese Acupuncture. The training ranges from basic 30-hour AACP-approved training courses run by AACP-approved trainers, enabling physiotherapists to use simple acupuncture techniques for pain relief, to courses leading to Advanced Membership for which a physiotherapist will have completed over 200 hours' training. The various levels of membership of the AACP are tied to the stage of training which the member has completed.

### Do acupuncturists hold a recognised qualification?

The Licentiate in Acupuncture (LicAc) or the Diploma in Acupuncture (DipAc) is the basic qualification held by most Traditional Acupuncturists in the UK. There are no formally recognised educational titles beyond this. Some colleges offer masters and doctorate programmes, and people may legitimately use the designatory letters MAc or DrAc after their names. However, titles such as 'professor' or 'doctor' gained in this way have no formal status, and the use of the title 'doctor' is expressly forbidden by the BAcC's Code of Ethics unless the member is registered with the General Medical Council.

### How do practitioners keep their skills and knowledge up-to-date?

Traditional Acupuncturists in the BAcC are currently involved in a pilot scheme of a practitioner-centred Continuing Professional Development (CPD) programme, which will be extended to the whole membership over the next two years, probably becoming mandatory in 2003. This involves broader development and the updating and maintenance of specific basic skills.

Medical Acupuncturists who are accredited members of the BMAS are required to do at least 30 hours of CPD every five years in order to remain a member. It also expects members as doctors to keep up-to-date in all medical areas relevant to their practice including acupuncture. The AACP encourages CPD by organising further training courses across the country and has an Education Officer charged with inspecting the basic courses, checking the intermediate courses and generally driving up the standard of practice throughout its membership. The AACP requires at least 10 hours of CPD every two years in order to remain on the register.

## Who monitors a practitioner's standards?

Most of the Codes that bind members of the professional bodies are voluntarily self-policed so the practitioner has to sign to abide by them each year as a condition of continued membership. Standards of clinical practice and the safety and hygiene of clinical premises are potentially subject to random inspection by local authorities or the professional bodies, depending on where the practitioner is based.

## What happens if a practitioner falls short of these standards?

If a complaint is made by a member of the public, or if the professional body becomes aware of a problem with someone's practice standards, there are investigative procedures to determine what action may be appropriate. The remit of investigating committees extends to ethical issues, health and safety, and the practitioner's own fitness to practise.

All of the major associations have formal procedures for dealing with professional conduct. Traditional Acupuncturists in the BAcC can be suspended or removed from membership or required to undertake further training or health examinations if a case against them is proven. Medical Acupuncturists are subject to the internal procedures of their acupuncture organisations but are also under

# Case history

Jane Jarrold, Acupuncture patient

I moved to England from Australia some years ago, and began to find it increasingly hard to cope with the harsh winter. Every year I suffered from a variety of respiratory infections, in fact I came down with every bug going, and felt low and miserable. Chest infections and flu would go on for weeks. I'd wake night after night drenched in sweat, and I constantly had to resort to antibiotics. I also suffered from terrible hay fever in the summer, and had to use inhalers and antihistamines. The doctors' view seemed to be that this situation would always be part of my life and was unlikely to change.

When I finally decided I'd had enough of orthodox medication, I consulted a homeopath, but a year of treatment produced no relief. I then saw a Western Herbalist, who helped a bit, but couldn't ease the hay fever, and specialists in allergies, respiratory problems, and asthma. I also saw a cranial osteopath for two years, and although I had some success with him, he was the one who eventually suggested acupuncture.

When I first met the acupuncturist she asked me for my whole life story, including questions about my family and medical history. We established that it was airborne allergens, such as house dust mites and pollen, that affected me. And we agreed that the aim of the acupuncture was to build up my immune system so that it could fight off airborne bugs, and to get my lung function up to its optimum level.

I have now been going to her for three years. Acupuncture can sometimes be slightly painful, especially if you have a dozen needles placed in parts of your body that are not naturally fleshy like your wrists. I experience a slightly peculiar feeling as the needles go in which I can only describe as a 'travelling' sensation. A needle inserted into my knee, for instance, can be felt right down in my toe. It's like a mild electric current. The needles are tailored to my individual needs, and the approach is holistic, focusing on my spleen, for example, as much as on my respiratory system.

Shortly after the first session, I came down with a horrendous case of tonsillitis that caused one whole side of my face to swell up. I was convinced that it was a direct result of the acupuncture, as the tonsil is a filter of the toxins that pass through the system, and that my first treatment had started this detoxification process moving. My therapist didn't deny this, but there is no way of finding out for sure.

I carried on with weekly acupuncture, and although I still caught colds and flu the first winter, I usually got over them at the same rate as a healthy person. I was fighting them rather than merely succumbing. The following winter was much better, and I was convinced that the acupuncture was helping. I had one short cold in November, and then nothing for the rest of the season. My hay fever was also vastly better in the summer.

I now go to my acupuncturist every week from September onwards, as autumn is the time I usually start to come down with infections, and I continue on through the winter. By April or May I am ready to stop treatment until the following autumn. This way I allow my body to take over fighting infection, instead of bombarding my system all the time. I feel very positive about the effect acupuncture has had on me; I can't really attribute my recovery to anything else.

the jurisdiction of their own regulatory bodies, the General Medical Council and the Chartered Society of Physiotherapy (CSP), by whom a case may be heard.

**Am I allowed to have access to my treatment records?**
Traditional Acupuncturists are not covered by the same legislation as doctors. Case notes remain their own property and are not legally available for inspection by you. Notes taken by a Medical Acupuncturist may, however, be available to you under the existing legislation.

**Are my treatment records open to inspection by anyone else?**
There are very few circumstances where case notes would be open to inspection without your express written approval. A Court of Law could require a practitioner to disclose your notes, but this rarely happens.

**Are my treatment and my case history confidential?**
All notes are entirely confidential, and the fact that you are having treatment is confidential. It would be unethical, for example, for a practitioner to tell a wife that her husband was having treatment, or to leave appointment books open in such a way that third parties could see who attended a clinic.

**Is there statutory regulation of acupuncture in the UK?**
At the moment there is no statutory regulation of acupuncture in the UK. Anyone may call themselves an acupuncturist without proper training. It is very important, therefore, to ensure that your acupuncturist is registered with a professional body.

Some Medical Acupuncturists are already statutorily regulated or registered by virtue of their main profession. Doctors, for example, are already regulated by the General Medical Council, to whom complaints can be made about any medical incompetence or professional misconduct. Physiotherapists belong to the Chartered Society of Physiotherapy (CSP) which, though not statutorily regulated, is a professional state-registered body that permits physiotherapists to work in the NHS. It also regulates professional conduct, public liability and insurance.

Without statutory regulation, the only controls exercised over Traditional Acupuncturists in the UK are those that are freely chosen by the profession itself in voluntary self-regulation, and through the licensing and registration procedures which are legally required of local authorities. The BAcC has for many years undertaken major public relations exercises to ensure that the public are aware of what to look for in a safe, well-trained and competent practitioner.

The House of Lords recommendation that acupuncture should be statutorily regulated as soon as possible was enthusiastically endorsed by the government and all the major acupuncture associations. Discussions are currently taking place between the Department of Health and all the major stakeholders in the acupuncture profession about how best to achieve this. The primary aim of legislation is to offer the public a guarantee of safety through sound practice and the highest possible standards of training.

### Can I get acupuncture treatment through the NHS?

There are no formal agreements with the NHS as a whole for the provision of acupuncture. Many Primary Care Groups and Primary Care Trusts have contracts with individual acupuncturists to provide a service to their areas, and some health authorities fund specific projects for addiction and substance abuse.

### Is Medical Acupuncture available on the NHS?

If your GP is also an acupuncturist you may be able to receive treatment free at your NHS surgery. At least two-thirds of physiotherapists practise acupuncture within the NHS, with the remainder in private practice.

## Can my GP refer me to an acupuncturist?

Many GPs work closely with complementary therapists in their area, and there are often good reciprocal referral procedures between GPs, osteopaths, chiropractors, acupuncturists and herbalists. Many GPs will refer you directly to a Traditional Acupuncturist but few are able to fund this treatment from their practice budgets.

It is becoming increasingly possible to be treated with Medical Acupuncture as more doctors are studying and using acupuncture. It is still not that easy to find acupuncture treatment on the NHS, however, and where it is available the  must come from the GP. Otherwise your GP may know of local medical acupuncturists who offer private treatment.

## What should I do if my GP refuses to make a referral?

Your GP does not have to refer you if they do not think that acupuncture is appropriate for your medical condition. However, your GP should discuss this decision with you, and if you and your GP cannot come to an agreement about whether homeopathic treatment is appropriate, there are several steps you can take:

- Request a second opinion; this would usually be from another GP at the practice.
- Complain under the NHS complaints procedure. Your local practice should provide you with information about making a complaint.
- Register with another GP. Your Primary Care Trust (Health Board in Scotland or Local Health Group in Wales) can provide you with a list of GPs in your area. You may wish to check with alternative GPs about their attitude towards acupuncture before registering. Suitably qualified GPs are able

to apply acupuncture directly in their work. You should check that they are registered with the British Medical Acupuncture Society so that you can be sure they are properly trained.

**If I have acupuncture outside the NHS, will my acupuncturist inform my GP?**

Acupuncturists are encouraged to keep your GP informed of treatment they have provided. However, they may only do so with your express consent.

**Can acupuncture be used during pregnancy and childbirth?**

There are several courses, both Traditional and Medical, which provide practitioners with postgraduate training in paediatric and obstetric acupuncture in addition to the skills that they acquired from their basic training. Babies and young children can be treated with needles or with gentle massage. Pregnant women can also be treated with care throughout pregnancy. Practitioners are trained to know which points should be avoided at the various stages of pregnancy, and any intervention should be kept to a minimum.

There are protocols for the most common problems in pregnancy (morning sickness, heartburn, etc.). There are also specific techniques designed to correct breech presentation in the last trimester. Late-stage needling is safe in the hands of practitioners with specialist training, as is the treatment of some of the late-stage complications in conjunction with other conventional treatments. Many practitioners now attend births and use acupuncture to assist in the stages of delivery.

Medical acupuncture is used at three NHS maternity units: Derriford Hospital in Plymouth, Warwick Maternity Hospital and UCLH Obstetric Hospital in London.

## Are all acupuncturists covered by insurance?

All acupuncturists belonging to professional bodies will either automatically have Professional Indemnity and Public Liability insurance as a part of their membership fees or have to provide evidence of insurance as a condition of membership. In all cases you should ask to see evidence of current insurance before treatment commences.

## Can I still give blood if I have had acupuncture?

Practitioners who belong to the three professional bodies can issue certificates that will enable you to give blood, should you choose to do so. Acupuncture delivered by other practitioners may be subject to discretionary rulings by the Blood Transfusion Service in your area.

## Do acupuncturists make home visits?

Medical Acupuncturists are generally unable to make home visits. Some Traditional Acupuncturists may be able to visit you at home, however, if your condition makes it impossible to attend normal clinics. 'Home visits' as a term covers everything from private houses to hospices, hospital wards and residential care facilities. The BAcC has strict rules about safety and hygienic procedure for such visits clearly laid out in its Code of Safe Practice.

## How can I complain if something goes wrong?

Each of the three major associations operate within guidelines for safe practice and standards of ethical behaviour. These are published as Codes by the professional associations and are available on request. If you are unable to resolve any problems directly with your practitioner, you can complain to their professional association. Your complaint will be investigated, and if upheld, the practitioner concerned may face penalties ranging from cautions and reprimands to suspension and removal from the register. In addition to their own internal procedures, members of the BMAS and AACP are also subject to the disciplinary procedures of their primary regulatory body and may face further action in serious cases.

## Where can I find further information?

### The British Acupuncture Council
63 Jeddo Road,
London W12 9HQ
Tel: 020 8735 0400
email: info@acupuncture.org.uk
www.acupuncture.org.uk

### The British Medical Acupuncture Society
12 Marbury House
Higher Whitley
Warrington
Cheshire WA4 4QW
Tel: 01925-730727
email: admin@medical-acupuncture.co.uk
www.medical-acupuncture.co.uk

### The Acupuncture Association of Chartered Physiotherapists
Mere Complementary Practice
Castle Street
Mere
Wiltshire BA12 6JE
Tel: 01747-861151
email: AACPsecretariat@btinternet.com
www.aacp.uk.com

# Homeopathy

### What is homeopathy?

Homeopathy is perhaps the most controversial of the five therapies looked at in this book. Some doctors remain very sceptical that homeopathic medicines – which are often chemically indistinguishable from water – could possibly have any effect beyond that of a placebo. On the other hand, homeopathy is quite widely practised inside the NHS, which runs five specialist homeopathic NHS hospitals in Bristol, Tunbridge Wells, Liverpool, London and Glasgow.

The principle behind homeopathy is that 'like cures like'. The belief is that a substance that produces certain symptoms in a person will be effective in treating an illness that has the same symptoms. To find remedies, a healthy person is given doses of a particular substance over a period of time until symptoms start to appear. These symptoms are then carefully recorded and the substance becomes the basis for a medicine that is used to treat an ill person who displays those symptoms.

In preparing the medicine, the substance is diluted in water. Often, the final remedy will be so dilute that there is no remaining trace of the original substance. However, homeopaths believe that the resulting solution is still able to have the necessary therapeutic effect.

### HISTORY

Homeopathic principles have been recognised in medicine since the fourth century. Hippocrates first described how a patient could be cured of an illness by being treated with a substance that caused the same symptoms of that illness. The principles of modern homeopathy were established in the eighteenth century when a chance observation by German practitioner Samuel Hahnemann led him to investigate the effects of various substances on himself and other healthy volunteers.

Hahnemann discovered that symptoms of illness could be treated by small doses of substances that caused similar symptoms in a healthy person. For example, Peruvian bark (quinine) given to a healthy person can cause dizziness and fever – the symptoms of malaria. This is the very disease it was used to cure. Hahnemann went on to test or 'prove' a large number of substances under the principle of 'like cures like'.

To avoid the toxic effects of the substances, Hahnemann repeatedly diluted the preparations. To his surprise he discovered that repeatedly diluting and vigorously shaking the preparation actually increased its potency. All homeopathic medicines available today are produced according to this process. They are very dilute and as a result are extremely safe.

Homeopathy was introduced into the UK in the early nineteenth century by Dr Frederick Quin, one of Hahnemann's students. Quin established the Homeopathic Society, the forerunner of today's Faculty of Homeopathy, in 1844. The opening of the Royal London Homeopathic Hospital (RLHH) followed soon after in 1849. Homeopathy is currently subject to voluntary self-regulation, and there are a number of professional associations representing homeopaths. The most important of these are the Faculty of Homeopathy and the Society of Homeopaths.

**How does homeopathy work?**

Nobody can explain exactly how or why homeopathy works. The high potency medicines are so dilute that under chemical analysis there is no measurable trace of the original substance left in the preparations. Homeopaths believe that the active agent imprints itself on the water molecules used to dilute the various substances. The water molecules are then thought to carry the 'memory' of the substance. However, opinion is divided over the mechanism of action, which has not yet been scientifically explained.

Nevertheless, homeopathy does appear to be effective for some conditions and it is a popular treatment in the UK. It is also believed that the homeopathic approach – treating the whole person and not just the localised symptoms of the disease – deals with the root cause of the problem rather than just its physical manifestation.

**What conditions can homeopathy treat?**

Homeopathy is a popular treatment for eczema, arthritis and premenstrual syndrome. It can also be used alongside conventional treatments. For example, if you have cancer, homeopathic medicines can be used to help you cope with the side-effects of chemotherapy and radiotherapy. Even in mechanical conditions such as fractures or injuries, homeopathy can help in the treatment of shock or trauma.

**Are there any conditions for which homeopathy is not appropriate?**

Homeopathy cannot repair permanently damaged tissue such as an aneurysm or a nerve destroyed by MS, or stimulate a process that lies outside the body's natural powers of recovery, such as the regeneration of glands that have failed, as, for example, in the pancreas of a diabetic patient. Homeopathy cannot provide a substitute for a missing endocrine secretion such as insulin or thyroxin, but if the condition that causes this is tackled in the early stages, homeopathy might help halt its progression.

**Is homeopathy safe and are there any possible side-effects?**

Homeopathic medicines are non-addictive and have very few side-effects, so under the supervision of a properly qualified and regulated practitioner they are considered safe to use for everyone, including babies, children and the elderly. The only side-effects that might be experienced are part of the 'healing reaction', which homeopaths regard as a sign that the medicine is beginning to work.

A review of the safety of homeopathy was conducted by practitioners associated with the Royal London Homeopathic

Hospital based on papers published between 1970 and 1995. It found that adverse effects in clinical trials were mild and transient and consisted mainly of headaches, tiredness, skin complaints and aggravation of symptoms.

## Is there research that shows that homeopathy really works?

There are Cochrane reviews (see p19) of the evidence for homeopathic treatment of asthma and influenza as well as the use of homeopathy to induce labour. The reviews found evidence that Oscillococcinum, a homeopatic remedy, had some effect on reducing the duration of illness for flu patients. It found no evidence that the treatment could prevent flu. There was not enough evidence to assess whether homeopathic treatments had any affect on asthma or on induction of labour.

Bandolier (see p19), which publishes information on evidence for clinical treatments, has found evidence that homeopathy can help recovery following surgery on the bowels (post-operative ileus). There have been few trials comparing homeopathic medicines with conventional treatments. A Bandolier review of such trials concluded that none had provided evidence of a homeopathic treatment being superior in outcomes to the orthodox treatment.

In 1997, the Lancet published a review of 89 clinical trials of homeopathy of which half found homeopathy to be more effective than a placebo. A wide variety of conditions were covered including asthma, rheumatoid arthritis, hay fever, glue ear, depression and pain of various types.

## What happens on a first visit?

A first session usually lasts longer than subsequent sessions because the homeopath will have to take a thorough history of your medical symptoms as well as detailed questions about your life in general. You may not realise the relevance of some of the questions about

# Case history

David Mundy, RSHom, Homeopath

I treat everyone from babies to the elderly, and see a variety of conditions, ranging from chronic problems such as asthma and migraine, to stress-related illnesses and acute problems such as influenza.

An initial consultation may last about two hours because I prescribe for the health of the whole person, not just for a particular symptom. As a homeopath I believe that a patient's various different complaints are actually manifestations of one imbalance. Our physical and emotional wellbeing are also intricately linked. Particular mental states may express themselves in the body (worry, for example, can result in a stomach ulcer). So, as well as details of a patient's current complaint and medical history, I need to know everything about their lives, their emotional state, how they react to things and how they interact with their environment.

Just as medicine classifies symptom complexes into 'diseases', homeopathy classifies a patient's mental, emotional and physical symptoms into 'remedy pictures'. This means that there is no one remedy for a particular disease. Six patients suffering from migraine may each require totally different remedies. Each patient is unique and finding the right remedy for the patient is a complex process.

In order to find out the healing properties in substances they are first tested or 'proved' on healthy volunteers to see exactly what physical and psychological changes they produce. A database is then built up and a 'picture' of the remedy emerges. Of course we cannot give toxic substances to volunteers, so the remedies are diluted until the original substance is harmless. Some argue that homeopathic remedies are so weak they can't be effective. However, my experience is that they will work if correctly matched to the patient's symptoms. The patient is sensitive to the remedy that heals them, rather like an allergy in reverse. We easily accept that minute amounts of an antigen such as pollen can cause a huge reaction in a susceptible person. In a similar way, a patient is sensitive to a remedy that is capable of curing them, but not to other remedies.

In acute disease the healing response is fast and the remedy may have to be given every two hours until the patient is well on the way to recovery. In chronic conditions, most homeopaths prefer to wait three to four weeks after a treatment in order to give the immune system time to react; and a series of remedies may be given as the patient progresses. However, only one remedy is given at a time and its action is assessed at each follow-up visit. If the patient has been unwell for a long time, the healing process will be slower.

The way that we assess improvement is based on the principle that in true healing, symptoms are observed to move in a centrifugal manner, and from above downwards and from more vital organs to less vital organs. Symptoms also disappear in the reverse order of their coming. Occasionally a healing crisis takes place in the form of a skin eruption or a fever, as the organism purifies itself.

Homeopaths believe that all symptoms are expressions of a compromised immune system doing its best to cope with stress. We read these symptoms and match our treatment accordingly with remedies that homeopaths have been using for over 200 years. The remedy aims to boost the immune system in order to help the patients heal themselves and, in the process, become more resistant to disease.

your lifestyle, eating habits, sleep patterns, medical history and state of mind, and it may appear that the homeopath is interested in matters that have little to do with the complaint which is bothering you. However, the practitioner uses this information to form an accurate assessment of which medicine to prescribe.

**How are homeopathic medicines prescribed?**

Homeopaths believe that symptoms of illness are evidence of the body's natural efforts to heal itself and all of these are used as clues to guide them to the correct homeopathic medicine.

Medicines are measured in potencies and can be prescribed in a number of different strengths, depending on your condition. The lower potencies have been diluted less than the higher potencies and, broadly speaking, are not as powerful. It is these medicines that can be bought over-the-counter. High potency medicines are usually only prescribed by experienced qualified homeopaths.

When medicines are given as a single dose it is common for the homeopath to wait a few weeks to observe the patient's response. Low potency medicines can be given in a single dose or repeated daily or more often, depending on the nature of the condition. Someone who has been ill a long time, for example, and whose body has been physically damaged, may need repeated doses of a medicine to stimulate their recuperative powers, whereas a normally healthy person may respond quickly to a high potency medicine.

**Is it safe to self-prescribe?**

Homeopathy is considered safe to self-prescribe and certain high potency medicines are available over-the-counter in chemists and health food shops. However, prescribing the right homeopathic medicine is a complex process that can take years of training and practice to perfect. Therefore, it is always best to take homeopathic medicines on the advice of a trained and registered homeopath.

## What do homeopathic medicines contain?

Homeopathic medicines are derived from a variety of natural substances, including plants, animals and minerals. For example, the remedy lachesis is derived from snake venom – an animal derivative; rhus tox from poison ivy – a plant; and nat mur from sodium chloride – a mineral.

## How are the therapeutic effects of the substances determined?

To determine their therapeutic effects, doses of a particular substance are given to volunteers over a period of time until symptoms begin to appear. These symptoms are then carefully recorded and the substance becomes the basis for a medicine that is used to treat an ill person who displays those symptoms.

## How will I feel after taking a medicine?

People respond to homeopathic medicines in different ways. You may feel an immediate surge of wellbeing, or you may suddenly feel very tired and need to rest for a day or so. Alternatively you may feel nothing at all. Sometimes the symptoms temporarily become worse; homeopaths estimate that this occurs in about 20 per cent of all patients. You may also experience symptoms of past illnesses from which you have never fully recovered. All these reactions are interpreted by homeopaths as a sign that a medicine is working and a process of self-healing has begun.

## How often is treatment needed?

As a general rule, if you have an acute condition, such as a cold, homeopaths may recommend frequent doses of homeopathic medicine for a short period of time. If you are undergoing homeopathic treatment for a chronic condition, such as arthritis, you might take a single dose of a medicine or be directed to take your medicine at regular intervals. It is quite usual to have an interval of up to three months between follow-up appointments.

## How much does a consultation cost?

Fees vary according to local market forces and the level of experience and reputation of the individual homeopathic practitioner concerned. Generally fees for a private consultation with a homeopath are likely to range from £30 to £150. Homeopaths usually charge more for initial consultations since these last longer than follow-up sessions. Consultations in London are more expensive than elsewhere. The cost of remedies is often included within the consultation but if purchased separately, the medicines themselves usually cost about £5.

## Can I have homeopathy at reduced rates?

A number of members of the Faculty of Homeopathy and the Society of Homeopaths offer their services at reduced rates for people on low incomes. The British Homeopathic Association publishes a list of homeopathic practitioners, dentists and vets, and this list indicates which practitioners offer lower rates. The listings in this guide tell you about homeopaths who provide low-cost clinics in your area.

## Can I get my private health insurers to pay for my homeopathy treatment?

An increasing number of health insurers allow you to claim back treatment fees for homeopathy. This is usually dependent on certain conditions, such as GP referral, so check the details of your policy. You should also check that your homeopath is on the insurer's approved list of practitioners. The level of cover may also vary according to the insurance company, the type of policy taken out and the level of premium paid.

## Will my homeopath belong to a professional body?

There are two types of homeopathy included in this guide.
• Homeopaths registered with The Faculty of Homeopathy are medically trained healthcare professionals, such as GPs.

- Homeopaths registered with the Society of Homeopaths will have taken a three-year full-time or four-year part-time degree course. However, they may have no other healthcare training.

## Where can I find a qualified homeopath?

The homeopaths listed in this guide are registered with either the Faculty of Homoepathy or the Society of Homeopaths and as such will be trained to the standards set out below and abide by a Code of Ethics. The British Homeopathic Association publishes a list of homeopaths registered with the Faculty of Homeopathy. The Society of Homeopaths publishes a register of its members.

## What questions should I ask before making an appointment with a homeopathic practitioner?

- Are they properly trained and a member of a recognised professional body?
- Do they have experience treating problems similar to yours?
- Are there any risks involved in treatment?
- Are there other treatment options available?
- How long is the treatment likely to last?
- Are they willing to discuss your condition with your GP if you request it?
- How much do they charge and do they offer concessionary rates?
- Do they have full professional indemnity and public liability insurance?
- Will they give you clear information about what your medicine contains, information about whether it is safe to take with any conventional medicine, and instructions on how to take it?

You should also make sure that:

- On the first consultation a full case history is taken. The consultation should last at least 40 minutes. If your practitioner does not speak English, make sure that there is a translator present.

# Case history

Lesley Ridout, Homeopathy patient

I used to have severe eczema, which I was born with, and it affected all the usual places, including the insides of my elbows, behind my knees and my ears. I also suffered from asthma and hay fever in the summer, both of which were hereditary. Throughout childhood I was profoundly itchy, then around the age of eighteen the eczema became really bad on my legs, manifesting itself in huge, red, raw patches. It was so embarrassing that I would completely cover up in summer, and the heat would aggravate the condition until it became infected.

I was sent to hospital where I was prescribed heavy-duty steroid creams and antibiotics. These would clear the problem up temporarily, but it always came back. Once I was sent to the Royal Free Hospital where my skin was exposed to ten different common household substances as part of a scratch test to identify what – if anything – I was allergic to. However, the only substance I tested positive to was nickel, which I hardly ever come into contact with. Then the same happened on another occasion, this time as part of a clinical trial. Many different substances were tested on my back, but nothing conclusive ever came back, and then the dermatology department lost everyone's notes!

I tried acupuncture for six months, but it only cleared up a tiny patch of the eczema. I also tried Chinese herbs, which made me feel sick, but did little else. I tried cutting various foods out of my diet, including wheat, dairy, alcohol and coffee. I even went on a fast, but nothing stopped it. Then a good friend of mine who is a homeopath recommended I try homeopathy, although she suggested I see another professional homeopath so that there was no conflict of interest. I was initially a bit sceptical, but very impressed by how thorough the homeopath's approach was. She not only wanted to know about my physical symptoms and medical history, but also, for example, about what made me happy or sad and whether I preferred hot or cold food. I don't remember a practitioner taking so much time to get the whole picture before. She didn't look at the eczema until towards the end of the appointment. Later that week I received some specially made-up remedies in the post. There were some unusual rules for taking them, including not smoking or eating for half an hour before or after taking them, nor could you use any kind of mint toothpaste, chewing gum or mints, as these things reduce their efficacy. I was also instructed to keep a diary of how I felt, noting any changes.

I carried on seeing my homeopath every week, and very quickly a patch of the scaly, raised red skin on my leg started to turn white. The real benefits took perhaps two months to show, by which time all the affected areas were rapidly healing. I saw the homeopath for six months, during which time I split up with my boyfriend of 12 years. It was the most stressful time, and I was fully expecting the eczema to come rushing back, but it didn't. Not only that, but my homeopath rang me every Friday night to check that I was OK and to give me her support. In fact, physically, I felt better than ever, with more energy too. After one and a half years I still see her on an occasional basis, when the eczema resurfaces a tiny bit, but generally this is just for 'maintenance' and prevention.

Perhaps the most important consideration is that you have a rapport with the practitioner, and feel that you can communicate with them. You should feel comfortable asking questions about your problems and your practitioner should be forthcoming about what the treatment will involve, how much it will cost and how payment should be made. It may be helpful to visit the premises so try and book your first appointment in person.

**What training do homeopaths have?**

All homeopaths registered with either the Faculty of Homeopathy or the Society of Homeopaths have received proper training in homeopathy.

Homeopaths who are Members of the Faculty of Homeopathy are medically trained healthcare professionals and will have undergone a minimum of three years intensive part-time training in homeopathy in addition to their medical training. They will have passed one or more of the Faculty's examinations.

Homeopaths registered with the Society of Homeopaths must attend a recognised course of three years full-time or four years part-time, which includes appropriate medical science education, followed by clinical supervision. For admission to the Society's Register there is a rigorously assessed registration development programme and a site visit of inspection to watch the practitioner at work.

Training programmes accredited by the Faculty of Homeopathy assume a knowledge of medical science and as a result training opportunities are only open to statutorily registered healthcare professionals.

However, anyone who has an interest in homeopathy can train to be a professional homeopath. Students should ensure that they train at a recognised college if they wish to be eligible to register with the Society of Homeopaths.

## What do all the letters mean?

Letters after a practitioner's name show the organisation the practitioner is registered with and the level of membership of that body.

The Faculty of Homeopathy has different levels of membership, depending on the homeopath's profession and depth of training in homeopathy.

**MFHom FFHom**  Homeopathic doctors who have passed the Faculty's Membership qualification are identified by the letters MFHom (Member of the Faculty of Homeopathy) or FFHom (Fellow of the Faculty of Homeopathy) after their name.

**LFHom**  This title is awarded to healthcare professionals who have passed the Faculty of Homeopathy's basic exam and are considered able to apply a basic knowledge of homeopathy in a way appropriate to their profession.

**VetMFHom VetFFHom**  Veterinary Members have the letters VetMFHom (Veterinary Member of the Faculty of Homeopathy) or VetFFHom (Veterinary Fellow of the Faculty of Homeopathy) after their name.

**DFHom(Dent) DFHom(Pharm)**  Dentists and pharmacists who have passed the Diploma of the Faculty of Homeopathy exam are able to apply an intermediate knowledge of homeopathy within the spheres of their profession. They are identified by the letters DFHom(Dent) and DFHom(Pharm) respectively. These Diplomas are the highest levels of qualification available to dentists and pharmacists and recognise their homeopathic skills applied within the bounds of dentistry or pharmacy.

The Society of Homeopaths has two levels of membership, depending on the training and the number of years in clinical practice.

**LHom**  Professional homeopaths who have trained at a recognised college for three years full-time or four years part-time are licensed to practise homeopathy by the Society and may use the phrase 'licensed member of the Society of Homeopaths working towards registration'.

**RSHom FSHom**  After a year licensed members of the Society of Homeopaths can apply for full registration. Practitioners need to complete a registration portfolio which may include additional case studies. These members are identified by the title RSHom (Registered Member of the Society of Homeopaths) or FSHom (Fellow of the Society of Homeopaths) after their name.

### How do homeopaths keep their skills and knowledge up-to-date?

Both the Faculty of Homeopathy and the Society of Homeopaths recommend minimum Continuing Professional Development requirements (CPD) for all registered practitioners. Professional development is important since it ensures that a practitioner's knowledge and skills are kept up-to-date. All Faculty members are required to keep a log of their Faculty-accredited CPD and this is validated every five years. CPD might include attending events, conferences and seminars as well as private study.

### Will a homeopath have access to my medical records?

If you are referred by your GP to a homeopathic hospital or specialist clinic, your doctor will provide any relevant information from your medical records needed by the homeopath. If you refer yourself to a private practitioner, you can ask your GP for any medical information that your homeopath may need to know, such as the results of clinical tests.

Practitioners will keep their own detailed records of your treatment. With very specific exceptions, you have a right to access your records wherever they are held. If treatment is provided under the NHS, your homeopath will provide a report to your GP informing them of assessment, treatment and any changes observed. This will form part of your medical records held by your GP.

**Is there statutory regulation of homeopathy in the UK?**

There is currently no statutory regulation of homeopathy in the UK. Anyone may still call themselves a homeopath without proper training. It is very important, therefore, to ensure that your homeopath is registered with a professional body.

The Faculty of Homeopathy is the only UK body that regulates the practice of homeopathy by statutorily registered healthcare professionals. Healthcare professionals are required to practice within the bounds of competence of their profession and their level of training and experience in homeopathy. If, for example, the GMC were to receive a complaint about the practice of homeopathy by a doctor, then the GMC would be likely to call on the Faculty to advise on their competence to practice in this field.

There is currently no single registering body for non-medically trained homeopaths. The Society of Homeopaths is the largest organisation regulating the practice of professional homeopaths. The various bodies representing professional homeopaths have set up the Council of Organisations Representing Homeopaths (CORH) and work is taking place with the aim of creating a single register of non-medically qualified homeopaths.

**Can I get homeopathy treatment through the NHS?**

Homeopathy is the only form of complementary medicine that has been continuously available on the NHS since it was established in 1948. Homeopathic medicine is practised in five specialist hospitals throughout the UK – in Bristol, Glasgow, Liverpool, London and Tunbridge Wells. However, you can only be treated at a homeopathic hospital if you have a referral from your GP or specialist.

Homeopathy is also practised in GP surgeries and in specialist clinics. It can sometimes feel like a struggle to obtain homeopathy on the NHS, particularly if your GP is unsympathetic or your health authority is not keen on funding it. Most people therefore refer themselves to a homeopath in private practice.

# Case history

Maria Crace, Homeopathy patient

My son was perfectly healthy until the age of eighteen months when he developed a urinary tract infection. I took him to the GP, who put him on antibiotics and ordered kidney abnormality tests. A month later he developed another infection, then a second and a third. The doctors put him on antibiotics for a year. The real trouble started, however, when they took him off them. After five days he had severe diarrhoea, followed by a bacterial infection, salmonella, and monthly ear infections. We were referred to an ear, nose and throat surgeon who suggested grommets and antibiotics. However, by this time I had heard about professional homeopathy and asked if we could try it. We agreed to give it three months.

On our first visit to the homeopath, my son was running a 40-degree temperature from an ear infection and was screaming. The homeopath popped a remedy into his mouth, and within minutes his temperature started to drop and he fell asleep while we discussed his medical history. After that, although he still had lots of ear infections, he responded to homeopathic treatment quickly. At one point he also had croup, and given his history we might have expected hospitalisation, but he recovered within days with homeopathic treatment.

When he started nursery he was still overreacting to every infection, and at the age of four and a half, began to have severe back pain. The paediatricians were concerned that this could be a sign of bone infection. All the tests were negative, nevertheless they recommended antibiotics and painkillers. I was determined not to go down this route again, and decided to try a homeopathic approach that included medical expertise. I knew that my son's problems were getting more complex, and that we needed to negotiate between a complementary approach and orthodox medical treatment. My GP referred us to a homeopathic hospital.

The medical homeopath we saw was concerned about the medical implications of my son's infections, and her approach – wanting to know about the nature of the organisms causing the infection and whether MRI and CAT scans had been performed – reassured me of her expertise. Her homeopathic treatment almost immediately relieved his pain and started to improve his health. However, because of the lack of resources, we couldn't get enough appointments, so I decided to go to a private medical homeopath.

As my son was still becoming ill every three weeks or so, we saw the new homeopath at least once a month and often had phone consultations with her. We also had a homeopathic kit for those frequent middle-of-the-night problems. However, although he was still prone to picking up any bug going, his health was improving all the time. After a year, when he was about five, his level of health had improved to such an extent that he was only missing the same amount of school as his classmates. The homeopathy was also great for accidents; he broke his leg and his toes, and we used a homeopathic remedy that quickly reduced the swelling.

Now aged thirteen, he gets the odd infection, but as the homeopath has gone deeper into treating the underlying causes of his ill health, which go back into our family history, she is clearing his system of potential triggers of illness. For example, since she has been treating him with remedies that relate to tubercular illness, he doesn't pick up chesty coughs and ear infections.

**Can my GP refer me to a homeopath?**

GPs are becoming increasingly aware of the benefits of homeopathy and may refer you to a homeopath. In the vast majority of areas GPs can refer patients to one of the NHS homeopathic hospitals. Your GP may also have the option of referring patients to a local NHS homeopathic clinic or to a homeopath in private practice. However, it is likely that you will have to pay for private treatment yourself.

**What should I do if my GP refuses to make a referral?**

Your GP does not have to refer you if they do not think that homeopathy is appropriate for your medical condition. However, your GP should discuss this decision with you, and if you and your GP cannot come to an agreement about whether homeopathic treatment is appropriate, there are several steps you can take:

- Request a second opinion; this would usually be from another GP at the practice.
- Complain under the NHS complaints procedure. Your local practice should provide you with information about making a complaint.
- Register with another GP. Your Primary Care Trust (Health Board in Scotland or Local Health Group in Wales) can provide you with a list of GPs in your area. You may wish to check with alternative GPs about their attitude towards homeopathy before registering. Suitably qualified GPs are able to apply homeopathy directly in their work. You should check that they are registered with the Faculty of Homeopathy so that you can be sure they are properly trained. The British Homeopathic Association can provide you with a list of GPs trained in homeopathy and you may be able to register with a homeopathic doctor in your area.

**Will my homeopath discuss my condition with my GP?**

If you have been referred on the NHS your homeopath will communicate with your GP to ensure they are kept up-to-date with your assessment and treatment. If you refer yourself to a homeopath privately, the practitioner is likely to encourage you to give them permission to communicate with the GP if necessary. However, they cannot do this without your consent.

**Can homeopathy be used safely during pregnancy and childbirth?**

Under the supervision of an appropriately qualified and regulated practitioner, homeopathy is a very safe form of medicine. It is often used to treat the minor health problems caused by the physical and emotional changes of pregnancy, such as morning sickness. It is also sometimes used to help with post-delivery problems such as the 'baby blues' and mastitis.

**Can homeopathy be used on animals?**

Animals can only be treated by a trained vet although owners may treat their own companion animals. Details of vets with the Faculty of Homeopathy's qualification VetMFHom or VetFFHom are included in the practitioner list distributed by the British Homeopathic Association. There is also an association of homeopathic veterinarians (British Association of Homeopathic Veterinary Surgeons) who may be contacted through the Faculty of Homeopathy and there is a range of books on how to treat your own domestic animals.

**What about dental care?**

Details of dentists with the Faculty's qualification DFHom(Dent) or LFHom(Dent) are included in the practitioner list distributed by the British Homeopathic Association. There is an association of homeopathic dentists (British Homeopathic Dental Association), who may be contacted through the Faculty of Homeopathy.

# Case history

Dr Sara Eames, Homeopath

I am a medically qualified homeopath and work mainly within the NHS at the Royal London Homeopathic Hospital, specialising in women and children's health. I am also Director of Education.

Today I am going to spend the morning in a children's clinic. I have two new patients and six patients coming for a follow-up visit. The new patients are brothers who have fairly severe asthma. They have needed hospital in-patient treatment a number of times and both take two different inhalers regularly. Their GP and their mother are concerned by their repeated hospitalisation and their long-term use of inhalers.

Although they are brothers, and have the same medical diagnosis, they have contrasting personalities, and their asthma presents itself in different ways. The older boy is quiet and tends to keep his feelings to himself. His first asthma attack was soon after his grandfather died. His attacks usually start in the daytime on hot days, and he has been rushed to hospital twice during seaside holidays. I prescribe him natrum muriaticum.

His younger brother is a lively, mischievous boy. He gets bored easily and is at his best when he is out of the house and on the move. He often catches colds that spread rapidly to his chest. His attacks are more common in the winter, especially when the weather is cold and damp. I prescribe tuberculinum. These brothers are a good example of how a homeopathic prescription is made on the basis of the overall personality of the patient and on their particular symptoms.

The children I see for follow-up visits have initially been referred variously for hyperactivity, glue-ear, Crohn's disease, recurrent tonsillitis and eczema. It is quite common, however, that during treatment we discover other problems, both physical and emotional, that can also be helped. So after treatment patients can seem generally better in themselves. Today the most dramatic change has been in the hyperactive boy who apparently began to improve after the first homeopathic dose. His mother has repeated it twice during the last four months when his behaviour started to deteriorate, again with good results.

The others are improving more slowly and a four-year-old girl with eczema is no better. There are over 2000 different homeopathic remedies, and even the most experienced homeopaths don't always find a helpful remedy with the first prescription. Sometimes it can take a few interviews to discover the information that will lead to a useful remedy. Homeopathy needs patience, both on the part of the practitioner and the patient, but in my experience will often effect a deeper and longer-lasting cure than that achieved by conventional treatment.

I also see a private patient, a 38-year-old woman with severe premenstrual tension and abdominal pain before and during her periods. She has not had any gynaecological investigations and is keen to start a family. The symptoms she describes suggest endometriosis, and I recommend asking her GP for a referral to a gynaecoclogist. In the meantime I need to study her case and consult some reference books before I decide what to prescribe. As I quite often do, I say that I will send her a remedy in a few days' time.

Problems such as mouth ulcers or bleeding gums can be self-treated with homeopathy but you should check with your dentist that these do not signify an underlying condition. Advice may also be given about the avoidance or removal of mercury fillings, and alternatives to antibiotics and painkillers.

## Do homeopaths make home visits?

Consultations normally take place at the practitioner's practice, although some homeopaths may offer to visit you at home if you are housebound. Often, practitioners will conduct follow-up consultations for minor conditions over the phone.

## Are homeopathic practitioners insured?

All homeopaths who are registered with the Faculty of Homeopathy and the Society of Homeopaths are required to have professional indemnity insurance.

## How can I complain if something goes wrong?

There are different complaints procedures depending on where and from whom you received treatment. These are:

**Faculty of Homeopathy**  A copy of the Disciplinary, Capability and Complaints policy is available through the Faculty of Homeopathy. Complaints should be made in writing and addressed to the Chairman of the Disciplinary and Professional Performance Committee.

**Society of Homeopaths**  If you have a complaint about a homeopath registered with the Society of Homeopaths, write in confidence to the Professional Conduct Officer. Policy is laid out in a leaflet called 'Expressing concerns, making complaints'.

**NHS GP Practices, Hospitals and Clinics**  These are required by law to have their own local complaints policy. Complaints about the practice of any doctor can be made directly to the General Medical Council.

**Where can I find further information?**

**The British Homeopathic Association
and the Faculty of Homeopathy**
15 Clerkenwell Close
London EC1R 0AA
Tel: 020 7566 7800 (BHA)
Tel: 020 7566 7810 (Faculty)
email: info@trusthomeopathy.org
website: www.trusthomeopathy.org

**Society of Homeopaths**
4a Artizan Road, Northampton NN1 4HU
Tel: 01604 621400
Email: info@homeopathy-soh.org.
Website: www.homeopathy-soh.org

**Homeopathic Hospitals**

**Bristol Homeopathic Hospital**
Cotharm Hill, Cotharm,
Bristol BS6 6JU
Tel: 0117 973 1231

**Royal London Homeopathic Hospital**
Great Ormond Street,
London WC1N 3HR
Tel: 020 7837 8833

**Department of Homeopathic Medicine**

The Old Swan Health Centre,
St Oswald's Street, Old Swan,
Liverpool L13 2BY
Tel: 0151 228 6808

**Glasgow Homeopathic Hospital**

1053 Great Western Road,
Glasgow G12 0XQ
Tel: 0141 211 1616

**Tunbridge Wells Homeopathic Hospital**

Church Road,
Tunbridge Wells,
Kent TN1 1JU
Tel: 01892 542977

# Osteopathy

## What is osteopathy?

Osteopathy is used to treat a variety of musculo-skeletal problems involving the bones, joints, muscles, ligaments and connective tissues, including those of the viscera. Osteopaths believe that when the body is in balance and working efficiently, it functions with the minimum of wear, stress and energy. However, mechanical problems occurring within the body can in turn create imbalances within the normal tension of the spine. This may affect the nervous and circulatory systems and lead to pain, disability and dysfunction.

Osteopaths employ a wide range of treatment methods according to the individual's age, physique and particular problem. Methods range from soft tissue 'massage' of muscles and ligaments, passive stretching and traction to joints and manipulative separation techniques (which patients often feel as a click) to improve joint mobility.

## HISTORY

Osteopathy originated in early nineteenth-century America when a trained doctor, Andrew Taylor-Still, sought to find a new method of treating illness by aiming to influence the blood supply to bodily organs and the body's nervous system. He believed this treatment to be a total system of medicine which would eventually replace conventional medical treatment. Still founded the first school of osteopathy in Missouri in 1892 after which the practice found its way to the UK. The British School of Osteopathy was founded in London in 1917.

Osteopathy was the first complementary therapy to be regulated by law and the General Osteopathic Council was set up in 1993 to protect patients from untrained and unauthorised practitioners. Today there are around 3000 osteopaths in the UK performing over 6 million patient consultations per year.

## How does it work?

Osteopaths apply treatment directly to your body with their hands, using joint manipulations to improve the range of motion of individual joints. You will often feel a 'click' as these manipulations are performed. Other stretching 'articulatory' techniques are employed to stretch rhythmically the ligaments of a joint by manually using the patient's limbs as levers. 'Soft tissue' manual techniques are another umbrella term used to describe a wide range of massage-style techniques.

Osteopaths believe that their particular method is more than just a series of manipulations and combine their knowledge of psycho-social factors with a range of different manual techniques to improve musculo-skeletal function, so influencing the function of the other body systems and the general wellbeing of the patient.

## What conditions do osteopaths treat?

Osteopaths most frequently treat spinal pain, from which four out of five people will suffer at some stage of their lives. But it is also used for the treatment of mechanical and functional problems throughout the entire body and in all age groups. Examples include:

- Muscle and joint pains in active and developing children.
- Sports-related injuries such as 'tennis elbow', 'pulled hamstring' or 'strained ankle'.
- Muscular pain and circulation problems associated with pregnancy.
- Work-related difficulties such as back problems as a result of poor posture.
- Problems in later life, for example osteoarthritic hips and knees.

Osteopathy is used to treat other problems of pain and function (such as headache, gastric pain, chest pain and gynaecological pain). These can be referred pain of a mechanical origin rather than due to an underlying illness (although this should be verified by your GP in the first instance).

## Can osteopathy treat chronic conditions?

Chronic conditions can be assessed and treated in the same way as acute ones. However, it is important to realise that in chronic conditions, tissue changes such as muscle spasm and joint restriction are more established and can be resistant to change.

## Who can benefit from osteopathic treatment?

Osteopathy is used to treat all age groups. A good osteopath will tailor each treatment to the individual and look at your physique and general health as well as the problem. For example, the correct level of treatment for a frail 75-year-old woman would be inappropriate for use on a 25-year-old sixteen-stone rugby player.

## Are there conditions for which osteopathy is not appropriate?

Some osteopathic techniques are not suitable for the treatment of recent fractures, rheumatoid arthritis, osteoporosis, cervical or thoracic myelopathy, or for women in the first three months of pregnancy.

## Is osteopathy safe and are there any possible side-effects?

Overzealous or inappropriate treatment can be harmful and your condition can be compounded if you are not thoroughly assessed or 'screened' at the time of your initial consultation. The risk to you is minimised in the hands of a properly trained and experienced clinician who is thorough in assessment and monitors progress carefully. At the end of an undergraduate degree programme, students undertake a clinical examination that is specifically designed to assess safety and competence to practise. However, during osteopathic training, the importance of knowing when not to treat is given great emphasis. Examples of these situations include:

- Following major trauma where there could be structural damage

- When pain is out of proportion to the clinical findings
- If you are too apprehensive or in too much pain
- Where there is known pathology such as tumour
- Severe osteoporosis
- Additionally, forceful manipulation should not be used on your neck if you have rheumatoid arthritis and if you have signs of nerve root entrapment, manipulation should not be used on the affected segments.

The most common side-effect from hands-on mechanical treatment is an increase in pain or soreness in the first 24 to 48 hours following treatment. If you are concerned about the level of your reaction to treatment, you should initially speak to your practitioner – particularly if your discomfort is unacceptable or if it lasts more than 48 hours. Proper management usually enables these side-effects to settle quickly.


**Is there research that shows that osteopathy really works?**

Although there is no single undisputed reference that demonstrates the effectiveness of osteopathic interventions for any particular group of ailments, there are many publications from around the world that report trials and evaluations of osteopathy and other physical treatment modalities for musculo-skeletal problems, especially lower back pain.

There are a number of systematic reviews of current literature, in particular, those carried out by the Clinical Standards Advisory Group. The Royal College of General Practitioners' Guidelines for the Treatment of Acute Low Back Pain show that there are indications for the use of manipulation. However, they do also acknowledge that the methodological quality of much of the research literature is poor.

Some evidence indicates that cervical manipulation for neck pain is safer than non-steroidal anti-inflammatory drugs (NSAIDs) which are often the conventional first-line treatment for similar musculo-skeletal problems, but other experts question the accuracy of this study. Since there are so many conditions that osteopaths treat and so many elements to the history-taking assessment, investigation, diagnosis, management and treatment of each of these, it is almost impossible to gain evidence either to support or refute elements for every aspect of the clinical intervention.

Evidence has been cited to support the effectiveness of osteopathy in treating the following conditions, however, other experts have questioned the reliability of these conclusions:

- Back pain (evidence for this condition is strongest)
- Chronic fatigue syndrome
- Headache
- Infantile colic
- Menopausal symptoms
- Neck pain
- Premenstrual tension

## What happens on a first visit?

At an initial assessment, osteopaths aim to diagnose your problem and gain an understanding of its underlying cause. Once this is established, it is easier to devise ways of avoiding relapses or recurrences.

Firstly, your osteopath will take a history of your problem. They will ask you questions about the nature of the pain and how it is affecting your life. These will be followed by in-depth questions about the range and extent of activities that you perform in your working and personal life. The osteopath will also need to know about other issues relating to your present and past general health since this can be relevant to conditions that can sometimes be mistaken for mechanical pain.

Following your medical history, the osteopath will examine you. You will probably need to undress to your underclothes so that the affected area can be examined in relation to your posture and movement as a whole. By the time the history and examination have been completed, the osteopath will generally have decided what is at fault, how they intend to treat the problem and whether extra investigations are necessary.

By the end of your initial consultation, you should have a good idea as to the cause of your problem and how your osteopath intends to treat it. You should also have been given advice about progress and when to return. In the majority of cases, the osteopath will begin the treatment straight away. Usually treatment is pleasant and rarely painful, although you may occasionally experience some minor discomfort. If at any stage you feel you are not ready for treatment, or if you would rather just have advice about your problem, you should make this clear.

### What does a treatment involve?

As well as joint manipulation, your treatment plan may include advice on posture, diet, lifestyle or stress, if the practitioner believes these are contributing to your problem. Osteopaths generally compile an informal programme for recovery. This might include exercises to do at home and appointments to return for treatment if this is needed. Your general day-to-day activities, whether during sport or leisure, can greatly affect your progress and your contribution to the treatment is just as important as that of the osteopath.

### Will I need an X-ray?

You might need an X-ray if, for example, you have had recent injuries or are an older patient where there may be a question relating to the extent of wear in your spine.

### How long does a treatment session last?

Osteopaths vary in the length of time they spend with you according to their style of practice and experience. Most first appointments are usually 45-60 minutes and subsequent appointments can range from 20 to 40 minutes, depending on your individual needs.

### How often is treatment needed?

It may not be possible at the outset to safely judge how many sessions will be needed for a given condition. As well as the effectiveness of treatment, your co-operation in such things as 'do's', 'don'ts' and exercise is an important factor in your recovery. For the management of acute spinal pain, an average number of treatments could be six sessions. It is, however, important for you and your practitioner to work out early on how many treatments should be given before you could reasonably expect to see some progress. For many conditions this would occur within three or four treatments, but longer may be required in the case of particularly chronic or complex cases such as chronic fatigue syndrome or asthma. You should be wary of entering into 'open-ended' or 'ongoing' plans of treatment unless you have a thorough understanding of the reasons for it.

### What will happen when I return for follow-up treatment?

Treatment at follow-up visits is quite different from the initial consultation. You will be asked questions regarding the progress of your symptoms and your ability to undertake certain tasks. You will usually be asked to undress to your underclothes to receive manual treatment. The mode of treatment may vary according to your response, as may the techniques used from one visit to another. The practitioner will make notes on each occasion so that your rate of progress can be monitored carefully. You may be given further advice on 'do's and don'ts' to help you avoid factors that could hamper your progress. Your osteopath should keep you informed of how treatment is progressing.

# Case history

Torben Hersborg, Osteopath specialising in sports injuries

I work from 9–7 in a typical day, which is pretty action-packed, and treat about 20 patients. I see a lot of back problems, particularly of the lower back, and also many knee problems and pulled hamstrings, as I treat many sports men and women.

I am most busy in the training season when athletes come in with pulled hamstrings, shin-splints and Achilles tendon problems.

Pulled hamstrings are very common and can be caused by sprinting, jumping, kicking a football, or anything that uses fast, explosive movement. Very often the hamstring is the weak link, weakened by a stiffness in other structures such as the sacroiliac joint. As the hamstring is attached to the pelvic bone it becomes elongated and taut, so that if you suddenly flick out your leg you can pull it.

There are many ways of treating a pulled hamstring, but the way I prefer to go about it is to loosen up the sacroiliac joint so that I can get the pelvic bone rotating and the hamstring relaxing. Sometimes it can be difficult to do this, as the hamstring is a delicate muscle. It is also usually impossible to persuade the athletes to stop training and competing during recovery. Very often the imbalance is caused by a leg length difference, so that when the athletes are running they are not running evenly. Most people have one leg longer than the other, and that's the way it should be, so I never measure leg length difference. Instead I test all the muscles while the patient is standing up to see where they function best.

I prefer a high-velocity approach, mainly because I know I can do it precisely. If you are very fast you can loosen up the joints before the muscles start reacting or guarding, which they tend to do particularly if a person is nervous because of their pain. So if I can get the joint loosened up, high velocity is in fact a much gentler technique. The sound that the joints make when they are manipulated is not the sound of anything breaking, but a release between two joint surfaces, similar to the sound of your tongue clicking against the roof of your mouth.

If I have 20 patients in one day, I probably see them for 20 minutes each. Treatment duration varies from patient to patient and according to injury, but the average person may have three or four treatments in the space of a fortnight, depending on how well they respond. But obviously that would not necessarily make them strong enough to compete in a sport such as sprinting.

I often attend competitions, such as the World Athletics Championships. The most I have ever had to treat a single athlete in one day during a competition is ten times. Another athlete suffered from lower back pain from a sacroiliac joint and wasn't able to support any weight at all. But twenty hours after we started treatment, he won a gold medal and has never had back pain since. Then there was the sprinter with a pulled hamstring whom I treated nine times in one day; she had three races that day. Ten days before the competition she couldn't walk. I saw her once a day leading up to the competition, and she ended up doing three personal bests in three races and won her first British title.

**I've heard that my condition may get worse before it gets better. Is this true?**

Sometimes you may experience a temporary exacerbation of your symptoms after treatment. This is the body's reaction to treatment, which precedes proper healing of the tissues. Some osteopaths may refer to this as 'the healing crisis'.

**Are there any different osteopathy techniques?**

Many osteopaths have special areas of interest in which they may be highly trained and experienced. Examples are sports injuries, cranial osteopathy, and the treatment of children. The Osteopathic Council does not have a register of special interests but it does help you to identify such practitioners. Some osteopaths use 'indirect techniques' which are very gentle and are particularly suitable for the elderly and children.

Cranial osteopathy is a very subtle and gentle approach and treats the whole body. It differs in that it recognises the importance of subtle mechanics at work within the head and the effect that those strains can have on influencing the health of the whole body. Most osteopaths have a working knowledge of the cranial approach, but only some choose to specialise in this field, which involves considerable postgraduate study. The gentle nature of cranial treatment makes it suitable for the treatment of children. It is particularly used in treating babies for colic or constant crying and for older children with behaviour difficulties, 'glue' ear, sinus problems and head injuries.

**How much does a consultation cost?**

Fees vary considerably according to geographical location, the practitioner's experience, the extent of the facilities provided and administrative back-up. You can expect to pay anything from £25 to £50. Some osteopaths charge more for the first consultation as this usually takes longer than follow-up appointments.

### Can I have osteopathy treatment at reduced rates?

Most osteopaths will endeavour to provide treatment for as wide a range of patients as possible. Some osteopaths will publish reduced rates for particular groups of patients, but many will assess them on individual need. A good strategy is to find the osteopath that suits you best and then ask if reduced rates are available at that practice. The listings at the end of this guide tell you which osteopaths do this.

### Can I get my private health insurers to pay for my osteopathy treatment?

These days most health insurance companies do cover osteopathy. However, the extent and conditions of cover vary enormously and you would be best advised to contact your health insurer prior to treatment. BUPA and PPP carry a list of practitioners who have 'specialist status', which requires at least five years' full-time experience and references from peers, general practitioners and consultants. The extent of cover varies considerably – from a fixed amount to the number of permitted visits – and each policy carries different rates of excess.

### Where can I find a qualified practitioner?

The osteopaths listed in this guide are all registered with the General Osteopathic Council, which carries a Code of Conduct and has an ethical complaints procedure. Osteopaths who are registered with the GOsC (see below) and practise within a Code of Ethics and Practice, have professional insurance, and have passed stringent academic and clinical assessments before being admitted to the register. The letters ADO, DO or BSC Ost after their name identify qualified practitioners. Some osteopaths listed in this guide may also be members of the British Osteopathic Association.

You can be referred by your GP under the NHS, or you can find a practitioner yourself. When choosing an osteopath, you need to make sure they are a registered member of the General Osteopathic Council.

## What questions should I ask before making an appointment with an osteopath?

- Are they properly trained and registered with the GOsC?
- Have they had experience in treating similar health problems to yours?
- What are the possible side-effects of the treatment?
- How long is the treatment likely to last?
- What other treatment options are available?
- How much will they charge and do they offer concessionary rates?
- Are they, where necessary, licensed or registered with the local authority to practise from the address where you see them?
- Are they properly insured?

You should also ask:

- How many years have they been in practice and is this full- or part-time?
- Are they registered with any major health insurance companies?
- Will they speak to you prior to the consultation?
- Are they involved in any teaching or other professional activity?

Perhaps the most important consideration is that you have a rapport with the practitioner, and feel that you can communicate with them. You should feel comfortable asking questions about your problems and your practitioner should be forthcoming about what the treatment will involve, how much it will cost and how payment should be made. Other questions might relate to the type of technique they practise. It may be helpful to visit the premises so try to book your first appointment in person.

## What training do osteopaths have?

Students train through a degree programme run by schools having 'recognised qualification' status. A list of schools that have been awarded this status is held by The General Osteopathic Council (see below). Graduates are not entitled to practise until they have registered with the GosC, who recommend the use of the title 'Registered Osteopath'. This allows registrants to distinguish themselves from any graduates who are not on the register during their transitional period. A degree course in osteopathy is generally four years full-time or five years part-time. The Diploma in Osteopathy has now been phased out although that does not mean that practitioners who hold this qualification are not as good as those with degrees, which are taken at GosC accredited colleges: it simply means that they have been practising for longer.

Osteopathy involves knowledge of basic medical sciences such as anatomy, physiology and biochemistry, a grounding in medical knowledge such as pathology, neurology and orthopaedics, and a focus on manipulation and clinical skills. Professionalism, ethics research and radiology are included in a long list of other subjects.

### What do all the letters mean?

**GOsC** your practitioner is registered with the General Osteopathic Council

**DO, BSc (Ost)** your practitioner has a degree or diploma in osteopathy

**ADO** your practitioner has an advanced diploma in osteopathy

**MLCOM, FLCOM** your practitioner has graduated from the London College of Osteopathic Medicine (13-month full-time post graduate course for doctors)

### How do osteopaths keep their skills and knowledge up-to-date?

As the process of regulating the profession was only completed in May 2000, the assessment of all practitioners currently on the register is up-to-date. In order to maintain these standards from this date forward, a system of Continuing Professional Development (CPD) is being put in place and this will be mandatory in order to maintain registration.

**Is there statutory regulation of osteopathy in the UK?**

The osteopathic profession was the first complementary therapy to achieve statutory regulation. The passing of the Osteopaths Act by Parliament in 1993 led to the creation of the Statutory Register in May 2000. The role of the General Osteopathic Council is to regulate, promote and develop the practice of osteopathy under the supervision of the Privy Council and the Department of Health. The opening of the Statutory Register has meant that the osteopathic profession has undergone a rigorous process of individual practitioner evaluation where each practitioner already practising before that date has had to complete a document known as a PPP (Personal Profile and Professional Portfolio) as a condition of entry to the Register. The PPP explores the length and depth of an osteopath's training and the way in which they have worked since qualifying. Patient profiles are explored, any courses that have been attended are analysed and answers to particular clinical scenarios invited. Osteopaths failing to meet the requirements of the PPP are unable to continue to call themselves osteopaths.

**Is osteopathy available on the NHS?**

Many GPs will refer you to an osteopath for treatment of chronic and acute back pain, neck and shoulder pains and for sporting injuries. Treatment is becoming more commonly available on the NHS.

**Can my GP refer me to an osteopath?**

Many GPs will refer you to osteopaths either by informally suggesting this route or by a formal referral letter. The General Medical Council welcomed the Osteopaths Act of Parliament passed in 1993 and attitudes towards osteopaths have changed enormously in recent years. If your GP refuses to make a referral, despite indications that osteopathy would be appropriate treatment for your medical condition, you can follow the procedure outlined in the section on homeopathy on page 76.

## Will the practitioner discuss my condition with my GP?

If you have been referred by your GP then your osteopath will always inform them of your treatment plan and keep them abreast of your treatment and progress. If you have self-referred to an osteopath, they may wish to discuss your condition with your GP but can only do so with your consent.

## Will my practitioner have access to my medical records?

An osteopath will not generally have access to your medical records and certainly cannot do so without your written consent. With the appropriate consent, however, access to certain medical information can be helpful, particularly X-ray, MRI and imaging reports.

## Can osteopathy be used during pregnancy?

Pregnant women at all stages of pregnancy may receive treatment, although particular care should be taken at 12 and 16 weeks when most natural miscarriages occur. Osteopathy can help minimise the effects of the changes that your body goes through during pregnancy. For instance, changes in posture as your baby grows can often result in back pain. Realignment of the spine and pelvis can help reduce the strain to your joints, shoulders, lower back and legs – the areas most affected during the later stages of pregnancy.

## What other services can an osteopath provide?

Practitioners can provide you with sick-leave certificates, liaise with your employer and produce medico-legal reports. Osteopaths can refer you for X-rays, MRI and bone density scans which are all common in osteopathic practice. Osteopaths can also refer you to consultants such as orthopaedic surgeons or neurologists if they think it is necessary.

# Case history

Jenny Freedland, Osteopathy patient

About three months ago I was due to be a bridesmaid at a friend's wedding, and my boyfriend and I travelled down to London a few days early so that I could help with the final preparations.

I am not a huge yoga fan, but that evening I was feeling slightly stiff after our long drive and decided to stretch my muscles. I got carried away and did a headstand, and as I came down, I felt something 'give' in my neck. I began to feel slightly strange, but put it out of my mind and flipped on the TV. Thirty minutes later, I was flat on my back in excruciating pain and unable to move a muscle.

I could barely sit up and couldn't move my neck or arms at all; and when I tried to walk my ears buzzed, my vision blurred and I fainted. This happened every time I stood up. It was terrifying. I thought I had broken my neck, and spent the night crying my eyes out.

The next morning my boyfriend called the hotel doctor. He assured me that I hadn't broken my neck, and explained that my muscles had gone into deep spasm as a result of severe strain on my neck. He said the fainting was a result of limited blood supply to my brain when I stood up, but not to worry – he could give me painkillers and muscle relaxants and I should begin to feel better in a week or two. I was beside myself. I had exactly one day and a night before I had to walk down the aisle, and I couldn't move a muscle.

The doctor then suggested I consult an osteopath. He referred me to a clinic around the corner from the hotel, and luckily the practitioner was able to come and see me, bringing her portable treatment table with her. She asked me some basic questions about my injury and more detailed questions about my family history and past problems, performed some neurological tests, and, at last, examined me. She almost immediately discovered that I had compressed the vertebrae in my neck, and confirmed that all the muscles in my neck and shoulder were in spasm as a result of the strain.

She spent about 20 minutes on a series of very gentle cranial techniques on my skull and neck, designed to realign and decompress my spine. She also did high-velocity manipulations on my lower back, which had seized up as a result of the extra stress and strain. She then started deep tissue work on my neck and shoulder muscles. The pain was excruciating and she kept at it for about half an hour, but slowly and surely the muscles began to relax.

By the end of the treatment the pain had gone and I could walk, move my head slightly, and my arms freely. She wrote a detailed report of her treatment and gave me copies – one for my GP, and another for an osteopath near my village who she suggested I saw for follow-up treatment.

She also gave me a series of exercises to loosen my neck, which I was to do as often as I could, and advised me to take it easy, but not to be inert. By the following afternoon I was by no means back to normal, but I wasn't in pain and made it to the wedding. I continued with the exercises and felt completely normal after about four days, and have had no problems since.

### Do osteopaths make home visits?

Most osteopaths will offer home visits where needed. However, it is generally acknowledged that it is most cost-effective for you to come to the practice if at all possible. Home visits are more expensive in terms of practitioner time, and the lack of adjustable treatment tables and other equipment can make the treatment at home less effective.

### Are all osteopaths covered by insurance?

All osteopaths are required to have professional indemnity insurance.

### How can I complain if something goes wrong?

If the situation allows, you should inform your osteopath of anything you are unhappy with. This gives the practitioner the opportunity to clarify, explain or rectify the situation.

If you feel your practitioner has been in breach of their professional or ethical rules, you should contact the General Osteopathic Council. The council has mechanisms in place to deal with such complaints in confidence.

### Where can I find further information?

### General Osteopathic Council

Osteopathy House
176 Tower Bridge Road
London SE1 3LU
Tel: 020 7357 6655
email: info@osteopathy.org.uk
www.osteopathy.org.uk

## British Osteopathic Association

Langham House West

Mill Street

Luton

Bedfordshire

LU1 2NA

Tel. 01582 488 455

email:boa@osteopathy.org

www.osteopathy.org

# Chiropractic

## What is chiropractic?

Chiropractic is a method of healing based on manipulation of the spine and other joints. A loss of normal function in the joints or spine can be the result of external factors such as accidents, stress, over-exertion or poor posture. However, chiropractic is concerned not just with skeletal mobility, but also with the nervous system. Practitioners believe that spinal displacement, muscle and joint problems can cause nerve irritation, which in turn disturbs the nervous system and leads to illness. Therefore, manipulation of the spine is thought to have a positive effect on the nervous system and even relieve apparently unrelated conditions such as asthma.

## HISTORY

The founder of chiropractic was a Canadian, Daniel Palmer. He had no orthodox medical training but a keen interest in anatomy and physiology. In 1895, Palmer cured a janitor of deafness with manipulation. The janitor told Palmer that he had lost his hearing seventeen years earlier just after he had felt something 'give' in his back. Palmer found a misaligned vertebra, which he adjusted, and shortly afterwards the janitor regained his hearing. Palmer then set out to develop the use of spinal adjustment to treat disease. His philosophy was that illness is essentially due to malfunction in the spine which affects the various organs of the body.

In 1897, Palmer founded the Palmer Institute and Chiropractic Infirmary in Iowa, USA. Palmer's son continued to develop the profession, and by the time of his death in 1961 chiropractic was the second largest healthcare system in the United States. In the UK, chiropractors have been practising since the early 1900s, when students of the Palmer Institute set up clinics here.

In 1925, the British Chiropractors' Association was formed with six members, making it the oldest chiropractic association in the world. It was also a founder member of the European Chiropractors Union, and together they set up in 1965 the first recognised chiropractic college outside the United States, the Anglo-European College of Chiropractic in Bournemouth. The BCA only accepts graduates from internationally recognised colleges of chiropractic.

In 1981, the British Chiropractors' Association changed its name to the British Chiropractic Association (BCA). The McTimoney Chiropractic College, which teaches the McTimoney approach to chiropractic, was founded by John McTimoney in 1972 and the McTimoney Chiropractic Association was formed soon afterwards and is soon to include in its membership members of the British Association of Applied Chiropractic, which practises the McTimoney-Corley technique. Between them the three associations have over 1500 members.

Over the last decade in the UK, the chiropractic profession has progressed from voluntary self-regulation by professional associations to the introduction of statutory regulation with the establishment of the General Chiropractic Council (GCC) in 1997.

**How does it work?**

Chiropractic is based on the principle that the body's well-being is dependent on the nervous system, centred in the spinal cord. The spinal cord runs within the spinal column from the brain, sending out 31 pairs of nerves that exit from between the vertebrae. These nerves form a complex network running through the joints, muscles and skin and affecting all body tissue. Accidents, stresses, over-exertion or general lifestyle factors can cause a joint or vertebra to lose its normal motion or function. This in turn can irritate areas of the nervous system, often the spinal nerve roots themselves, causing pain, discomfort or even disease.

Chiropractic is based on a whole body assessment of the individual. As well as looking at the mechanical disorders of the joints and skeleton, chiropractors will also look at your general well-being and quality of life. Chiropractors also believe that chiropractic plays an important role in maintaining and improving health, rather than just offering symptomatic pain relief.

Chiropractors use their manipulative skills to remove nerve interference and restore normal mobility. By doing so, they assist the body's healing process, thus allowing the body to function as efficiently as possible.

## What conditions do chiropractors treat?

Chiropractic is claimed to be beneficial for people with a wide range of musculo-skeletal conditions including:

- Back pain
- Sciatica
- Tension headaches
- Migraine
- Neck, shoulder and arm pains
- Knee, ankle and foot pains
- Sports injuries
- Repetitive strain injury (RSI)
- Whiplash injuries
- Many other joint and muscle disorders

Practitioners say that people who have had chiropractic treatment for one or more of these conditions often find that, because of the direct connection between the nervous system and all the organs and tissues of the body, other conditions such as asthma, painful periods or constipation improve. Some also maintain that it can relieve infantile colic.

## Can chiropractic treat chronic conditions?

Chiropractic is claimed to be effective in treating chronic conditions like five-year-old neck injuries. Age-related aches and pains such as reduced mobility and stiffness might also be the direct result of conditions such as arthritis or of falls and accidents. Chiropractic can help these by working with your body to re-align the skeleton and stimulate the nervous system. Progress of treatment is usually slower with a long-standing problem.

### Who can benefit from chiropractic treatment?
Chiropractic is suitable for most age groups. Your chiropractor will tailor each treatment to you, the individual, not just to your symptoms.

### Are there conditions for which chiropractic is not appropriate?
Some chiropractic techniques are not suitable for the treatment of recent fractures or severe osteoarthritis. Chiropractic is also not appropriate for a range of conditions including osteoporosis, which may affect people in later life. The importance of knowing when not to treat is given great emphasis during chiropractic training.

### Is chiropractic safe and are there any possible side-effects?
Inappropriate treatment can be harmful and your condition can be compounded if you are not thoroughly assessed at the time of your initial consultation. The risk to you is minimised in the hands of a properly trained and experienced practitioner who is thorough in assessment and monitors progress carefully.

The frequency of serious side-effects (such as stroke, bone fracture or nerve damage) is unknown. Some research has shown that chiropractic is one of the safest and most effective forms of treatment available for a wide array of nerve-, spine- and muscle-associated problems throughout the body, although this is not conclusive. Mild and transient side-effects are experienced by about half of all patients receiving treatment. Your chiropractor will discuss fully any concerns you may have regarding treatment, giving you a full appraisal of your case.

# Case history

Gabrielle Swait, McTimoney Chiropractor

My first appointment of the day is a new patient, Mr Baxter. From the outset I can see that walking is causing him pain and he is unable to straighten his back. I ask him some important questions to ensure that he doesn't have any signs of a serious spinal problem that it would be inappropriate for me to treat. I also check that his general health is good and examine his lifestyle for the cause of his symptoms.

Mr Baxter drives a lot for his job and leads a rather sedentary life. His pain is located on the right side of his back just above the buttock, and in an area down the back of his thigh. It only began yesterday when he bent down to the fridge. This seems an innocuous movement to have caused such acute pain, and I suspect he may already have had some weakness in that region. The only accident he can remember was two years ago when he fell onto his right knee. He recovered quickly, but, the fall may have jarred his back, although he felt no pain at the time. He has had no serious illnesses and no other symptoms.

I spend a few minutes explaining McTimoney chiropractic and then use my model spine to explain that his pain could arise from small joints either side of his lumbar vertebrae, or from the larger sacroiliac joints at the back of his pelvis. Both could refer pain down his leg. A more serious possibility is the compression of the nerves that exit the spinal cord between the lumbar vertebrae and travel down into the legs (some of these form the sciatic nerve). This can occur when one of the shock-absorbing discs between the vertebrae is damaged.

I carry out routine health checks, such as blood pressure, and these are normal. I then run some neurological tests to check his reflexes, strength and skin sensation, as compression of a spinal nerve usually causes some weakness of the leg muscles and a reduction in skin sensitivity. Again these are normal. Orthopaedic tests designed to stress the discs and nerves do not reproduce his pain, but similar tests on the right sacroiliac joint do, suggesting that this is the origin of his symptoms.

I run my fingertips down his spine. His posture is poor and there are a number of areas where his spine curves. He is in too much pain to lie on his back so I check the alignment of as many individual bones as possible while he lies on his side and front, making adjustments to his neck and spine. I would usually check other joints, as misalignment in one area can soon cause changes elsewhere, but these will have to wait until his next visit. The most significant misalignment is at the back of his pelvis where a bony prominence feels higher on the right side than the left. I make a small adjustment which brings the bony points level.

At the end of the treatment Mr Baxter sits up relatively easily. I explain the adjustments made and that I suspect this problem has been building up for some time and may require a short course of treatment. The pattern suggests a gradual process of his body trying to compensate for an earlier misalignment rather than a recent injury. His fall is a possible cause, but so are poor posture and body use, and I outline ways of improving these. I recommend gentle mobility and no strenuous activity. As he leaves he is walking cautiously but in a much more upright position.

**Is there research that shows that chiropractic really works?**

There are Cochrane reviews (see p19) of the effectiveness of spinal manipulation for the treatment of dysmenorrhoea – painful menstrual cramps – and for asthma. In both cases, the reviewers found insufficient evidence to demonstrate that the treatments worked. In the case of dysmenorrhoea studies that found an effect were done on low sample sizes. In contrast the only study with an adequate sample size found no evidence of improvement

Bandolier, the publisher of information on evidence-based medicine (see p19), has reviewed the evidence for chiropractic as a treatment for headaches and for lower back pain. It found limited evidence that chiropractic could reduce the frequency and intensity of migraines. On lower back pain, it concluded, from a 'small, poor quality set of trials', that there was some evidence of reduction in short-term pain. It did not find sufficient evidence to demonstrate any long-term improvement.

In 1995, the *British Medical Journal* published a report on the follow-up of a Medical Research Council trial, conducted in 1990, on the techniques employed by BCA chiropractors. It concluded that patients with low back pain treated in a chiropractic setting derived more benefit and long-term satisfaction than those treated in NHS hospitals with a variety of treatments. Other studies from the US and Scandinavia have not found chiropractic to be superior to other treatments. Nevertheless, the Royal College of General Practitioners now recommends that manipulative treatments such as chiropractic should be considered for patients who need additional help with pain relief or who are failing to return to work because of lower back pain.

There are studies that have suggested chiropractic is an effective treatment for chronic fatigue syndrome, infantile colic and menopausal symptoms, but in all these cases other trials have found that chiropractic is not effective.

## What happens on a first visit?

A chiropractor begins a first consultation with a discussion of your symptoms, medical history, lifestyle and posture.

After taking your case history, the chiropractor will undertake a full clinical examination to confirm any initial ideas they may have about your problem. You will normally be asked to undress as far as your underwear, and female patients will be offered a gown to wear for this part of the consultation as well as for any subsequent treatments. If it is necessary for diagnosis, you may be offered either an X-ray or sent for further diagnostic or laboratory tests such as a scan or blood tests. After they are satisfied that they have all the information relating to your case, your practitioner will then move on to the treatment.

## What does a treatment involve?

Before beginning treatment, your chiropractor will discuss their findings. They will also address any concerns you may have. You will be asked to lie on a specially designed treatment table. The chiropractor will then begin treatment using a range of techniques from gentle stretching and mobilising of muscles and joints to very specific manipulation of a vertebra or joint that is not functioning normally.

At the end of your treatment your chiropractor may, when appropriate, give postural, exercise and lifestyle advice to minimise the recurrence of any problems in the future.

## Will I need an X-ray?

X-rays may be necessary, although not in all cases. You may need an X-ray if you have had recent injuries, are an older patient where there may be a question relating to your bone density, or if you have had unusual examination findings or a history of other serious conditions, such as psoriasis, arthritis, osteoporosis or ankylosing spondylitis. If the examination identifies underlying disease, or a condition for which chiropractic is inappropriate, the chiropractor will immediately refer you to a GP or consultant.

Many chiropractors are qualified to take and interpret X-rays, operating under strict guidelines for the use of ionising radiation. The BCA employs a Radiation Protection Advisor to inspect the X-ray installations of all its members on a regular basis.

### How long does a treatment session last?

This depends on the technique used, but in general the first treatment will usually take between 30 and 60 minutes, depending on the patient. This is because the chiropractor will need to take a detailed medical history, perform an assessment and conduct the treatment. Subsequent treatments may take between 15 minutes and half an hour, depending on what needs to be done in that session.

### How often is treatment needed?

Your treatment plan will be tailored to suit you individually. The number of sessions needed varies considerably depending on a variety of factors including your age, the nature and duration of your problem.

You may feel immediate relief, or you may need several treatments before you start to respond. Once you feel better, you do not need to visit a chiropractor again. You may be advised to return for regular check-ups if you have had serious injuries or if you have long-term problems as a result of wear and tear to your joints. Your chiropractor will discuss with you how to maintain your progress and will evaluate and reassess your treatment as it continues.

Some chiropractors believe that chiropractic also has an important role in maintaining function and improving your health. As a result, some chiropractors may suggest that you return regularly for check-ups in a similar way to visiting the dentist – commonly every three months – even though you may not be in any pain.

**What will happen when I return for follow-up treatment?**

Follow-up treatments are usually quite different to the initial consultation. First your chiropractor will ask you about your progress. If you need manual treatment, you will be asked to undress to your underclothes. Your rate of progress will be measured through careful note-taking and you will probably be given further advice on lifestyle changes, for example, to maintain your progress. Your chiropractor should keep you informed about how your treatment is progressing.

**Are there any different chiropractic techniques?**

There are a number of different chiropractic techniques in use in the UK today involving the manipulation of joints and work on muscle and tissue to stretch and relax the muscles. One of the most common is the high-velocity low-amplitude thrust. This aims to push the joint beyond its normal range of movement (though within its physical capacity) to adjust it back into place. There is sometimes an audible 'crack' in the joint when the adjustment is made. This is merely the sound of gas bubbles in the joint fluid popping due to the release of pressure and not the bones cracking, as many first-time patients believe. The thrusts are short and sharp, and not at all painful, although there may be some minor short-term discomfort.

Another commonly used technique is blocking, a 'no force' adjustment which involves placing triangular wedges under the pelvic bones while you are lying down to allow the body's own mechanisms to rebalance and realign as appropriate. Other techniques include thrusts such as 'toggles', which rely on speed and light force to toggle the vertebrae into the correct position, and the use of an activator, a hand-held mechanical device that delivers a controlled thrust to the joint.

Some practitioners, predominantly McTimoney chiropractors, use only light force adjustments – although BCA chiropractors

# Case history

Matthew Chapman, Chiropractic patient

For the past seven years, I have suffered on and off from a dull ache in my lumbar area, sometimes accompanied by a sharp twinge down one leg. It used to go away after a week of taking painkillers, but in July this year it got so bad I could barely support my upper body.

My doctor gave me painkillers, and when they didn't help, diagnosed inflammation of the sciatic nerve, and said that my muscles had gone into spasm. He recommended a chiropractor.

When I first went I could barely walk, and the chiropractor didn't mince his words. If I didn't seek treatment now, it could get a lot worse. On the second appointment I saw the X-rays. The problem muscles were no longer supporting my back, and my weight was unevenly distributed, causing one of my discs in the lumbar region to bulge out, pressing on the sciatic nerve running through my buttocks and down my legs. Where the disc had worn away it was only half its usual thickness. The chiropractor tried to lift my leg to test my reflexes, but only got to 10 degrees before I was screaming. When he tested my Achilles reflex, I had no response, signalling bad nerve damage.

He then told me to take three weeks off work, and to use an ice pack to bring down the swelling that was pressing on the sciatic nerve. He also advised me to stand or lie down, but not to sit, as this tightened the nerve, making it rub against the disc.

At first I saw him twice-weekly. We worked with a couple of different 'no force' techniques. As my hips were slightly twisted, he put wedges under them, while I lay on my front, and stretched me using the wedges to create the right torsion. The treatment table is designed so that while part of it moves, the rest of your body remains still; this way muscles can be stretched without affecting the rest of you. He used ultrasound on my damaged nerves and hamstrings, encouraging them to stretch, thus making me more supple and able to distribute my weight more evenly. He also manipulated the tops of my thighs near the pubic bone with his fingers.

The timing of the sessions was crucial. Sessions in mid-afternoon left me in severe pain the next day. When we moved them to nine o'clock in the morning, I felt fine. We attributed this to the fact that I kept on moving throughout the rest of the day, effectively 'warming down' from the chiropractic stretches.

After four sessions, I felt some improvement, but this was short-lived, as I went back to work and had a relapse. I had to start from scratch. After treatment picked up again, I was careful only to work for a couple of hours a day, and actually found that this (limited) activity helped. During the night the disc swells as it absorbs water, but when you get up, your weight squeezes the water out, and the disc shrinks slightly, reducing the pressure on the nerve. Five weeks after the initial pain, I was back at work. My back hurt a little in the early morning and again in the afternoon, but this was generally because I was using underdeveloped back muscles, and was soon rectified by special exercises.

I now see my chiropractor every ten days, and can raise my legs to 60 degrees. In the last three weeks I have felt almost back to normal, provided I don't overdo it. I imagine I will need another couple of months of treatment, but progress is good; I can even detect feeling coming back into the Achilles tendon.

will also use light force adjustments where clinically appropriate. They maintain that problems in one area of the body may actually be caused in another area entirely. A problem with the alignment of the pelvis or low back, for example, may cause compensatory problems in the neck and shoulders. They use only light force techniques to realign and adjust the skeleton in order to stimulate the body's own self-healing mechanism. Light force adjustments use light, swift and dextrous movements to adjust each joint that needs it. A McTimoney treatment is more likely to involve manipulation of the pelvis and mobilisation of the arms and cranium.

**I've heard that my condition may get worse before it gets better. Is this true?**

After a treatment you can sometimes feel worse before you feel better as your body adjusts to its new alignment. This may manifest as aching or stiffness as your muscles get used to positional changes. The area or seat of pain may change, or you may find that previous aches recur as your body settles down after treatment. Generally this lasts for no longer than 24–48 hours, and your chiropractor will make sure you understand the range of reactions before you commence treatment.

Your practitioner will also advise you on how to minimise any effects by taking particular care immediately after you have been adjusted. Spinal disc problems may appear to flare up in the early stages of treatment and where an underlying inflammation is already present, the condition may initially seem to worsen. Treatment to the neck may make you feel light-headed and, less frequently, result in a short-lived headache.

**How much does a consultation cost?**

The first consultation and treatment will generally cost in the range of £30 to £55, and subsequent treatments in the range of

£25 to £40. Prices may vary based on geographical location, experience of the chiropractor, and the extent of the facilities provided and administrative back-up.

**Can I have chiropractic treatment at reduced rates?**

Most chiropractors will do their best to offer reduced rates for those unable to pay the full cost of treatment. Some chiropractors will publish reduced rates for particular groups, but many will assess on individual need. If you cannot afford the full cost of treatment, you should find the chiropractor that suits you best and then enquire about the possibility of a reduced rate at that practice.

**Can I get my private health insurers to pay for my chiropractic treatment?**

Many private health insurance companies will now pay for chiropractic treatment. However, the extent and condition of cover varies enormously and you should check with your health insurer. BUPA and PPP carry a list of practitioners who have 'specialist status'. This requires at least five years' full-time experience and references from peers, GPs and consultants. You should be aware that the extent of cover varies considerably, from a fixed amount to the number of permitted visits, and each policy carries different rates of excess.

**Where can I find a qualified chiropractor?**

All chiropractors listed in this guide are registered with the GCC, which means that they are properly qualified. The GCC publishes the register in which all chiropractors must appear. You may want to ask your practitioner for their registration number before making an appointment to assure yourself of this fact. Anyone who calls themselves a chiropractor but who is not registered with the GCC is breaking the law. However, the GCC is policing all chiropractors to ensure that anyone advertising as a chiropractor is registered.

The BCA and MCA also publish registers of their practitioner members. You can contact them directly for details of practitioners in your area.

## What questions should I ask before making an appointment with a chiropractor?

- Are they properly trained and registered with the GCC?
- Have they had experience in treating similar health problems to yours?
- What are the possible side-effects of the treatment?
- How long is the treatment likely to last?
- What other treatment options are available?
- How much will they charge and do they offer concessionary rates?
- Are they, where necessary, licensed or registered with the local authority to practise from the address where you see them?
- Are they properly insured?

You should also ask:

- How many years have they been in practice and is this full- or part-time?
- Are they registered with any major health insurance companies?
- Will they speak to you prior to the consultation?
- Are they involved in any teaching or other professional activity?

Perhaps the most important consideration is that you have a rapport with the practitioner, and feel that you can communicate with them. You should feel comfortable asking questions about your problems and your practitioner should be forthcoming about what the treatment will involve, how much it will cost and how payment should be made. Other questions might relate to the type of technique they practise. It may be helpful to visit the premises so try to book your first appointment in person.

## What training will my chiropractor have?

The title of chiropractor is protected by law and as a result only practitioners who are registered with the GCC can call themselves a chiropractor. The GCC has set the standards of education in chiropractic and in future all chiropractors must have graduated from an accredited institution before being accepted onto the Register. There are four accredited institutions in the UK; two are independent colleges, whose courses are validated by UK universities, and two are university-based courses.

Chiropractic training covers a variety of subjects including life sciences, biomechanics, clinical medicine and differential diagnosis. Practitioners also undergo practical training in adjustment and supervised clinical training, where they have hands-on practice in treating patients. Graduates who are members of the British Chiropractic Association and the McTimoney Chiropractic Association undertake an additional year of supervised training as a requirement of membership.

## What do all the letters mean?

**BAAC**  British Association of Applied Chiropractic
**BCA**  British Chiropractic Association
**GCC**  General Chiropractic Council
**MCA**  McTimoney Chiropractic Association

## How do chiropractors keep their skills and knowledge up-to-date?

The General Chiropractic Council will be introducing a mandatory requirement for chiropractors to undertake Continuing Professional Development (CPD) as a requirement for re-registration on an annual basis.

# Case history

Tim Hutchful, BCA Chiropractor

I trained at the Anglo European College of Chiropractic for four years, and have been in practice for eleven years. I currently work with two other full-time chiropractors.

Our first patient is booked in for 8.00am. I usually allow about 15 minutes for current patients, which gives me enough time to chat to them about their progress before I treat them.

My first patient today is a 70-year-old folk dancer who had a hip replacement three years ago and suffers from lower back pain. Her treatment involves lying on two wedges placed at different heights on each side of the pelvis to correct pelvic rotation. It is a passive treatment, the only force is the patient's own body weight. She responds well and I see her every three months to manage her condition.

I usually have at least one new patient a day. Before the consultation, they fill out a questionnaire about their personal and medical history, and then a revised Oswestry or a Vernon Mior questionnaire, which assesses the initial severity of their complaint, and monitors recovery.

I then ask for the history and nature of the pain and whether any symptoms preceded it, or whether it has caused new symptoms. I also ask whether they have had any investigations done, such as X-rays, MRI scans or blood tests, and if there has been any diagnosis and treatment.

I examine the patient starting off with blood pressure, pulse, etc. If it is a lower back complaint, I ask them to stand while I do a postural assessment. I also get them to walk and to do a few simple movements both standing and sitting to measure their gross movement. I then palpitate their spine to check segmental movement, and put different pressures on it to see if they help or aggravate the condition.

I then check reflexes (each spinal reflex is associated with a spinal nerve), and I look for any neurological deficit in the dermatomes. (These are the areas of skin and muscle that are supplied by a particular nerve, for example the nerve that comes out of the spine at the third lumbar vertebra supplies the skin around the knee, so a problem with the back may manifest itself with knee pain.) I test for nerve root function and muscle strength. After the examination and diagnosis, I'll explain the treatment options to the patient and agree a treatment plan.

My new patient today is a 40-year-old hosiery worker who has come in with pain in his shoulders and neck that has been getting worse over the last six months. He has very restricted movement in his shoulders and they are unusually warm. He also suffers from psoriasis. I suggest an X-ray, and ask his GP for two blood tests: the first is to determine how inflamed the condition is, the second is an antigen marker for arthritis. There is sometimes a link between psoriasis and a type of inflammatory arthritis. I will not treat the patient until we have the results of these tests.

During the afternoon I see a young woman who has had a chronic lower back problem for five years following a riding accident. She lies on her left side with pressure applied to the lower back, and her joint lets out an audible 'click' as it is stretched. This is the sound of nitrogen being released from the joint and not, as some think, the joint 'being put back in place'.

Before I go home I develop X-rays and reply to patient enquiries. I get home at about 8.45. Even though it's a long day, it's a rewarding job that I enjoy.

**Is there statutory regulation of chiropractic in the UK?**

Chiropractic was the second complementary therapy to achieve statutory regulation. The Chiropractors Act received Royal Assent in July 1994. As a result, the General Chiropractic Council (GCC) was appointed in January 1997, and the statutory register was opened in June 1999. It is now illegal for anyone not registered to call themselves a chiropractor.

**Can I get chiropractic treatment through the NHS?**

Although some Primary Care Groups and Trusts do purchase chiropractic for their patients, chiropractic is not widely available through the NHS.

**Will my chiropractor discuss my condition with my GP?**

If you have been referred by your GP, your chiropractor will always inform them of your treatment plan and any progress you make. If you have self-referred, however, your chiropractor will only discuss your condition with your GP if you have given them permission to do so. If your chiropractor discovers or suspects a problem that requires medical investigation, they will refer you to your GP. Wherever possible your chiropractor will work in co-operation with your GP.

**Will my chiropractor have access to my medical records?**

Your chiropractor may be able to gain access to your medical records with your permission and that of your GP. However, this would be impossible without your consent. Chiropractors keep their own medical records of your treatments. The few chiropractors operating within the NHS will provide a report to your GP informing them of their assessment, their treatment and any changes that they have observed. This will form part of your medical records held by your GP.

**Do I need a referral from my doctor to visit a chiropractor?**

Chiropractors are viewed as primary health care professionals under new legislation, so you do not need a referral from your doctor in order to see a chiropractor. However, your GP is still free to refer you to a chiropractor if they choose to do so. With your permission, your chiropractor may also write to your doctor to keep them informed of your progress.

**Are all chiropractors covered by insurance?**

All chiropractors are required to have professional indemnity insurance.

**Do chiropractors make home visits?**

In an emergency, contact your GP, who will visit you at home. You may find a chiropractor who will make home visits, but generally chiropractors will need you to visit them at their clinic, where they will have the appropriate treatment table and equipment to assess and adjust you properly.

**Can chiropractic be used during pregnancy? Is it suitable for children?**

Chiropractic can be used successfully throughout pregnancy, although particular care should be taken between 12 and 16 weeks when most natural miscarriages occur. Depending on how your body responds to pregnancy and on any pre-existing conditions, treatment could involve monthly visits until the last four weeks of pregnancy, when weekly visits might be advised. Treatment during pregnancy usually involves lying on both the back and the stomach, depending on which is most comfortable, on the special treatment table that allows support in all positions. Your chiropractor will discuss a treatment plan with you for the duration of your pregnancy.

The aches and pains associated with the changes your body undergoes during pregnancy may be helped by chiropractic treatment. For instance, the changes in posture as you adapt your stance to accommodate your growing baby can often cause back pain. Realignment of the spine and pelvis can help take some of the strain off your joints, shoulders, lower back and legs, the areas usually most affected by your changing posture.

Another change that occurs naturally in pregnancy is the softening of your ligaments. While this process is perfect for giving birth, it does mean that your joints come under additional stress. Your chiropractor may offer you advice on posture, some simple stretch exercises, and advice on how to lift and carry to prevent injury.

Chiropractic employs a range of techniques suitable for people of any age, including babies and children. The majority of chiropractors will adjust children and babies using low-impact or low-force techniques. However, you may need to check with your practitioner first to see if they are comfortable treating children. Some chiropractors will concentrate their practice around very young babies and children.

**Am I too old for chiropractic?**

Although chiropractic is suitable for most age groups, older people suffering from the effects of osteoporosis are not advised to seek chiropractic treatment. However, many fit older people find that chiropractic helps them maintain their mobility as well as retain their health and wellbeing, especially with a low-force or no-force approach that puts no additional pressures on the body.

By working with your body to re-align the skeleton and stimulate the nervous system, helping the body to regain its natural balance, chiropractors claim treatment may help a range of conditions. These include back, neck and joint pain, migraines and headaches, although the evidence supporting it is not uniform. Chiropractors also claim to help alleviate the pain and problems caused by the following conditions:

- Arthritis – osteoarthritis and rheumatoid arthritis
- Poor circulation – particularly in the legs, feet and hands
- The after-effects of operations, accidents, falls and bumps
- Dental and denture-associated pain
- General symptoms of declining health, including poor mobility

Although chiropractic cannot reverse the effects of arthritis or degenerative diseases, by improving the function of the joints treatment can help to reduce further damage and keep you active and fit.

**How can I complain if something goes wrong?**
If you are dissatisfied with chiropractic care, you should seek further advice from the General Chiropractic Council, which enforces a strict Code of Conduct. The GCC has a published complaints procedure by which all chiropractors must abide. In the event of malpractice the GCC has the power to suspend registration or remove a chiropractor from the register, which would deny them the right to practise legally in the UK.

However, most problems are best resolved when they arise, and if the situation allows, you are encouraged to talk informally to your chiropractor. This gives the practitioner the opportunity to clarify, explain or rectify the situation. Alternatively, you could contact the relevant professional association who will try to resolve the complaint in conjunction with the chiropractor.

# Case history

Jill Harris, McTimoney Chiropractic patient

About five years ago I had an accident when riding my bike. I had just come downhill at a fair speed when a dog ran into me, causing me to fly over the handlebars and land heavily. I fractured my pelvis, four ribs and my skull, and damaged my inner ear (I still have a permanent ringing in my ear as a result). The right side of my face was also paralysed from damage to the nerve-endings. Although everything eventually healed, I was left with severe neck pain and headaches. These were caused by the top of my spine being thrown out of alignment and by the flow of blood to my brain being restricted. The headaches were so bad that I would wake up hourly in the night to move my head in order to maintain the flow of blood.

When I was still in hospital, the doctors recommended I saw the hospital physiotherapist. I was suffering from lower back pain at the time, and the doctors believed it had been caused by the accident aggravating an existing deterioration of the spine. I made some progress with this problem, but the headaches persisted and were acutely painful.

Over the years I saw a number of different practitioners, including an osteopath, a cranial osteopath and a chiropractor. I also had Indian head massage. The chiropractor eased the pain a little, but I found the approach somewhat distressingly forceful. Then six months ago the pain got very bad again, possibly as a result of the natural progression of the condition, or perhaps because I wasn't receiving regular treatment, and it was at this point that I heard about McTimoney chiropractic and decided to give it a go.

At the first appointment, the chiropractor not only asked me about my accident, but also asked if I had any other problems. Perhaps significantly I had had a hysterectomy a year after the accident as they had found a cyst on my ovary and on my breast, and the chiropractor suggested that my body had stopped functioning efficiently as a result of the accident. This general consultation, which included a physical examination and a mild treatment, lasted over an hour.

I now find the treatment with my chiropractor wonderfully relaxing, in fact sometimes so much so that I am practically a zombie for the rest of the day! The treatment takes place mostly on her table, and consists of a series of quick movements that 'twist' and 'toggle' the joints with a very light touch. She also effects a light pressure on my head and face, and gives my neck and shoulders a pleasant deep fingertip massage. She pulls and kneads my joints and limbs, and works down each side of my spine and legs. There is never any pain.

She has also given me some lifestyle advice: the type of bed and the number of pillows I use for example; explaining how I should exercise when going to the gym; and how not to use breaststroke in the swimming pool because of the way it causes the neck to strain.

The treatment has been really effective so far. I have lost that constant pain in the back of my head, and the headaches have gone. However, I know that I have to be careful, and that they may return if I do something to throw my neck out of alignment. I am still stuck with the rushing sound in my inner ear, which gets worse if I am ill, but that's a condition I have to learn to live with.

**What other services can a chiropractor provide?**

As registered health professionals, chiropractors can supply you with sick-leave certificates and produce medico-legal reports. Chiropractors can refer you for X-rays or other scans, such as bone density scans. They can also refer you to a consultant if they think it necessary.

**Where can I find further information?**

**General Chiropractic Council**
344-354 Gray's Inn Road,
London, WC1X 8BP
Tel: 020 7713 5155
E-mail enquiries@gcc-uk.org
www.gcc-uk.org

**British Chiropractic Association**
Blagrave House
17 Blagrave Street
Reading
Berkshire, RG1 1QB
Tel 0118 950 5950
E-mail enquiries@chiropractic-uk.co.uk
www.chiropractic-uk.co.uk

**McTimoney Chiropractic Association**
21 High Street
Eynsham, Oxon OX29 4HE
Tel: 01865 880974
E-mail admin@mctimoney-chiropractic.org
www.mctimoney-chiropractic.org

# The herbal profession

Of all complementary therapies, herbal medicine is perhaps the closest to orthodox modern medicine. The modern pharmaceutical industry has grown out of the use of medicinal plants and many modern pharmaceuticals are derived from plants – for example, aspirin comes from willow bark.

Whereas pharmaceutical drugs are generally prescribed singly for a particular symptom, traditional herbal medicines use whole plant extracts that contain hundreds of plant constituents and are generally prescribed in combination to create complex individual formulas for each patient.

It is important to remember that although many herbal remedies are safe to self-prescribe, some can be very potent and may not be appropriate for treating your particular health problems. It is generally advisable therefore to consult a qualified herbalist. You may also want to inform your GP that you are taking herbal medicine, especially if you are taking any other medication.

There are three broad groupings of professional herbal practice in the UK: Western herbal medicine, Chinese herbal medicine and Ayurvedic medicine, based on herbal traditions from Europe and North America, China and India. Other herbal traditions practised in the UK are Kanpo (Japanese medicine) and Tibetan Medicine. Although all forms of herbal medicine use plant-based therapies, each discipline is based on its own distinct therapeutic principles and medicinal preparations.

**How do herbal medicines differ from pharmaceutical drugs?**

Herbal medicines are produced from the whole plant or parts of the plant such as the root, leaf, flower, bark or berry. Herbalists may use plants either in their raw form as dried herbs for infusions or simply processed into tinctures, capsules or tablets. Unlike pharmaceutical drugs which are generally based on a single active constituent with a particular biochemical target, a herbal medicine may contain hundreds of complex molecules with various pharmacological effects.

Herbalists believe the chemical complexity of whole plant medicines produces a more balanced medicine that is more easily absorbed, used and excreted by the body with less likelihood of side-effects. There is increasing evidence that synergistic interactions between chemical constituents of whole plant extracts enhance their effectiveness as well as reduce unwanted side-effects.

**Will the herbalist tell me what is in my herbal prescription?**
It is important to know what is in the medicine you are taking. All herbalists should be happy to tell you the contents of your herbal prescription and explain why each of the herbs has been chosen.

**Do herbal medicines have a shelf-life?**
Pre-packaged herbal products bought over-the-counter should have an expiry date on the container. Those supplied by your practitioner may not. Provided herbal medicines are stored in dark conditions that are cool and dry, tinctures and tablets should last for about three years and dried herbs and powdered herbs in capsules should last for about 6 to 18 months.

**What else do herbalists do?**
In addition to prescribing herbal medication, a herbalist will also provide advice on other aspects of your physical and emotional health, including healthy diet, lifestyle, exercise and methods for stress management. The common aim of the herbal disciplines is to improve health and vitality as well as provide relief from symptoms.

**Is herbal medicine safe and are there any possible side-effects?**

Just because herbal medicines are natural, it does not automatically mean that they are harmless. Although herbs are freely available over the counter, it is advisable to consult a professionally trained and registered herbalist for help with treating complex or longstanding health problems, especially if you are pregnant, breastfeeding or already taking other medication. Some herbs can have potentially harmful interactions with conventional drugs, e.g. St John's wort reduces the effectiveness of immuno-suppressant drugs. There are also certain medical conditions where particular herbs should be avoided, e.g. liquorice with high blood pressure. It is important, therefore, to inform your herbalist of any conventional drugs you are taking while also informing your GP about any herbal medicines being taken.

There have been very few reports of serious adverse reactions to prescribed herbal medicines. Most reported adverse reactions have involved self-prescribed herbs bought over-the-counter or from a source other than a qualified herbal practitioner. The main causes of adverse reactions were due to:

- Misuse or overdosing with self-medicated products
- Misidentification of the herb
- Contamination with heavy metals, pesticides, radiation, micro-organisms and toxins
- Adulterations of the original plant material by other plant species with known toxicity
- Substitution with synthetic substances such as steroids
- Interactions with pharmaceutical drugs

When self-prescribing it is therefore advisable to stick to the recommended dose and not combine herbal medicines with other medications. If symptoms persist or you experience any side-effects, consult your doctor or qualified practitioner. Herbal medicines prescribed by professionally trained herbal practitioners are generally safe. Occasionally patients report mild side-effects such as nausea, headaches and diarrhoea. These may be resolved when the dose is either reduced or the medicine changed.

## Can I take herbal medicines long-term?

Very little is known about the safety of long-term use of herbal medicines and more clinical trials are needed to ascertain this. The fact that herbal medicines have been in use for thousands of years is often cited in their defence but it is not advisable to take the same herbal remedy for long periods without supervision.

## Will herbal medicines interact with medicines from my doctor?

There are some known interactions between herbs and pharmaceutical drugs that may be harmful. If you are taking any of the following medications, particular caution is necessary and herbs should only be taken under the supervision of a qualified practitioner:

- Diabetic medication (insulin and oral antidiabetic drugs)
- Anti-coagulants (warfarin, heparin, aspirin)
- Beta-blockers
- Heart drugs (particularly digoxin)
- Steroids
- HIV medication
- Immuno-suppressive medication
- Anti-hypertensives
- Anti-depressants
- Anti-fungals
- Anti-malarials
- Diuretics
- Anti-epileptics

- Asthma medication
- Anti-psychotics
- Cancer drugs

## Is there any research evidence that shows that herbal medicine is effective?

Many of the therapeutic properties of herbal medicines have now been substantiated by scientific research. There is a large body of laboratory and animal research confirming the pharmacological effects of many plant extracts such as anti-inflammatory, anti-microbial and anti-oxidant effects. Many human research studies have also confirmed specific therapeutic effects of particular herbs such as the anti-microbial and cholesterol-lowering properties of garlic[1], the anti-stress properties of ginseng and the liver protective effects of milk thistle and artichoke[2]. Increasingly, randomised clinical trials are providing more evidence of the effectiveness of herbal medicines[3]. For example, a systematic review of 23 randomised clinical trials investigating St John's wort (*Hypericum perforatum*) for the treatment of depression was published in the *British Medical Journal* in 1996[4]. It was concluded that *Hypericum* was superior to placebo and therapeutically equivalent to other anti-depressants in the treatment of mild to moderate depression but with fewer side-effects.

Evidence has been reported that herbal medicines can be effective for the following conditions:
- Alzheimer's disease
- Anxiety

[1] *Ernst E. et al. (1985) Garlic and blood lipids BMJ 291:139*

[2] *Raman A & Houghton PJ (1995) Ginseng, Pharm. Journal 254: 150-1*

[3] *Ernst E. (2000) Herbal Medicines: where is the evidence? BMJ 321: 395-6*

[4] *Linde K et al. (1996) St Johns wort for depression: an overview and meta-analysis of randomised clinical trials. BMJ 313:253-8*

- Atopic eczema
- Back pain
- Benign prostatic hyperplasia (enlarged prostate)
- Congestive heart failure
- Constipation
- Depression
- Headache and Migraine (prevention of)
- Hepatitis
- Herpes Simplex
- Herpes Zoster and post-herpetic neuralgia
- Hypercholesterolemia (high cholesterol)
- Irritable bowel syndrome
- Intermittent claudication
- Insomnia
- Nausea & vomiting (motion sickness, postoperative, pregnancy)
- Osteoarthritis
- Premenstrual syndrome
- Rheumatoid arthritis
- Upper respiratory tract infection

**What training do the different herbalists have?**

The different herbal practitioner associations represented in this guide have various training requirements for membership. However, all meet the core standards of training and clinical competence set down by the European Herbal Practitioners Association (EHPA). An independent accreditation board monitors the training standards in the institutions whose graduates join EHPA member organisations.

**What questions should I ask before making an appointment with a herbal practitioner?**

- What type of herbal medicine do they practise (Western, Chinese, Ayurvedic etc.)?

- Are they a member of a recognised professional body such as the National Institute of Medical Herbalists, etc?
- Do they have experience in treating similar health problems to yours?
- Are there any risks involved in treatment?
- Are they willing to discuss your condition with your GP if you request it?
- How much do they charge and do they offer concessionary rates?
- How long is the treatment likely to last?
- Do they have full professional indemnity and public liability insurance?
- Will they give you clear information about what your medicine contains, information about whether it is safe to take with any conventional medicine, and instructions on how to take it?

You should also make sure that:

- On the first consultation a full case history is taken. The consultation should last at least 40 minutes. If your practitioner does not speak English, make sure that there is a translator present.
- Any pre-packed herbs or patent remedies have a list of ingredients, written in English, and have a sell-by date on the label.

Perhaps the most important consideration is that you have a rapport with the practitioner, and feel that you can communicate with them. You should feel comfortable asking questions about your problems and your practitioner should be forthcoming about what the treatment will involve, how much it will cost and how payment should be made. It may be helpful to visit the premises so try to book your first appointment in person.

### What do all the letters mean?
**AMH**  Association of Master Herbalists
**AMAUK**  Ayurvedic Medical Association UK
**EHPA**  European Herbal Practitioners Association

**NIMH**  National Institute of Medical Herbalists
**IRCH**  International Register of Consultant Herbalists
**RCHM**  Register of Chinese Herbal Medicine

### How do herbalists keep their skills and knowledge up-to-date?

All herbalists should undertake regular Continuing Professional
Development (CPD) to keep their skills and knowledge up-to-date.
All practitioners who are members of associations affiliated with
the EHPA are required to undertake CPD seminars and courses. It is
up to each body to decide its own guidelines. Some associations,
such as the National Institute of Medical Herbalists, require
practitioners to have a mentor during their first year of practise in
addition to attending CPD seminars.

### Is there statutory regulation of the herbal profession in the UK?

The British Medical Association and the Department of Health have
both endorsed statutory self-regulation as a more appropriate
method of regulation for the herbal profession as it offers the
public greater protection against unscrupulous, unqualified
practitioners. Statutory self-regulation will mean that practitioners
are obliged to conform to compulsory standards of training, ethics,
professional codes of practice and disciplinary procedures.

The European Herbal Practitioners Association (EHPA) was
founded in 1993 to improve the provision of herbal medicine in the
UK and Europe. It brings together the major UK herbal practitioner
organisations and aims to set common standards across the profession
while promoting the development of each distinct herbal tradition.
Along with the Department of Health, the EHPA is preparing the
ground for the statutory self-regulation of herbal medicine.

The EHPA estimates that the herbal profession will become
statutorily registered by 2004. Statutory regulation may be
necessary for herbalists to maintain their rights to access all herbal
medicines, which are otherwise likely to be restricted by European

and UK Medicines Law. It will also make their position in the European Community more secure, since at present practising as a professional (non-doctor) herbalist is against the law in many member states. Statutory registration will enable herbalists to work more closely with other health professionals within the NHS and will give increased security to members of the public who wish to consult a herbalist. A herbalist may lose their state registration if found in breech of their professional code of conduct.

## Do all UK herbal associations belong to the EHPA?

Not all UK herbal practitioner associations belong to the EHPA: there is no legal obligation to become a member. Only those bodies that are members of the EHPA are represented in the guide. Membership of the EHPA confirms an association's commitment to statutory self-regulation for the herbal profession.

## Which UK herbal practitioner associations are members of the EHPA?

**Ayurvedic medicine** Ayurvedic Medical Association UK

**Chinese medicine** The Register of Chinese Herbal Medicine, The Association of Traditional Chinese Medicine (UK), The Tara Association of Tibetan Medicine

**Western herbal medicine** Association of Master Herbalists, International Register of Consultant Herbalists, National Institute of Medical Herbalists, College of Practitioners of Phytotherapy, Unified Register of Herbal Practitioners

## Can herbal medicine be used during pregnancy and breastfeeding? Is it suitable for children?

Some herbalists may prescribe herbal medicines to treat common problems associated with pregnancy, such as morning sickness and mild postnatal depression. To be absolutely safe, pregnant or breastfeeding women should avoid herbal medicines because there is no conclusive evidence that they are completely safe. There is some evidence to suggest that plant chemicals from herbs taken by nursing mothers may be transferred to breast milk.

Many herbal medicines can be used safely and effectively for children. However, children require much smaller doses than adults, and not all herbal medicines taken by adults are suitable for children. Herbal medicines should only be given to young children on the advice of a qualified herbal practitioner and it is advisable to inform your GP.

## Is it safe to self-prescribe?

Self-diagnosis and self-treatment with herbs can be inappropriate for some health problems. There is a great deal of information available on herbal medicines but much of it can be misleading or inaccurate. This has led to the popular misconception that all natural medicines are completely harmless. Herbal remedies may be safe and effective for treating minor ailments but more complex or longstanding health problems will need professional advice to ensure safe and effective treatment. If you are pregnant, breast feeding or taking any other medication, you should only take herbal medicine under professional guidance.

## Basic guidelines for buying herbal medicines over-the-counter:

**1.** Always buy herbs from a specialist supplier who can give you accurate and detailed information about the products they are selling.

**2.** Avoid cheap or discounted herbal products: they may be old or of poor quality. If the deal looks 'too good to be true', it generally is.

**3.** Do not buy dried herbs stored in clear glass (unless you know they have been kept in the dark, which may be difficult to establish) or herbs exposed to heat or sunlight. Good quality aromatic herbs should have a distinctive smell and bright colour.

**4.** When buying herbal capsules, tablets or tinctures over-the-counter, only select products with the following information on the label:

- The names of all the ingredients in the product and their amounts in weight contained in each tablet or capsule.
- The ratio of herb in tinctures (e.g. 1:3 = 1 part herb to 3 parts liquid) and percentage of alcohol.
- The recommended daily dosage.
- Expiry date, batch number and name and address of the supplier.

## Should I tell my doctor that I am taking herbal medicines?

You should tell your GP if you are taking herbal medicines so that they can take this into account when prescribing your medication. Many doctors are becoming increasingly aware that many of their patients are consulting herbal practitioners and self-medicating with herbal medicines and vitamin supplements and are starting to take a more integrative approach to healthcare. Your herbalist should be willing to discuss any concerns about herb-drug interactions or any other safety issues that your doctor may have.

## Where can I find further information?

### European Herbal Practitioners Association

45a Corsica Street,
London N5 1JT.
Tel: 020 7354 5067
Email: info@euroherb.com
www.euroherb.com

### Medicines Control Agency

Market Towers,
1 Nine Elms Lane,
London SW8 5NQ.
Tel: 020 7273 0000

# Western herbal medicine

### What is western herbal medicine?

Western herbal medicine, sometimes known as phytotherapy, is the use of medicinal plants in the treatment of disease. After a fall in popularity with the rise in modern western medicine, herbal medicine is once again popular. It is estimated that nearly 4 million people in the UK are spending in excess of £200 million a year on over-the-counter herbal products. Although self-medication accounts for much of the spending on herbal medicines, the public are increasingly consulting herbal practitioners for professional herbal treatment.

There are currently over 1000 qualified herbal practitioners in the UK working in a variety of settings, such as clinics attached to health food shops, complementary medicine clinics and professional herbal medicine training clinics. Approximately 10 per cent work within an NHS setting such as a GP surgery or specialist hospital department. However, the majority of practitioners see patients on a private, fee-paying basis.

Western herbalists take a holistic approach to treatment that focuses on all aspects of a patient's physical and emotional health rather than simply the illness they present with. They aim to establish the cause of disease as well as addressing the patient's symptoms. Central to the practice of western herbal medicine is the recognition of a 'vital' curative energy within the body. Practitioners believe that this enables the body to cleanse, repair and heal itself, thus maintaining a balanced state of health. Herbal medicines are given to support the body's inherent ability to correct internal imbalances as well as providing relief from symptoms.

Herbal practice involves more than simply prescribing herbal remedies. The development of a therapeutic relationship that enables the development of a positive attitude to health is integral to herbal practice. Practitioners will work with patients to develop a treatment strategy that incorporates elements of self-help and empowers the patient to play an active part both in their own recovery and in the prevention of future illness.

## HISTORY

Humans have used medicines made from plants for thousands of years. Traces of medicinal plants have been found at Neolithic sites, and Egyptian writings dated around 1500BC detail the use of many common herbs such as myrrh, garlic, fennel, juniper and thyme that are still used by herbalists today. Herbal knowledge from ancient Egyptian, Middle Eastern and Indian civilisations was absorbed into the European herbal tradition and expanded by the Greek and Roman civilisations. The therapeutic ideas of physicians such as Hippocrates, Dioscorides and Galen formed the basis of both western herbal and medical practice until the eighteenth century.

In the mid-nineteenth century a new system of herbal medicine called 'Botanic Medicine' was imported to Britain from North America. It combined the healing traditions of the Native American Indians and the herbal knowledge of the first European settlers to North America with modern scientific medical techniques. This new wave of Botanic Medicine started a new movement of professional herbal medicine in England that saw the foundation of the National Association of Medical Herbalists in 1864. Its aims were to promote professionalism in herbal practice and encourage education and scientific research in Herbal Medicine. In 1945 it was renamed the National Institute of Medical Herbalists (NIMH) and is the main governing body for the profession today. Modern day herbalists receive a thorough training in botanical and medical science and combine elements of traditional herbal practice with medical diagnostic principles and the latest scientific research.

## How does it work?

Herbalists employ the therapeutic actions of plants in the form of both foods and as more concentrated herbal medicines. Foods such as fruit, vegetables, cereals and pulses provide essential nutrients, which maintain good health. Certain foods can assist the normal functioning of the body (e.g. prunes promote elimination) and many culinary herbs such as fennel and peppermint can help improve digestive processes.

In a more concentrated form, specific herbs have pharmacological actions similar to prescription medicines and can be used for treating, preventing or alleviating the symptoms of disease. Herbal medicines vary in potency. Those that are very gentle in action (such as marshmallow root and chamomile) can be taken safely in fairly large amounts. The more potent herbs (such as burdock root and goldenseal) are taken in moderate doses and the highly potent herbs (for example belladonna) can be consumed only in very small doses. The prescription of potentially toxic herbs, such as belladonna, is regulated by law and as a result they cannot be purchased over-the-counter.

## What conditions can western herbal medicine treat?

Western herbal medicine is a popular treatment for a wide variety of physical and emotional health problems including arthritic joint pain, digestive disorders such as gastritis and indigestion, skin diseases such as acne and eczema, respiratory problems such as asthma and bronchitis, menopausal problems such as hot flushes, gynecological problems such as premenstrual syndrome or irregular and painful periods, and stress-related problems such as insomnia and headaches.

Herbal medicine may be used to treat patients of all ages and may also be used alongside essential orthodox medical treatments in order to support immune, digestive and other bodily functions and minimise the side-effects of drugs.

**Are there any conditions for which western herbal treatment is not appropriate?**

Potentially life-threatening conditions such as cancer, insulin-dependent diabetes, HIV and highly infectious (notifiable) diseases such as measles and tuberculosis must receive conventional treatment from registered medical practitioners. However, complementary herbal treatment may be given alongside conventional treatment once the condition has been stabilised. There are a number of herbs which may be combined to support the immune system and practitioners have reported good responses in patients with conditions such as AIDS and MS.

**Is there research that shows that western herbal medicine really works?**

The vast majority of research into herbal medicines has been conducted on single herbs and does not entirely represent the therapeutic approach of the modern western herbalist, who may use various combinations of herbs individually selected for each patient. Despite the existence of hundreds of years of historical and empirical evidence of their safety and effectiveness in clinical practice, more formal controlled trials to study the prescriptions used by modern western herbalists are needed to satisfy the scientific world fully. However, systematic reviews of randomised controlled trials support the use of many herbs such as: echinacea for the prevention of upper respiratory tract and other infections, feverfew for preventing migraines, devil's claw for osteoarthritis and lower back pain, peppermint oil for irritable bowel syndrome and headaches, kava for anxiety, St John's wort for depression, saw palmetto for enlarged prostate, ginkgo for dementia, valerian for insomnia, chaste berry for premenstrual syndrome, horse-chestnut for chronic venous insufficiency and ginger for nausea and vomiting.

# Case history

Peter Jackson-Maine, Western herbalist

When a new patient comes to me, my first move is to take down a detailed patient history. This includes general information, from their occupation and marital status, to information on their lifestyle, stress factors, diet, exercise and recreational habits (whether they smoke or drink for example). I then ask for the details of the current symptoms and the history of the presenting complaint, of other current symptoms, whether seemingly connected or not, and of any other diagnosis – medical or complementary. I also enquire about their medical history, whether they are receiving other treatments or are on any medication, and their family health history.

I perform vital checks such as blood pressure if appropriate, and an iridology analysis (the diagnosis of illness/imbalance in the body through examining markings in the iris), as I believe some form of holistic diagnosis is essential. Iridology, however, is controversial, and not usual to western herbal practice.

My patient Mary is an example of someone suffering from an extreme case of the type of generalised, seemingly medically undiagnosable condition that is on the increase. There is in all cases an extreme environmental sensitivity and low resistance. It is very like what is generally called 'chronic fatigue syndrome'.

Mary came to me two years ago. She had been diagnosed as suffering from mercury poisoning from fillings in her teeth, and had had them removed and redone without any improvement to her health. A hair analysis had shown that the mercury was still in her system, and that mineral levels were deficient.

Her symptoms were also consistent with systemic candidosis, the disruption of the natural balance of gut flora by a yeast infection. The problem with both diagnoses was that very few medical professionals recognise either of them, so they remain largely unverifiable by orthodox means. However, she was obviously extremely debilitated, and several major systems and organs were malfunctioning acutely.

Her wide-ranging symptoms included: extreme anxiety, menstrual disruption, painful ovulation, PMT, pain in her side, and a host of unspecifiable symptoms, including a 'fluttering' sensation inside her head. Her pupils were abnormally dilated, and to different extents – the right wider than the left, suggesting profound instability of the central nervous system, and there was a rapid fluctuation of pupil size.

She had already made several changes in her diet and had been regularly performing a naturopathic liver cleanse. I decided to treat her nervous system first, using a blend of nervine herbs, and within a month it had stabilised, and the fluttering sensation was briefly reduced. Then, after learning that mercury was often found to be concentrated in the pituitary gland, and taking into account her menstrual and hormonal symptoms, I decided to use *Angelica sinensis*, a hormone regulator thought to work chiefly upon the pituitary. The result was impressive, and several of her symptoms began to decline noticeably.

The pain in her right flank, however, continued to flare up, and suggested gallstones or inflammation of the gall bladder, but every time we used the relevant herbs the pain worsened. I left it alone for a while, and then gave her a little dandelion root, and later added milk thistle and gentian root. She is tolerating this well, and her pains have subsided.

## What happens on a first visit?

Your first consultation should take about an hour. Your practitioner should conduct a full case history and carry out any necessary clinical examinations. You will be asked about any health problems, past medical history, family history, diet and general lifestyle. Your pulse rate and blood pressure should be checked and you will probably be asked about your sleep patterns, appetite, digestion, bowel and bladder function. Your practitioner may ask you about your levels of stress and the state of your emotional health and aims to take all aspects of your health into account. Herbalists consider nutrition to be important to health and so they are also likely to discuss dietary and other lifestyle changes. Your practitioner should give some indication of the expected length of the treatment and how many visits you may need to make.

Sometimes your herbal prescription will be dispensed by the practitioner directly after the consultation. However, not all herbalists have a dispensary on the premises. In these cases arrangements are made for medicines to be posted to you, or for you to collect your medicines later.

## How do western herbal practitioners choose which herbs to prescribe?

Herbs are prescribed according to their known pharmacological actions, their affinity for particular organs and tissues as well as the traditional properties of tastes and temperatures attributed to each plant. For example, bitter herbs are seen as cooling and detoxifying, pungent, spicy herbs as heating and stimulating and aromatic herbs as warming and relaxing. Although herbs may be prescribed singly, the majority of herbalists prefer to use herbs in combination according to the needs of the individual patient.

### How often is treatment needed?

The frequency and length of treatment will depend on you and the type of health problem you have. For long-standing health problems such as osteoarthritis your herbal practitioner may want to see you on a monthly basis to monitor your progress and adjust your prescription to take account of any changes in your condition. For more acute conditions such as colds and coughs you may only need to visit your practitioner once or twice. At your first appointment, your herbalist will usually arrange a follow-up appointment for two to four weeks time and should also tell you how many visits they think necessary.

### What types of herbal preparations are used in western herbal medicine?

Western herbalists use herbal preparations as close to their natural state as possible and will prescribe the lowest therapeutic dosage possible for you. The choice of herbs and type of preparations will depend on your condition but a typical prescription will contain about five or six different herbs. These are combined to make a highly complex and individualised formula.

Herbal medicines are usually dispensed as alcohol-based liquid medicines called tinctures or fluid extracts. Fluid extracts are more concentrated than tinctures and your prescription may contain a mixture of the two. Herbal medicines may also be prescribed as syrups, fresh herb juices, tablets, as dried herbs for teas or in powdered form as capsules. Herbal creams, ointments and infused oils may also be prescribed for external use.

### Why do western herbalists mainly prescribe herbal tinctures?

There are several advantages to using herbal tinctures rather than capsules or tablets:

- Herbal tinctures are traditional preparations which have been tried and tested for hundreds of years.

- Tinctures have undergone minimal processing (unlike tablets) and contain a chemical make-up that is close to that of the original plant.
- Alcohol is an excellent medium for extracting certain plant constituents and is also a good preservative.
- Tinctures are concentrated whole plant extracts, so only small doses are required (unlike powders and teas).
- Liquids are easier to swallow and provide greater dosage flexibility than capsules and tablets.
- Any number of herbal tinctures can be combined easily to create individual formulas.
- Experience has shown that liquid herbal medicines are rapidly and easily absorbed.
- Tinctures have a very long shelf life.

However, the presence of alcohol in tinctures may not be suitable for some patients.

### Where do the herbs come from?

Traditionally herbalists have used the plants available to them locally, and many of the herbs in use today still come from the wild. Some herbalists grow their own herbs but most buy from small specialist organic growers and manufacturers of traditional herbal remedies. The majority of herbs sold commercially in the West are imported from Eastern European countries although many herbs come from France, Spain, Holland, Egypt, China, India, America and the UK. Manufacturers may purchase their raw material from herb importers or directly from growers in the country of origin. Many herbs are now bought via large wholesale markets in Germany which in turn buy from producers all over the world. Increasingly, herbs are being cultivated by professional growers, although the majority of herbs on the world market are still collected from the wild.

### Will the herbal medicine taste unpleasant?

Most herbal tinctures have a distinctive taste which you may find unappealing at first. However, when preparing a prescription, a skilled practitioner will incorporate particular herbs to help improve the flavour. Some herbal medicines will be prescribed specifically for their bitter taste as this is thought to stimulate the production of digestive enzymes throughout the gastro-intestinal tract, which helps to improve appetite and digestive function. Generally, the taste of herbal teas is not unpleasant and herbal capsules and tablets are tasteless but are not generally available in complex tailor-made prescriptions.

### I have heard my condition can get worse before it gets better. Is this true?

Some health problems such as skin diseases may appear to get worse during treatment. This is often referred to as a 'healing crisis'. Some practitioners view this as a positive sign that the body is detoxifying and may encourage you to stick with the treatment for several days or weeks. Other practitioners may consider it to be a negative reaction and advise a change of prescription. If symptoms worsen, you should always contact your herbalist or your GP for advice.

### How much does a consultation cost?

There are no set charges and the cost of your herbal treatment will depend on factors such as geographical location, the length of your consultation and the experience of your practitioner. Generally, first consultations range from between £20 and £50 with second treatments varying between £15 and £35. The medicines cost extra and prices vary, although on average a week's supply of herbal tincture is around £5.

# Case history

April Lively, Western herbal medicine patient

I was brought up with herbal medicine, so it has never been an alien concept to me. However, when I turned to it as an adult, I wasn't initially confident that it could help.

In 1986, after a year of marriage, my husband left me for someone else. I was devastated, and went to my GP soon afterwards with what he diagnosed as the symptoms of delayed shock. I started to develop raised red acne and lumpy cyst-like growths on my face. My weight ballooned from eight-and-a-half to eleven-and-a-half stone, although I wasn't actually eating more than usual. And my legs became so bloated that I had to wear size eight shoes instead of size five. As I was working as a model, this turn of events was disastrous. I also had no energy and was depressed. I felt as if my body was slowly being poisoned.

I tried all sorts of remedies, including over-the-counter herbal tablets, and eventually consulted a private GP. He diagnosed an underactive thyroid gland and prescribed thyroxin, but even the maximum dose did nothing for me. He also put me on slimming pills, and when these made me restless and disturbed my sleep, added sleeping tablets to the cocktail of drugs, all of which seemed to intensify the sensation of being poisoned.

I then consulted an endocrinologist who diagnosed polycystic ovaries, describing them as a 'condition' rather than an illness, a result of how my body worked and the chemicals it produced. He prescribed a low-hormone dose of the Pill, which I took for a year without result, and then told me there was nothing else he could do.

I visited a homeopath, and over a long period he did improve my acne slightly, but admitted he could only offer limited help. I also consulted a gynaecologist, who confirmed my fear that my polycystic ovaries might mean that I would never be able to have children. This news only added to the stress caused by my condition, and the stress seemed to exacerbate my symptoms. I felt as if my body was going berserk.

It was at this point that I heard about a local herbalist and decided to go and see him. After taking down a detailed history, the herbalist told me that my polycystic ovaries were an indication of severe hormonal problems, aggravated by a badly functioning liver. As the liver filters toxins from the body, I was congested with poisons that my body could not eliminate. Encouraged by this diagnosis, I decided to give his treatment six months. I know there are no 'quick fixes' in herbal medicine; you have to treat the underlying cause, and progress is gradual but steady.

The treatment consisted of dietary advice and a combination of herbs made up at the clinic into a medicine that I took by the teaspoon. After a month I felt a bit brighter, I had more energy and my feelings of hopelessness receded. After a few months, the painful lumps on my face were less red and angry, and my skin really began to clear. And then something miraculous happened, I met someone and got married. I am now six months pregnant, have had no morning sickness at all, and feel really fit.

In my mind there is no doubt that the herbal treatment helped reduce the cysts and improved my hormone function, and I have nothing but praise for my herbalist. Despite the expense and time involved, I have come to see my monthly appointments with him as a worthwhile investment, a way of looking after myself that is as fundamental as cleaning my teeth.

## Can I see a western herbal practitioner at reduced rates?

There is no official list of practitioners who are prepared to reduce their fees for those on low incomes. However, most practitioners will reduce their charges if you cannot afford treatment, but you will have to negotiate this directly with them.

## Can I get my private health insurers to pay for my western herbal medicine?

Some private insurance schemes will pay for herbal medicine. Insurance companies are becoming increasingly aware that there is a demand for certain complementary therapies to be included in medical insurance schemes. The best thing to do is to check your policy with your insurance company.

## Will my practitioner belong to a professional body?

At the moment, anybody can practise as a herbalist in the UK without adequate training or membership of a professional body. You should always check that your chosen practitioner is a member of a credible professional association affiliated with the European Herbal Practitioners Association (EHPA).

In the UK these are:

- The Association of Master Herbalists
- The College of Practitioners of Phytotherapy
- The International Register of Consultant Herbalists
- The National Institute of Medical Herbalists (NIMH), which is the largest professional body for western herbalists
- Unified Register of Herbal Practitioners

## Where can I find a qualified western herbalist?

The western herbalists listed in this guide will be registered with the organisations that are members of the EHPA and as such will be fully trained and abide by a Professional Code of Ethics.

Professional associations affiliated with the EHPA all publish registers of qualified practitioners. You can contact the associations directly for a list of practitioners in your area.

**What questions should I ask before making an appointment with a western herbal practitioner?**

As well as the questions outlined on p133, you should ensure that:

- Your practitioner is properly trained and a member of the Association of Master Herbalists, the International Register of Consultant Herbalists, the National Institute of Medical Herbalists, College of Practitioners of Phytotherapy or Unified Register of Herbal Practitioners.

**What training do western herbal practitioners have?**

Levels of professional training vary between the different associations of herbal practitioners. However, the EHPA has set minimum training standards that are equivalent to degree level. In order to join any herbal association affiliated with the EHPA, your practitioner must meet these standards. As anyone can legally practise as a herbalist without proper training, you should make sure that your herbalist is a member of an appropriate body. Training for members of the NIMH is particularly thorough in the medical sciences and clinical skills. Currently there are five universities that run degree courses that lead to membership of the NIMH.

Your practitioner should have undertaken at least three years' professional training at one of several accredited colleges. Training includes the study of botany, biochemistry, pharmacology, anatomy, physiology, clinical medicine, pathology, diagnosis, research methods, nutrition, herbal therapeutics and extensive supervised clinical training. You can contact the EHPA for details of accredited colleges.

## Can I get herbal treatment on the NHS?

The provision of herbal medicine in the NHS is very limited across the UK and is only available in a few hospitals and Primary Care Centres. A recent study of the provision of complementary therapies in the NHS found that herbal medicine is the least commonly provided of all complementary therapies.

## Will my herbal practitioner discuss my condition with my GP?

In cases where a patient is taking a lot of medication, or where children are being treated, or the practitioner feels it is appropriate to liaise with other healthcare professionals, they may ask your permission to write to your GP. Communication with your GP will help your herbal practitioner to integrate your herbal treatment with any other medical treatment you may be having. It also keeps your GP updated with your treatment and progress. However, your herbalist will not contact your GP without your permission.

## Will my herbal practitioner have access to my medical records?

Sometimes it may be helpful for your herbalist to see your medical records in order to make decisions about your herbal treatment. However, your practitioner can only access your medical records if you sign a consent form giving them permission.

## Do I need a referral from my doctor to visit a western herbalist?

You do not need a referral from your doctor to visit a western herbalist. Anyone may self-refer by contacting a local practitioner and making an appointment.

### Are all herbal practitioners covered by insurance?

All herbalists who are constituent members of the EHPA are fully insured with professional indemnity and public liability insurance.

### Do herbal practitioners make home visits?

Some practitioners are happy to make home visits and others are not. It is up to the individual practitioner and needs to be discussed on a case-by-case basis.

### How can I make a complaint about a practitioner?

All complaints that cannot be dealt with directly with the practitioner concerned should be addressed in writing to the relevant professional body. All bodies affiliated to the EHPA will soon have a common Code of Ethics. If your practitioner is shown to be in breach of the code, they may be suspended or struck off the register completely.

### Where can I find more information?

### The National Institute of Medical Herbalists

56 Longbrook Street
Exeter
Devon EX4 6AH.
Tel: 01392 426022
Email: nimh@ukexeter.freeserve.co.uk
www.nimh.org.uk

### The Association of Master Herbalists

3 Maple Cottages
Broadgate
Walkington
E Yorkshire HU17 8RW
Tel: 01482 887352

**The International Register of Consultant Herbalists**

32 King Edward Road

Swansea SA1 4LL

Tel: 01792 655886

Email: office@irch.org

www.irch.org

**The College of Practitioners of Phytotherapy**

Bucksteep Manor

Bodle Street Green

Hailsham

Sussex BN27 4RJ

Tel: 01323 834800

**Unified Register of Herbal Practitioners**

58 Fairmantle Street

Truro

Cornwall TR1 2EG

Tel: 01872 222699

# Chinese herbal medicine

## What is Chinese herbal medicine?

Chinese herbal medicine is a system of healing that has been practised in China and other Far Eastern countries for over 2000 years. It uses plant materials, and in certain cases animal and mineral substances, combining them into formulae that are tailor-made for each patient's individual condition. Chinese herbal medicine is part of a wider tradition of Chinese medicine which includes acupuncture and is sometimes used in conjunction with it.

Chinese herbal medicine is part of Traditional Chinese medicine, and uses the same unique diagnostic and therapeutic approach. Therapeutic principles are based on the concepts of yin and yang and of Qi (pronounced Chee), which is a form of energy that flows through distinct channels in the body. Disease is seen as an imbalance of yin and yang which affects the free flow of Qi.

## HISTORY

A number of important texts such as the Tang Materia Medica, with detailed anatomical drawings and illustrated lists of hundreds of individual herbs and herbal remedies, have emerged from China during the last two centuries.

Currently, Traditional Chinese medicine exists alongside western medicine in China. The two are considered complementary and are often used together. Chinese herbal medicine has been in the UK since the Chinese community became established, but it was not until the 1980s that it gained wider popularity.

In 1987, the Register of Chinese Herbal Medicine (RCHM) was set up to regulate the practice of Chinese herbal medicine in the UK and currently has around 400 registered members. The RCHM is a member organisation of the European Herbal Practitioners Association (EHPA), and is working towards statutory regulation.

### How does it work?

Traditional Chinese medicine believes that good health depends on the balance of the body's energy or Qi. Too much or too little activity in one of the 12 meridians or energy channels is believed to be the cause of illness. Two opposing forces – yin, the passive force, and yang, the active force – are believed to regulate mood. The five basic elements of Chinese philosophy – fire, water, earth, matter and wood – are believed to play a vital role in your well-being and are critical aids to diagnosis. Practitioners also often use terms such as 'hot', 'cold', 'damp' or 'dry' to describe symptoms.

Herbs, and often acupuncture, are used to help to rebalance your Qi and to treat your condition. Herbs are not prescribed to treat symptoms, but rather each herbal formula is designed to treat you as an individual. When making a diagnosis, your herbalist will take into account your constitution, lifestyle, emotional state and the level and duration of your condition.

### What conditions can Chinese herbal medicine treat?

Chinese herbal medicine is a popular treatment for a number of acute and chronic conditions including skin diseases such as eczema and psoriasis, gynaecological conditions such as premenstrual tension and irregular periods, respiratory disorders such as asthma and bronchitis and digestive disorders such as gastritis and indigestion. Chinese herbal medicines are often used alongside orthodox medical treatment in order to support immune, digestive and other bodily functions.

### Are there any medical conditions that are not suitable for Chinese herbal treatment?

Potentially life-threatening conditions such as cancer, insulin-dependent diabetes, HIV and highly infectious (notifiable) diseases such as measles and tuberculosis must be treated by a registered medical practitioner. However, Chinese herbal medicine can complement your medical treatment once your condition is stable. Herbs are often used in conjunction with acupuncture to help relieve the symptoms of some chronic conditions such as cancer.

## Is there research that shows that Chinese herbal medicine really works?

A great deal of research has been conducted on Chinese medicine in China and elsewhere in the Far East, and supports the practice of herbal medicine in state hospitals throughout China. However, much of this research is not regarded as methodologically sound in the West.

One of the few studies in the UK tested 37 children with severe eczema at a practice in Soho, London. A double-blind placebo-controlled trial found that over 60 per cent showed significant clinical improvement with no side-effects. However, a second, more recent trial which replicated the study found that the results were negative and suggested that the formula used in it may have been responsible for severe side-effects.

## What happens on a first visit?

Your first visit to a Chinese herbalist is likely to last around an hour, but definitely no less than 40 minutes. Your practitioner should take a detailed patient history which will involve asking questions about your past medical history, family history, diet and general lifestyle. You will also be asked about your symptoms, any pain you may have, sleep patterns, sensitivity to hot and cold, eating and bladder and bowel function. This will be followed by a clinical examination.

A practitioner of Chinese herbal medicine relies on sight, touch and smell for diagnostic information, taking into account your appearance, size, shape and general demeanour. The colour, coating and condition of your tongue will also be noted and you pulses will be taken. Tongue diagnosis and pulse-taking are considered the

# Case history

Maurice Lavenant, Chinese herbalist

I usually see 8–13 patients a day, depending on the kind of treatment I am providing. A first herbal consultation may take up to 90 minutes. I always take a comprehensive patient history, as most complaints from patients result from practitioners missing an important detail. Together with mundane details like date of birth, I always ask where a patient was born, as this can be significant, especially if they were born abroad and experienced a different climate. I also make an account of their height, weight, general health, sleep, energy levels, appetite, digestion, bowel movements and urination. I find out about their diet, what their body temperature is like (sweaty or cold), and about their emotional state.

For the medical history, I ask whether the patient has had any surgery, fractures, broken bones, recurrent illnesses or a history of disease. Do they have headaches, earaches, sinusitis, chest or back pain? Are they on any medication? With women, I ask what age menstruation began and for details of any pregnancies, abortions, gynaecological problems or STDs. Often patients forget details, so I ask the questions again but in a different way – this is the traditional Chinese method. I then take down a description of the current problem.

Then I examine the tongue and take pulses in both wrists, and I may refer a patient to their GP or a clinic for a liver function test (this usually produces same-day results). I will also prescribe Chinese herbs and/or acupuncture, and usually book a further appointment for six weeks' time to see how the patient is responding.

I recently treated a man in his early seventies who had been experiencing pain around his umbilicus and in his bowel for a week. It was usually triggered by eating, and relieved by a bowel movement. He had been hospitalised five years earlier with suspected gallstones, but this had never been confirmed or treated. He was worried that this pain signalled the return of the problem, and might result in the removal of his gallbladder. I gave him acupuncture for pain relief, and herbs to unblock the stagnation of food that I believe had occurred in a pocket in his intestinal tract. The clue to this diagnosis lay in the thick yellow coating on his tongue signifying problems in the gut. I saw the patient a week later and he was feeling much better.

A woman in her late forties with severe arthritis came to see me. It had begun in her lower back in childhood, and then spread to her neck and shoulders. She also suffered from eczema, which had been exacerbated by orthodox treatment. She had had surgery on a prolapsed disc, and was experiencing constant severe pain over her right scapula, and shooting pains down her back and into her left buttock. Her system seemed very low and depleted, and the cannabis she smoked as a painkiller wasn't helping. She was weepy, and saw herself as inherently vulnerable.

I treated her with herbs, and some acupuncture, and she soon experienced pain relief and an improvement to her skin. Her menstrual cycle is also longer, which is a good indication of improving health. She has a less 'fuzzy head', is not so cold and sweaty, her energy levels are higher and her asthma has improved.

Although the patient initially came to me for arthritis, she also reported other improvements, and this is the way Chinese herbal medicine should work. The herbalist should take all symptoms into account and treat the whole person. The focus is on the main symptom, but others should also improve.

most important part of the examination as these reveal any imbalances of Qi. They will also look closely at your eyes, which reveal the state of Shen[1]. Your herbalist will also listen to your breathing, speech and cough, and may also palpate the parts of your body where you have pain or touch your skin where you have a rash.

You will be prescribed a selection of raw herbs according to your condition. These may be prescribed as a tea (your practitioner will give you instructions on how to prepare it), or in powder, pill, capsule or tincture form. Creams are also used topically for skin conditions. At the end of your first consultation you should be given an indication of the expected length of the treatment and how many visits you will need to make.

**How do practitioners choose which herbs to prescribe?**
Chinese herbs are ascribed qualities such as 'cooling' (yin) or 'stimulating' (yang). Your practitioner chooses herbs according to the deficiencies or excesses of yin or yang. Your constitution, lifestyle, emotional state and the level and duration of the condition will also be taken into account.

**What substances are used in Chinese herbal medicine?**
In addition to herbs, Chinese medicine has traditionally also used some mineral and animal ingredients. However, in the UK the vast majority of herbal formulae are made up of plant materials. The most commonly used substances include barks, roots, berries, leaves, twigs, seeds, pips, fruits and flowers. Several formulae have been found to contain toxic heavy metals or have been adulterated with prescription drugs: both are illegal in the UK.

---

[1] In Chinese traditional medicine, Shen is believed to be the power behind your personality, guiding the emotions and ruling the organs.

---

**Where do the herbs come from?**

The majority of Chinese herbs come from China or Taiwan. Suppliers buy in bulk from wholesalers and sell herbs to practitioners in the UK. The quality of herbal medicines may vary, especially where they are being imported and where it is easy for suppliers to substitute cheaper herbs for expensive ones. The RCHM has a list of approved suppliers who must meet quality control standards that have been agreed with the RCHM.

**Will the herbs taste unpleasant?**

Some people find the taste and smell of the herbs extremely unpleasant. If this is likely to deter the patient, the practitioner may instead prescribe pills, capsules or tinctures.

**How often is treatment needed?**

The frequency and length of treatment depends on your condition. For instance, an acute condition such as a cold will need less treatment than a long-standing condition such as wheat intolerance. In the early stages of treatment it may be necessary to see the practitioner every week for a month or so. After the initial course of treatment, however, you may only need to return once a month.

**I've heard that my condition may get worse before it gets better. Is this true?**

The Chinese tradition does not adhere to the idea that a condition is likely to get worse before it gets better. In general, any aggravation would be an indication that the treatment approach was not appropriate. In certain cases some symptoms may appear to worsen temporarily, but the practitioner will warn you about such a possibility and explain what you can expect with further treatment.

## How much does a consultation cost?

There are no set charges for Chinese herbal medicine and fees vary according to the level of your practitioner's experience, whether they have administrative support and where they are located – practitioners usually charge more in London. As a guideline, an initial consultation with a Chinese herbalist is likely to cost between £25 and £35. However, you need to remember that you pay for your herbs separately. In the case of teas the cost is likely to be in the region of £10 to £20 for a week's supply.

## Can I have Chinese herbal treatment at reduced rates?

There is no official list of practitioners who reduce their fees for those on low incomes but many will do so if you have a real need. You will need to negotiate this with your chosen practitioner.

## Can I get my private health insurers to pay for my Chinese herbal medicine?

Generally the answer is that they will not. Some insurance schemes do cover acupuncture, but very few will pay for Chinese herbal medicine. However insurance companies are becoming increasingly aware that there is a demand for complementary therapies to be included in medical insurance schemes. The best advice is to contact your insurance company directly.

## Will my Chinese herbalist belong to a professional body?

Anybody can practise as a herbalist in the UK without adequate training or membership of a professional body and you should always check that your practitioner belongs to a credible professional association. The RCHM regulates the practice of Chinese herbal medicine in the UK. It is a member organisation of the EHPA, which is working towards statutory regulation.

### Where can I find a qualified Chinese herbalist?

The Chinese herbalists listed in this guide belong to the RCHM and as such are properly qualified. To be certain of this, you should check that your chosen practitioner has the letters MRCHM after their name. This means that they are members of the RCHM. The RCHM publishes a list of its members and you can contact them directly for a list of practitioners in your area.

### What questions should I ask before making an appointment with a Chinese herbalist?

As well as the questions outlined on p133, you should ensure that:

- Your practitioner is properly trained and a member of the Register of Chinese Herbal Medicine (RCHM) or another professional association that adheres to a strict Code of Ethics and Professional Conduct.
- On the first consultation a full case history is taken. The consultation should last at least 40 minutes. If your practitioner does not speak English, make sure that there is a translator present.

### What training do Chinese herbalists have?

All herbal associations represented in this guide abide by the minimum training standards laid down by the EHPA. Members of the RCHM are qualified in Chinese medicine, and often in acupuncture, and will have studied for up to four years at one of several accredited independent colleges throughout the UK. All members have a thorough grounding in the principles and theory of traditional Chinese medicine, and will have studied anatomy, physiology, pathology and some pharmacology as part of their training. They will achieve either a Diploma or a Bachelor of Science degree. You can contact the RCHM for details of accredited colleges.

# Case history

Liz Wilson, Chinese herbal medicine patient

I started taking Chinese herbal medicine in 1996 after doing the rounds of orthodox medical treatment from the age of 15, when I began to show symptoms of candidiasis. Candida albicans, a common yeast infection which resides in the gut (where it is balanced out in a healthy person by good intestinal flora), can interfere with the immune system in a number of ways and cause a variety of disorders. Some acquire candida infections because of compromised immunity (caused by large doses of antibiotics, a bad diet, or a major operation), but I inherited a susceptibility to yeast infection from my mother.

During my early teens I was often bloated and constipated after eating, had many colds, was frequently run down, and had painful periods that lasted for ten days. But it was not until my mother came across it in a book, that we realised the 'yeast connection' to our shared problem.

I saw various doctors and specialists over the next few years, cut out many food types and tried a variety of medicines, but I never felt any better. I experienced a range of attitudes, from the mildly sympathetic but patronising (suggesting that my symptoms were all part and parcel of being a woman), to the insulting (one doctor suggested I was suffering from 'food addiction').

I then consulted an eminent traditional Chinese herbalist. From the outset his approach was holistic. He wanted to know how I slept, what I ate, what foods I craved, whether I got angry, anxious or tired, and what I dreamt about. Then he asked for information about my physical state, including my menstrual cycle, exercise regime, and whether I smoked, drank or took drugs. He asked whether I was a 'hot' or 'cold' person, and whether I had cold extremities and was sensitive to changes in temperature. He also examined my tongue, as a good indicator of general health, and took my pulse to ascertain my energy levels.

He confirmed the candida explanation, explaining that my constitution was 'damp' and unable to cope with foods that promoted the accumulation of mould in the gut, including dairy products, and suggested I eliminate them. He prescribed a herbal powder designed to help my immune system fight infection by itself, and loose dried anti-fungal herbs to be boiled up and drunk as a tea. At first the taste was so dreadful I wasn't sure I could manage, but as the herbs have begun to bring about a recovery, I now barely notice the taste.

I saw my herbalist once a month for a year. Progress was initially slow, but gradually my symptoms abated. Five years on, I see him twice a year. On each visit he examines my tongue and pulse, we discuss my progress, and he asks whether there have been any significant changes in my lifestyle. He then alters my prescription accordingly. (These constant alterations are also necessary to prevent the candida spores from becoming 'immune' to the herbs used to combat them.) As well as the herbs, I take a number of vitamin and mineral supplements, and eat lots of sesame seeds, which are high in calcium.

I am now fitter and healthier than many of my peers, and no longer suffer from cystitis and thrush. I still get tired and run down quickly, but as long as I look after myself, I can lead a relatively normal life. I'm probably never going to be free from candida, and am still dependent on Chinese herbal medicine, but I don't believe any treatment could ever 'cure' me without seriously compromising my immune system.

### Can I get herbal treatment on the NHS?

Some GP practices are funded to provide some forms of complementary medicine but currently very few practices will pay for Chinese herbal medicine.

### Do I need a referral from my doctor to visit a Chinese herbal practitioner?

No. Anyone can self-refer by contacting a local practitioner and making an appointment.

### Will the practitioner discuss my condition with my GP?

In cases where you are taking a lot of medication, or where children are being treated, or if your practitioner feels it is appropriate or necessary, they may ask your permission to write to your GP. Your herbalist should always be prepared to discuss your treatment with your GP if you ask them to.

### Will the practitioner have access to my medical records?

Sometimes your herbalist may need to see your medical records to make a decision about your treatment. However, they can only access your medical records if you sign a consent form giving your permission.

### Are all herbal practitioners covered by insurance?

All members of the RCHM are fully insured with professional indemnity and public liability insurance.

### Do Chinese herbal practitioners make home visits?

Some practitioners are happy to make home visits and others are not. It is up to the individual practitioner and needs to be discussed on an individual basis.

## How can I make a complaint about a Chinese herbalist?

All complaints that cannot be dealt with directly by your practitioner should be addressed in writing to the RCHM. If your practitioner is found to be in breach of the associations' Codes of Conduct and Ethics, they can be disciplined or struck off the register completely.

## Will my medicine contain animal products?

Some Chinese remedies do contain animal products. Commonly used animal products include fossilised ox bones, deer antlers and buffalo horn. Chinese herbal remedies may also contain mineral material from the shells of shellfish. Currently these ingredients have food status, and discussions are under way as to their position in relation to forthcoming changes in European law relating to traditional medicines. Most practitioners would not prescribe animal products without telling you first, but you should ask what your formula contains if you do not wish to take animal products.

## What about endangered species?

Traditionally, Chinese herbal medicine has contained some plant or animal ingredients that are now on a list of endangered species. The RCHM have strict rules in force that prohibits the use of any endangered animal or plant material. Any practitioner found to be in breach of this policy would face disciplinary action and any supplier who breached the Code would be removed from its list of approved suppliers.

## Is it true that some Chinese herbal ointments contain steroids?

Some Chinese herbal creams sold in the UK for skin diseases have in the past been found to contain steroids. This is illegal and it is strictly against RCHM policy for any practitioner to prescribe substances containing steroids or other pharmaceutical drugs, or to use any supplier who has been found to supply such products. Any practitioner found to be in breach of this policy would face disciplinary action and any supplier who breached the Code would be removed from its list of approved suppliers.

## Where can I find further information?

### The Register of Chinese Herbal Medicine
Office 5
Ferndale Business Centre
1 Exeter St
Norwich, NR2 4BQ
Tel: 01603 623994
Email: herbmed@rchm.co.uk
www.rchm.co.uk

# Ayurvedic medicine

## What is Ayurvedic medicine?

Ayurvedic medicine is an ancient system of healing that originated in India and Sri Lanka. Although it is relatively unknown in the West, it is practised widely in the Indian subcontinent, often in combination with orthodox methods of treatment. Ayurveda, like Chinese medicine, treats the whole person rather than just the disease. As is often the case with holistic medicine, Ayurveda draws on spiritual and philosophical approaches to illness and uses nutrition and yoga to help bring your health back into balance.

## HISTORY

Ayurveda, meaning 'the science of life', has been practised as a medical system of healing for more than 5000 years. It is believed that originally wise men called Rishis or Siddhars acquired Ayurvedic knowledge through meditation. Later the Ayurvedic Medical System was written down but it was still firmly believed to be divinely inspired. Ayurveda spread to the UK in the mid-1970s with the arrival of Asian immigrants into the country.

The Ayurvedic Medical Association UK (AMA UK) maintains a register of qualified Ayurvedic practitioners in the country. There are currently about 25 to 30 qualified Ayurvedic physicians registered with them. Most are based in London but they can also be found in areas with large Asian communities such as Leicester, Birmingham and Bradford.

## How does it work?

Ayurveda views a person as a unique individual made up of five primary elements: ether (space), air, fire, water and earth. According to Ayurvedic principles, it is the interaction between these elements, in both the external world and within our own physical body, which determines the state of our physical and mental health.

Any imbalance between these elements results in illness and disorder.

The human body is made up of three principal types of energy-forces or 'doshas' known as vata, pitta, and kapha. Their influence affects all mechanisms of the body. Most individuals have a predominant dosha which determines their body type and temperament. Environment, lifestyle and external forces such as chemicals and bacteria can cause an imbalance in these three forces, which then leads to disease.

Many people turn to Ayurveda as a natural system of medicine and way of life. Because it offers medicine, diet, yoga, exercise and meditation, Ayurveda can be used as a form of preventative medicine as well as a healing therapy.

**What conditions can Ayurveda treat?**

Ayurveda is commonly used to treat chronic illnesses like arthritis, eczema, psoriasis, hormonal imbalances, premenstrual syndrome, rheumatism, blood pressure, migraine, stroke, stress-related and sexual problems. Practitioners also claim to have had good results with conditions such as multiple sclerosis and ME.

**Can Ayurveda be used to treat chronic conditions?**

In addition to chronic conditions such as arthritis, eczema and hormonal problems, Ayurveda can also be used to treat chronic rheumatism, blood pressure and migraine.

**Are there any conditions for which Ayurvedic medicine is not appropriate?**

Serious conditions that are potentially life-threatening or require surgery should not be treated solely with Ayurveda. Examples of these would be cancer, insulin-dependent diabetes, HIV or tuberculosis. However, once your condition has stabilised Ayurveda can complement your treatment, since there are a number of remedies that are thought to support the immune system. You must always make sure, however, that you inform your GP if you are taking herbs alongside conventional medication.

### Is there research that shows that Ayurvedic medicine really works?

In the West, Ayurvedic preparations and treatments have not been subjected to critical clinical studies. However, in India, the specific Ayurvedic preparation Mentat, which was formulated to treat common behavioural and mental disorders including memory impairment and speech defects, has undergone extensive clinical trials. In Bombay, researchers and practitioners in children's hospitals undertook a number of different studies and treated children with speech problems with Mentat. They found that in all trials, between 22 per cent and 90 per cent of children showed marked improvement.

### What happens on a first visit?

Your first consultation should take between 40 minutes and an hour, depending on the nature or severity of your problem. The first thing that an Ayurvedic practitioner will do is to establish your predominant dosha. While acknowledging that no single individual will display a single dosha, the practitioner believes that your dominant dosha affects your entire physical, mental and spiritual well-being.

Having established your dosha type the practitioner will feel your pulse, which is used as a diagnostic tool. In Ayurvedic medicine, three pulses at different points just above your wrist indicate the state of your three doshas. Any abnormalities in your pulses indicates imbalances in your system and will give the practitioner their first clue about what type of condition they may have to treat you for.

You will probably be asked a number of questions, initially

# Case history

Daphne Gillingham, Ayurvedic patient

In January 1999, I sprained my sacroiliac joint. This was initially misdiagnosed, but eventually identified by a chiropractor, who told me I had a pelvic tilt as a result of childbirth (25 years earlier). He manipulated my pelvis back into place, and gave me a chiropractic belt. My GP then prescribed diazepam as a muscle relaxant for the pain and I took it for 13 months.

I spent most of this period off work and bed-ridden, but eventually asked my GP if I could return to work. He expressed doubts, but agreed to take me off diazepam over a month. At first I felt fine, but in May 2000, two weeks after coming off completely, I experienced full-blown withdrawal, including panic attacks, palpitations, 'jelly' legs, pins and needles, a feeling like an electric current running through me, and feet as heavy as lead. In addition, because diazepam affects the central nervous system and overrides messages sent from the brain to the muscles, when you come off it, the muscles are unable to respond normally. So the muscles in my back were very weak, and I was pulling them all the time, even by simply turning over in bed, and was soon bed-ridden again.

My GP suggested I go back on diazepam, reassuring me that I was not 'an addictive person'. By this time I was feeling suicidal, but when a support helpline and a kinesiologist backed my GP, telling me there was no homeopathic or herbal substitute, I started taking diazepam again.

In May 2001, however, I began, over a five-month period, to take myself off it, and experienced no withdrawal. I also changed my GP, and started seeing an osteopath for my stiffness, and because my pelvis remained slightly twisted. However, I still had problems relating to a damaged central nervous system, the legacy of the diazepam: high blood pressure; sensitivity to noise and light; spasms around my genital area; acute headaches; stress (I thought I was never going to recover); and erratic sleep. The osteopath then recommended an Ayurvedic practitioner, and it was through him that I discovered what the diazepam had caused. I had severe nerve damage, and as a result everything was exaggerated, including my feelings of hopelessness.

I started to see the Ayurvedic therapist once a week, and from the outset he focused on my mental state and my physical condition, stressing that my mind and spirit needed to recover before my body could heal. He used a combination of medicines and marmatherapy (Indian acupuncture) to get my body back into balance. He also told me that the 'vata' aspect of my personality had been thrown off balance, causing anxiety, and emphasised the importance of positive thinking, literally 'changing one's thoughts'. This was difficult, as I was often tearful. However, after a month I felt I had stabilised. I had fewer tearful days, and although I was still having physical problems (muscle spasms), I knew that chronic problems take longer to respond.

My therapist is currently using massage to improve my lymphatic system, which is congested due to the effect of the diazepam on my liver function. He also hopes to improve my swollen ankles and poor circulation by stimulating lymphatic drainage and excess fluid absorption. I will revisit my osteopath once my physical symptoms have settled, and he is optimistic that he can fix my twisted pelvis; I can already hold myself and keep my head up better. The important thing is not to set unrealistic goals or put time limits on treatment.

about your family medical history. You will then be asked detailed questions about your health, diet, lifestyle and social behaviour such as relationships, drinking, smoking and sex. This enables the practitioner to make meaningful connections between the information you have given them and their own reading of your pulses. Finally, you will be asked questions concerning your particular condition or complaint. An astute practitioner will probably already have a very good idea of the nature of your problem, but your own appraisal and input are important in assisting diagnosis and deciding on effective treatment.

After you have described your symptoms, the practitioner will conduct a physical examination. This may include looking at your eyes, nose, tongue, hair, nails, feet and skin. The tongue is particularly important in Ayurvedic diagnosis. It is believed that parts of the tongue correspond to different organs in the body. The practitioner may also ask for a detailed description of the colour, quantity and frequency of your urine and bowel movements.

After diagnosis, the next step is to work out an appropriate course of treatment. This will be tailored to your individual condition and is likely to be based on diet, medication and any necessary lifestyle changes.

**What does the treatment involve?**
Exercise is likely to be a significant feature of your Ayurvedic treatment. Any exercise programme will be tailor-made to suit you and your level of fitness or health. Yoga is particularly recommended, not primarily for getting and keeping fit, but for balancing the body's energy centres and bringing body, mind and spirit into harmony and symmetry. Herbal medicines, the only medication in the Ayurvedic system, may be prescribed. In the UK your practitioner will probably use single herbs. These will need to be boiled in water and drunk as a tea, or they may be given in powder, tablet or syrup form. You will

also be offered an internal and external detoxification and cleansing programme known as 'panchakarma' (see below).

### What substances are used in Ayurvedic medicine?

Ayurvedic products are prepared from plants using all their component parts such as the bark, root, fruit, leaf and seeds. Internal preparations are given in powder, tablet, syrup and decoction form, where plants are boiled in water and the fluid drained off and drunk. External preparations are administered as pastes, oils and creams. In India and Sri Lanka, purified minerals, animal substances and metals are mixed with these preparations. In Europe, however, Ayurvedic practice does not use animal substances in its medicines.

### Where do the herbs come from?

Most of the plants come mainly from the mountains of Sri Lanka and India and are then imported to the UK. Suppliers buy from wholesalers who in turn sell the herbs to practitioners in the UK. You should make sure that your practitioner is a member of the AMA, so that you can be sure that your herbs have come from a reputable supplier.

### Will the herbal medicine taste unpleasant?

Many people find the taste of the herbal 'teas' extremely unpleasant. For this reason many practitioners in the UK will prescribe powders, tablets and syrups rather than boiled herbs.

### How often is treatment needed?

Following the first consultation your practitioner will decide how often you should visit them. In most cases you may be asked to make weekly or fortnightly visits over a period of two to three months. Once your condition is under control, you may not have to visit the practitioner again, although they may recommend that you visit every six months to maintain good health.

## What is 'panchakarma'?

Anyone suffering from a disease or complaint will have toxins in their system. Since the accumulation of toxins may slow down the healing process, they need to be eliminated by a qualified practitioner. Before detoxification, oil massage and a steam bath help to eliminate impurities through the skin. The cleansing techniques involve the use of mild laxatives and enemas. These procedures are best undertaken early in the morning and on an empty stomach.

Panchakarma is available in the UK, but the techniques used are not as extreme as those performed in India. Although the level of purging is not taken to the same lengths that it is in Asia, however, in some cases mild laxatives and enemas may be appropriate. Panchakarma is always preceded by a preparatory procedure including herbs, advice on diet and lifestyle which allows your practitioner to determine what level of panchakarma you can cope with.

## Is fasting part of Ayurvedic treatment?

Fasting is central to Ayurveda. Practitioners believe that it is particularly helpful in the treatment of both mental and physical problems, that it plays an important role in controlling certain diseases and that it can solve certain health problems. Should fasting be recommended, you should always inform your GP and follow your practitioner's instructions.

There are three different types of fast:
- Total fasting, where you eat or drink nothing at all
- A liquid fast, where you take only liquids such as juice, coconut water, milk, etc.
- A fruit and vegetable fast, where you can only have fruit and vegetable preparations.

### Will I have to change my diet?

A basic ideology of Ayurveda is that the best way to achieve lasting health is to eat the right kinds of food for your dosha type. It is believed that eating the wrong kinds of food can lead to poor health in general. Ayurveda recommends a vegetarian and high quality diet, though it acknowledges that non-vegetarian food may be appropriate in certain circumstances. The same dietary rules are not prescribed for everyone and your unique constitution will be taken into account.

### I've heard that my condition may get worse before it gets better. Is this true?

This is not usually the case with Ayurveda, although patients treated with the cleansing method known as 'panchakarma' before any chronic conditions are addressed may experience mild short-term reactions. Occasionally, patients may feel tired as a result of the treatment, but this is a temporary effect. Practitioners claim that Ayurvedic medicines are easily assimilated with relatively few side-effects and that they are non-addictive and so may be used over a long period of time.

### Are there any specialisms within Ayurvedic medicine?

Orthopaedic bone-mending is one such field in the Ayurvedic system. Special plasters are made up from herbs and minerals to speed up the healing process. Similar techniques can be used to treat snake bites and insect bites.

### Are toxic substances used in Ayurvedic medicine?

Some preparations have been found to contain metals and minerals such as arsenic and mercury. Although these types of herbal preparation are not generally available in the West, there is evidence that remedies from Asia contaminated with heavy metals have sometimes found their way into this country. It is vital, therefore, that you consult a qualified practitioner who uses

# Case history

Dr Namasivayam, Ayurvedic practitioner

On meeting a new patient, I usually spend a little time telling them about Ayurveda, and I give them a form to fill out that helps me identify what category they fall into in Ayurvedic terms. I note the way they move, walk and react, and whether they are tense or calm – such information can provide valuable clues to diagnosis and treatment. Obviously if they have a visible problem such as acne, I can pick this up immediately and I already know what the imbalance in their system is. However, they may still reveal more about the problem by talking to me about it. I ask for details of their problem and any previous treatment, and for general information about their health and family medical history, including whether they suffer from headaches or have breathing problems. I also ask why they decided on Ayurveda.

I then take their pulse in each wrist at three different points, an Ayurvedic technique for locating imbalances. I check their eyes, tongue, skin, hair and nails, and palpate their abdomen and legs, feeling for any tender points, and I look for tension in their neck, back and the backs of their legs. Usually this whole process, which takes around 25 minutes, allows me to make a diagnosis. Then I ask about the patient's lifestyle and give advice on making useful changes to it, like waking up earlier or altering their diet, if necessary. I also prescribe one or a combination of treatments. These include herbs; panchakarma, an oil massage which relieves congestion and toxic buildup; an Ayurvedic steam bath, which patients can have at the clinic; and Shirodhara, which is a technique of dropping warm oil on to the forehead to calm the system in the brain. I also might recommend marmatherapy, which is similar to (and a predecessor of) Chinese acupuncture.

Recently I treated a woman in her early fifties who had been suffering from chronic psoriasis for 28 years. Her menopause had started and she was in a state of hormonal and emotional flux, and her skin problem made her embarrassed and self-conscious. She had tried orthodox medications and light treatment without success.

I told her that she was suffering from pitta aggravation – which relates to the hormones and the skin – and that I could help her, but that it could take months. I advised her to cut out alcohol and smoking, and to increase her water intake to help cleanse her skin. I prescribed herbs and an oil-based cream. I also administered marmatherapy. To begin with there was no change, but by the sixth week her skin was a little better. This change gave my patient the confidence to continue. I then began panchakarma, and after ten months her skin was very much clearer.

I also saw a woman in her twenties who had polycystic ovaries. She had tried hormone treatment, but hadn't had any success, and was feeling self-conscious about her facial and body hair. Again it was a problem with pitta imbalance. I advised her about her diet, prescribed herbs and marmatherapy, and within two months she appeared to be responding to treatment. The pain in her abdomen had started to recede, her bad periods improved, and the hair growth had thinned. She then announced that she was pregnant, which seemed to me to be a reaction to the Ayurveda unblocking her system. At this point, I advised her to cease treatment, preferring to 'observe' her progress by phone interviews alone.

trustworthy suppliers before embarking on a course of treatment.

Although Ayurveda commonly uses some mineral and herbal combinations, most western qualified practitioners use single herbs in a limited number of combinations. The Ayurvedic Medical Association guides its members to ensure that all preparations are safe and effective and are prescribed according to your individual needs.

### How much does a consultation cost?

There are no set charges and costs vary depending on the experience of the practitioner, their geographical location and the length of the consultation. On average, expect to pay £35 to £50 for the first consultation. The average cost of a month's prescription of pills, herbs, powders and decoctions is £10 to £15.

### Can I have Ayurvedic treatment at reduced rates?

You would need to negotiate this with your chosen practitioner. This guide tells you about practitioners who are prepared to reduce their fees for those on low incomes.

### Can I get my private health insurers to pay for my Ayurvedic treatment?

Ayurvedic medicine is not as well established as other complementary therapies in the UK. It is unlikely that you could claim back treatment fees from your health insurer.

### What training do Ayurvedic practitioners have?

In India and Sri Lanka, the degree course in Ayurveda consists of full-time study for five to six years in a hospital environment. Practitioners trained in this way carry the title BAMS or DAMS after their name. After passing the final examination, graduates must complete a year's compulsory service as an Internee Medical Officer in an Ayurvedic General Hospital attached to the teaching university. They can then register themselves as a qualified Ayurvedic Medical Practitioner with the Ayurvedic Medical

Council, which is the government-controlled regulatory body.

During their training period, they are taught philosophy, materia medica, Ayurvedic pharmacology, clinical medicine, gynaecology, obstetrics, paediatrics, toxicology surgery, anatomy and physiology. Although all these subjects are taught according to the Ayurvedic system, they run parallel to the orthodox western medical syllabus. In India and Sri Lanka, Ayurvedic practitioners may also perform minor surgery.

In the UK, training standards are laid down by the European Herbal Practitioner Association (EHPA) and are currently equivalent to degree level. Students train at The College of Ayurveda in Milton Keynes for a Postgraduate Diploma in Ayurvedic Medicine (PGDAM). The diploma teaches the theoretical principles and philosophy of Ayurveda and its practical implications using an integrated approach. Students also learn how to administer panchakarma. The course is managed by the Ayurvedic Medical Association UK and the college is accredited by the British Council for Complementary Medicine.

## Will my practitioner belong to a professional body?

At the moment, anybody can practise Ayurvedic medicine in the UK without adequate training or membership of a professional body. You should check that your practitioner is a member of the Ayurvedic Medical Association (AMA UK).

## What do all the letters mean?

**AMA UK** your practitioner is a member of the AMA UK, the only body that represents practitioners of Ayurvedic medicine in the UK.

**BAMS** your practitioner is a Bachelor of Ayurvedic Medicine.

**DAMS** your practitioner has a Diploma or Degree of Ayurvedic Medicine or Surgery.

**PGDAM** your practitioner has a postgraduate Diploma in Ayurvedic Medicine.

## How do practitioners keep their skills and knowledge up to date?

Continuing Professional Development (CPD) is currently being developed according to EHPA guidelines. Seminars and courses for practitioners will take place through the College of Ayurveda in Milton Keynes and will be compulsory. The Association will maintain records of those in practice, and any practitioners failing to meet the requirements for maintaining their standards will be disciplined by the AMA UK.

## Where can I find a qualified practitioner?

The practitioners listed in this guide are all members of AMA UK and as such will be fully trained and abide by a Code of Ethics. You can also contact The Ayrvedic Medical Association directly for a list of local qualified practitioners in your area.

## What questions should I ask before making an appointment with an Ayurvedic practitioner?

As well as the questions outlined on p133, you should ensure that:

- Your practitioner is properly qualified. (An Ayurvedic practitioner will carry the title BAMS or DAMS, after their name and you should always check with the Ayurvedic Medical Association whether a practitioner is registered with them.)
- On the first consultation a full case history is taken. The consultation should last at least 40 minutes. If your practitioner does not speak English, make sure that there is a translator present.

## Can I have Ayurvedic treatment on the NHS?

Ayurvedic treatment is not available on the NHS.

### Will the practitioner discuss my condition with my GP?

Ayurvedic practitioners are keen to work alongside the orthodox medical profession and as a result may wish to write to your GP. However, they can only do so with your express permission.

### Will my practitioner have access to my medical records?

If you have been referred by your GP, your Ayurvedic practitioner will most probably want to communicate with them and keep them abreast of your treatment and progress. However, your practitioner cannot do so without your consent.

### Do I need a referral from my GP to visit an Ayurvedic practitioner?

Although you are able to refer yourself to an Ayurvedic practitioner, your GP is able to make a referral if they feel that Ayurveda would be of help to your condition.

### Can Ayurvedic treatment be used during pregnancy? Is it suitable for children?

Although there is no evidence to show that Ayurvedic medicines are harmful during pregnancy, pregnant women should be advised to abstain from using certain remedies, particularly those that have a mildly laxative effect on the system.

Preparations are available specifically for infants and children, and these will have been specially modified.

### Are Ayurvedic practitioners covered by insurance?

If your practitioner is a member of the AMC, they will be covered by the appropriate insurance.

### Do Ayurvedic practitioners ever make home visits?

Practitioners may make home visits if they have the time or the patient is local or bed-bound, but, on the whole, home visits are rare.

### How do I make a complaint about an Ayurvedic practitioner?

The Ayurvedic Medical Association has its own ethics committee which will take any complaints against a registered practitioner very seriously. Complaints should be made in writing to the AMA UK which will thoroughly investigate any complaint. If the practitioner is found to be in breach of the Code of Conduct and Ethics, they may be disciplined or struck off the register.

### Where can I find further information?

### Ayurvedic Medical Association UK

59 Dulverton Road
Selsdon
South Croydon
Surrey
CR2 8PJ
Tel. 020 8682 3876 before 2pm
Email: dr_nsmoorthy@hotmail.com

### College of Ayurveda

20 Annes Grove,
Great Linford,
Milton Keynes
MK14 5DR]
Tel 01908 664 518
Email: mauroos@ayurvedacollege.co.uk

# Section Three:
# **The Practitioners**

# How to use the data

In this section of the book we list over 6000 practitioners together with information designed to help you chose a practitioner best suited to your needs. The practitioners listed in this guide are all members of organisations that maintain a register of members; set educational standards and require members to graduate from an accredited college; run a continuing professional development programme; require members to abide by codes of conduct, ethics and practice; run a complaints system and disciplinary procedure accessible to the public; require members to take out professional indemnity insurance.

Practitioners are listed by geographical region, county and then alphabetically by town and postcode within that county. For instance, if you live in Canterbury, Kent, look up Kent in the South East section. Practitioners will be listed alphabetically by town. Each practitioner may have two or three different postcodes listed. These indicate other practices the therapist works from, not necessarily in the same town.

For each practitioner we tell you the name of the organisation they are a member of, which will be one of the following:

| | |
|---|---|
| **Traditional Chinese Acupuncture** | British Acupuncture Council (BAcC), (see p42) |
| **Western Medical Acupuncture** | British Medical Acupuncture Society (BMAS), Acupuncture Association of Chartered Physiotherapists (AAC), (see p42) |
| **Medical Homeopathy** | Faculty of Homeopathy (FH), (see p71) |
| **Professional Homeopathy** | Society of Homeopaths (SH), (see p71) |
| **Osteopathy** | General Osteopathic Council (GOsC), (see p95) |

| | |
|---|---|
| **Chiropractic** | General Chiropractic Council (GCC), (see p117) |
| **Western Herbal Medicine** | National Institute of Medical Herbalists (NIMH), Association of Master Herbalists (ASH), International Register of Consultant Herbalists (IRCH), (see p133) |
| **Chinese Herbal Medicine** | Register of Chinese Herbal Medicine (RCHM), (see p133) |
| **Ayurvedic Medicine** | Ayurvedic Medical Association UK (AMA UK), (see p 133) |

## Where the practitioner works

This icon shows whether the practitioner works from a private clinic. This will either be purpose-built or converted from an existing building.

This icon shows whether the practitioner works privately from their home. The practitioner should ideally have a separate room in their house dedicated solely for the purpose of their work (for example it should not double up as a spare room or study).

This icon shows whether the therapist works alongside other CAM practitioners. If they do, it may mean that you will have access to other forms of complementary therapies at the same site, for example, reflexology and massage, as well as acupuncture or herbal medicine.

## Relationships with orthodox medicine

Practitioners vary in their relationship to doctors and orthodox medicine. Some work closely with GPs and other doctors. Others tend to have less contact with orthodox medicine and may see themselves more as an alternative. We tell you whether a practitioner receives referrals from GPs or doctors working in the NHS. It does not mean a practitioner is any better because they get these referrals, but it does suggest they have developed good working relationships with GPs. We also asked practitioners whether they communicated with a patient's GP, assuming the patient gives permission. We believe that all practitioners should do this although few actually do consistently. One of the greatest risks in visiting a complementary therapist is that a more serious condition may go undiagnosed. We tell you which practitioners indicated that they regularly do write to patient's GPs. If your practitioner does not, we suggest you encourage them to do so. If not, you should talk to your GP about any complementary therapies you are receiving.

 This icon shows that the practitioner has taken referrals through the NHS in the last six months. This suggests that they have developed good working relationships with GPs.

 This icon shows whether the practitioner communicated with their patient's GPs for over a third of the cases they treated. It is important to ensure that if your practitioner cannot make a proper diagnosis or suspects that you have a serious condition that requires orthodox treatment, they will refer you to a GP or specialist. It is also important that the practitioner does not claim to be able to cure your condition, and that they will refer you elsewhere after 5 – 6 weeks if you are not responding to treatment.

**Equipment on site**

 This icon shows you which Osteopath and Chiropractic clinics have X-ray facilities on site. This could mean that should you need an X-ray for diagnostic purposes, the practitioner will not have to refer you elsewhere. Practices that have this are also likely to be larger.

**Out of hours service**

 This icon shows you whether you will be able to visit your practitioner outside normal working hours: a practitioner may conduct a late clinic on a Tuesday evening for example.

## Fees

We give you the practitioner's fees for the first consultation and treatment (which usually takes longer and so costs more) and for the second and subsequent treatments. These can range from less than £25 to more than £50.

 This icon shows you whether your practitioner offers a sliding scale of fees or runs a subsidised clinic. In cases of genuine hardship, most practitioners will offer you a reduced rate.

## Training

The following icons are for acupuncture only and help you to differentiate the different types of acupuncturists. Some medical acupuncturists might be medically qualified but have less than 100 hours of training. All TCM acupuncturists should have trained for more than 1200 hours (see p47).

 Your practitioner has trained for more than 1200 hours. This means that they are most likely to practice Traditional Chinese Medicine (see p47)

 Your practitioner has done between 501 and 1200 hours of training.

 Your practitioner has done between 101-500 hours of training

 Your practitioner has done less than 100 hours training. This means that they will practice Medical acupuncture (see p47).

## Contact details

We give you the contact details for the practitioner's main practice, but the icons will show the type of practices they operate from – either from home, or in a clinic and whether they practice alongside other complementary practitioners. Some practitioners may operate from two addresses, for example, they may work at a clinic one day a week and from a private address at other times. Where the practitioner has not supplied their postcode or phone number, you should contact their member organisation for contact details.

# East

Bedfordshire
Cambridgeshire (inc. Peterborough)
Essex
Norfolk
Suffolk

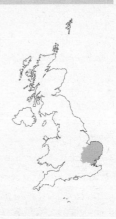

## Acupuncture

### BEDFORDSHIRE

**Kate Abrahams AACP**
● O ⊕ ⊕ ✿ ⓐ
**Fees:** £36–45; Second visit: £31–40
Bedford MK44
01234 378996

**Joan Biddle BAcC**
● ✿ ●
**Fees:** £36–45; Second visit: £21–30
Bedford MK45
01525 753937

**Alison Chick AACP**
● ⊕ ⊕ ✿ ●
**Fees:** £26–35; Second visit: £21–30
Bedford MK45
01525 841845

**Frederick J Steele BAcC**
● ⓝ ✿ ●
**Fees:** £26–35; Second visit: £21–30
Bedford MK41
01234 355937

**Li-Jun Dan BAcC**
● ⓝ ✿ ●
**Fees:** £26–35; Second visit: £31–40
Luton LU4
01582 495040

**Rachael De Vere Marfleet BAcC**
O ✿ ●
**Fees:** £36–45; Second visit: £21–30
Luton LU2
01582 411223

### CAMBRIDGESHIRE

**Francois De Menthon BAcC**
● ⊕ ⊕ © ✿ ●
**Fees:** £36–45; Second visit: £21–30
Cambridge CB2, Guildford GU1
01223 315541

**Alan Hext BAcC**
● ●
**Fees:** >£55; Second visit: £21–30
Cambridge CB1
01223 323473

**Christopher J Low BAcC**
● ⊕ ●
**Fees:** £46–55; Second visit: £31–40
Cambridge CB1
01223 415117

**Peter White BAcC**
● O ⊕ ✿ ●
**Fees:** £36–45; Second visit: £21–30
Cambridge CB1
01223 890832

**Matthew Kent BAcC**
🌐 🌐 🌐 🌐
**Fees:** £36–45; Second visit: £21–30
Ely CB7
01353 664476

**Wendy Goodman BAcC**
🌐 🌐 🌐
**Fees:** £26–35; Second visit: £21–30
Huntingdon PE29
01480 455221

**Garry Hares BAcC**
🌐 🌐 🌐 🌐
**Fees:** £46–55; Second visit: £21–30
Huntingdon PE28
01487 830877

**Phwoc T Huynh BAcC**
🌐 🌐 🌐 🌐 🌐
**Fees:** £26–35; Second visit: £21–30
Huntingdon PE21
01480 432869

**Carol Qirreh BAcC**
🌐 🌐 🌐
**Fees:** £36–45; Second visit: £21–30
Huntingdon PE28
01487 841733

**Stewart Menzies BAcC, BMAS,**
🌐 🌐 🌐
**Fees:** £46–55; Second visit: £21–30
Peterborough PE6
01733 252086

**J Longbottom AACP**
🌐 🌐 🌐
**Fees:** £26–35; Second visit: £31–40
St Neots PE19
01480 394715

**Lynn Pearce AACP**
🌐 🌐 🌐 🌐
**Fees:** £26–35; Second visit: £31–40
St Neots PE19
01480 394715

**Marilyn Clarke AACP**
🌐 🌐 🌐 🌐
**Fees:** £36–45; Second visit: £41–50
Wisbech PE14
01945 881332

## ESSEX

**S Kumaresan AACP**
🌐 🌐 🌐
**Fees:** £26–35; Second visit: £31–40
Benfleet SS7
01268 747349

**Godfrey Bartlett BAcC**
🌐 🌐 🌐 🌐 🌐 🌐
**Fees:** £26–35; Second visit: £21–30
Brentwood CM14
01277 223894

**Gillian Kelly BAcC**
🌐 🌐 🌐 🌐
**Fees:** £36–45; Second visit: £21–30
Brentwood CM15
01277 260080

**Margie Bell AACP**
🌐 🌐 🌐 🌐 🌐
**Fees:** £26–35; Second visit: £21–30
Burnham-on-Crouch CM0
01621 782194

**A Buillard-Meaden AACP**
🌐 🌐 🌐 🌐 🌐
**Fees:** £36–45; Second visit: £21–30
Chelmsford CM3
01245 325037

**Craig Fowlie AACP**
🌐 🌐 🌐 🌐
**Fees:** £26–35
Chelmsford CM3
01245 325037

**A Shapland BAcC**
🌐 🌐 🌐 🌐 🌐
**Fees:** <£25; Second visit: £21–30
Chelmsford CM1
01245 347277

**D Tatapudi AACP**
🌐 🌐 🌐 🌐 🌐
**Fees:** £26–35; Second visit: £21–30
Chelmsford CM5
01992 523753

**Hong Van Trinh BAcC**
🌐 🌐 🌐 🌐 🌐
**Fees:** <£25; Second visit: £21–30
Chelmsford CM1, London SW3,
London NW8
01245 257085

# Acupuncture

**Helen Yin Muey Tanner BAcC**
⊕ ⊕ ✿ ⊛
Fees: <£25; Second visit: £21–30
Chigwell IG7
020 8491 0648

**Andrew Cornelius BAcC, AACP**
⊕ ⊕ ⊘ ✿ ⊛
Fees: £26–35; Second visit: £21–30
Epping CM16
01992 561112

**Diana Cornelius AACP**
⊕ ⊕ ✿ ⊛
Fees: £26–35; Second visit: £21–30
Epping CM16
01992 561112

**E Longton BAcC**
O ✿ ⊛
Fees: £26–35; Second visit: £21–30
Epping CM16
01992 572594

**A Dharmalingam BAcC**
O ✿ ⊛
Fees: £26–35
Grays RM16
01375 383627

**Linda Culleton BAcC**
⊕ O ⊕ ✿ ⊛
Fees: £26–35; Second visit: £21–30
Harlow CM17,Stansted CM24
01279 438444

**Ahamed Lebbe AACP**
O ⊘ ⊛
Fees: £36–45; Second visit: £31–40
Ilford IG2
020 8518 2460

**Catriona Guiver AACP**
⊕ ⊘ ✿ ⊛
Fees: £26–35; Second visit: £21–30
Ingatestone CM4
01277 652770

**Christine Hayes AACP**
⊕ ⊘ ✿ ⊛
Fees: £26–35; Second visit: £21–30
Leigh-on-Sea SS9
01702 558069

**Anna Yang BAcC**
⊕ O ✿
Fees: £26–35; Second visit: £21–30
Leigh-on-Sea SS9
01702 482178

**David Kelsey BAcC**
O ⊕ ✿ ⊛
Fees: £26–35; Second visit: £21–30
Saffron Walden CB10
01799 521496

**Eveline Jacobs BAcC**
⊕ ⊕ ⊛ ✿ ⊛
Fees: £26–35; Second visit: £21–30
Southend-on-Sea SS3
01702 297265

**Anh Nga Phan BAcC**
⊕ ⊛ ✿ ⊛
Fees: £26–35; Second visit: £21–30
Southend-on-Sea SS1,
Billericay CM12, Loughton IG10
01702 390305

**M Voigts BAcC**
⊕ ⊕ ✿ ⊛
Fees: £26–35; Second visit: £21–30
Southend-on-Sea SS1
01702 582485

**Hubert Van Griensven BAcC, AACP**
⊕ ⊕ ⊛
Fees: £26–35; Second visit: £21–30
Westcliff-on-Sea SS0
01702 343785

**John Brown Lee BAcC**
⊕ O ⊕ ✿ ⊛
Fees: £26–35; Second visit: £21–30
Wickford SS11
01268 451663

**Jac Snape AACP**
⊕ ⊘ ✿ ⊛
Fees: £26–35; Second visit: £31–40
Wickford SS12
01268 561696

**Jennifer Linstead BAcC**
⊕ O ⊕ ✿ ⊛
Fees: <£25; Second visit: <£20
Wivenhoe CO7
01206 827355

## NORFOLK

**Kate Stewart BAcC**
⊕ ⊕ ⊕
Fees: £26–35; Second visit: £21–30
Downham Market PE38
01366 383840

**Andrew Latter BAcC**
⊕ O ⊕ ✹ ⊕
Fees: <£25; Second visit: £21–30
Fakenham NR21
01328 856601

**Roger Brown BAcC**
⊕ O ⊕ ✹ ⊕
Fees: £26–35; Second visit: £21–30
Norwich NR7
01603 415715

**Ann Chandler AACP**
⊕ ⊕ ⊕
Fees: £26–35; Second visit: £31–40
Norwich NR6
01603 408012

**Stephen Ellis BAcC**
⊕ ⊕ ⊕ ✹ ⊕
Fees: £26–35; Second visit: £21–30
Norwich NR6
01603 429276

**Alexandra Everington BAcC**
O ⊘ ⊕
Fees: £36–45; Second visit: £21–30
Norwich NR9
01362 850922

**Lynne Fanning AACP**
⊕ ⊕ ⊕ ⊘ ⊕
Fees: £36–45; Second visit: £31–40
Norwich NR6
01603 421321

**Nicholas J Hurn BAcC**
⊕ ⊕ ⊕ ⊕ ✹ ⊕
Fees: £46–55; Second visit: £21–30
Norwich NR1
01603 630226

**Elaine Munting AACP**
O ⊕ ✹
Fees: £36–45; Second visit: £31–40
Norwich NR15
01508 550523

**Graham Palmer BAcC**
⊕ ⊕ ✹ ⊕
Fees: <£25
Norwich NR3
01603 660792

**E Palmer AACP**
⊕ ⊕ ⊘ ✹ ⊕
Fees: £26–35; Second visit: £21–30
Norwich NR9, Norwich NR9
01603 872335

**A Pointer AACP**
⊕ ✹ ⊕
Fees: £26–35; Second visit: £31–40
Norwich NR10
01603 891276

**John Sampson BMAS**
⊕ ⊕ ⊘ ⊕
Fees: <£25; Second visit: <£20
Norwich NR14
01508 494343

**Jodie Williams BAcC**
⊕ ⊕ ⊕ ✹ ⊕
Fees: £26–35; Second visit: £21–30
Norwich NR14
01508 570122

**Richard Lamb BAcC**
⊕ ⊕
Fees: £26–35
Sheringham NR26
01263 823724

## SUFFOLK

**Sue Hooker BAcC**
⊕ ⊕ ⊕ ⊕
Fees: £26–35; Second visit: £21–30
Beccles NR34
01502 712505

**Dorothy Baker BAcC**
⊕ ⊕ ✹ ⊕
Fees: £26–35
Bury St Edmunds IP33
01284 704228

**Zara Hansen AACP**
⊕ ⊕ ✹ ⊕
Fees: £36–45; Second visit: £21–30
Bury St Edmunds IP33
01284 748200

# Acupuncture

**Dulchand Nathoo BAcC**
✪ O ⊕ 🅐 🅦 ❋ 🆐
**Fees:** £36–45; Second visit: £21–30
Bury St Edmunds IP32,Eye IP23
01284 763529

**Lena Tettelaar AACP**
✪ 🅦 ❋ 🅑
**Fees:** £26–35; Second visit: £21–30
Felixstowe IP11
07932 172958

**Barbara Jameson BAcC**
O ⒠ ❋ 🆐
**Fees:** £26–35; Second visit: £21–30
Ipswich IP1
01473 745646

**Philip Hodson BAcC**
✪ O 🆐
**Fees:** £26–35; Second visit: £21–30
Newmarket CB8
01638 667589

**Richard Graham BAcC**
✪ O ⊕ ⊕ ⒠ ❋ 🆐
**Fees:** £36–45; Second visit: £21–30
Sudbury CO10,Felixstowe IP11,
Woodbridge IP12
01787 210005

**Julie Iveson AACP**
✪ ⊘ ❋ 🆐
**Fees:** £26–35; Second visit: £31–40
Sudbury CO10
01787 374964

# Homeopathy

**BEDFORDSHIRE**

**Stephanie Field RSHom**
O 🅦 ❋
**Fees:** £46–55; Second visit: £31–40
Bedford MK43
01234 826407

**Fiona Dry MFHom**
✪ O ⊕ 🅦 ⊘ ⒠ ❋
**Fees:** >£55; Second visit: £20–30
Leighton Buzzard LU7
01525 373721

**Rosemary Nightingale RSHom**
O 🅦
**Fees:** £36–45; Second visit: £20–30
Leighton Buzzard LU7
01525 379224

**CAMBRIDGESHIRE**

**Pauline Dawber RSHom**
✪ O ⊕ ⊕ 🅦 ⊘ ❋
**Fees:** £46–55; Second visit: £20–30
Cambridge CB2
01223 842075

**Angela Gardner RSHom**
✪ ⒠ ❋
**Fees:** £25–35; Second visit: <£20
Cambridge CB2
01223 840091

**Brigitte Haworth RSHom**
O 🅦 ❋
**Fees:** £36–45; Second visit: £20–30
Cambridge CB2
01223 570575

**Ann Massing RSHom**
✪ ⊕ ⊕ 🅦 ⒠ ❋
**Fees:** £25–35; Second visit: £20–30
Cambridge CB1,Cambridge CB2
01223 313005

**Jennifer Boyle MFHom**
O 🅦 ⊘
**Fees:** >£55; Second visit: £41–50
Huntingdon PE28
01487 822409

**Stewart Menzies MFHom**
O ⊕ 🅦 ⊘ ❋
**Fees:** >£55; Second visit: £31–40
Peterborough PE6
01733 252086

## ESSEX

**Kathryn Meader RSHom**
⊕ ⓔ ✿
Fees: £36–45; Second visit: £20–30
Billericay CM11
01268 272757

**Susan Barber RSHom**
O ⓔ
Fees: £46–55; Second visit: £20–30
Brentwood CM15
01277 234035

**Linda Lemmon RSHom**
⊕ O ⊕ ⓝ ⓔ ✿
Fees: £36–45; Second visit: £20–30
Brentwood CM14,Brentwood CM13
01277 223308

**Gillian Gardner RSHom**
O ⓝ ✿
Fees: £36–45; Second visit: £20–30
Chelmsford CM2
01245 472604

**Jean Turfkruyer RSHom**
⊕ O ⊕ ⓝ ⊘ ⓔ ✿
Fees: £46–55; Second visit: £31–40
Chelmsford CM1
01621 782845

**Imogen Gosling RSHom**
⊕ O ⊕ ⓔ ✿
Fees: £36–45; Second visit: £20–30
Colchester CO5
01206 383436

**Susan Hyett RSHom**
O ⓝ ✿
Fees: £25–35; Second visit: <£20
Colchester CO2
01206 546319

**Richard Laing MFHom**
⊕ O ⓝ ⊘ ⓔ ✿
Fees: £46–55; Second visit: £20–30
Colchester CO2
01206 575581

**B O Taylor MFHom**
⊕ O ⊕ ⓝ ⊘
Fees: >£55; Second visit: £41–50
Colchester CO6,Cambridge CB4
01787 224876

**Anne Preece RSHom**
O ⊕ ⓝ ⓔ ✿
Fees: £36–45; Second visit: £20–30
Dunmow CM6,Braintree CM7
01371 873902

**Erica Wyld RSHom**
⊕ O ⊕ ⓝ
Fees: £46–55; Second visit: £20–30
Ilford IG4
020 8550 9722

**Julia Chilver RSHom**
⊕ O ⊕ ⓝ ⊘ ⓔ ✿
Fees: £36–45; Second visit: £20–30
Maldon CM9,Maldon CM9
01621 850633

**Brenda O'Brien RSHom**
⊕ ⊕ ⓝ ⓔ ✿
Fees: £36–45; Second visit: £20–30
Maldon CM9,Colchester CO7
01621 851741

**Lesley Carlisle RSHom**
⊕ O ⊕ ⊕ ⓝ ⓔ ✿
Fees: >£55; Second visit: £31–40
North Weald CM16
01992 579333

**S Z Haider MFHom**
O ⊕ ⊕ ⓝ ⊘ ✿
Fees: £46–55; Second visit: £20–30
Romford RM2
01708 444461

**Roger Savage RSHom**
⊕ ⊕ ⓝ ✿
Fees: >£55; Second visit: £41–50
Saffron Walden CB11
01799 524442

**D Frostick RSHom**
⊕ ⓝ ✿
Fees: £25–35; Second visit: <£20
Stanford-le-Hope SS17
01375 360626

## NORFOLK

**Diane Pitman RSHom**
⊕ ⊕ ⓝ ⓔ
Fees: £36–45; Second visit: £20–30
Dereham NR19
01760 722621

# Homeopathy

**Rachael Heap RSHom**
⊕ O ⊕ ⊛ ❀
Fees: £36–45; Second visit: £20–30
Harleston IP20,Norwich NR14
01379 853860

**Stephen Gordon RSHom**
⊕ ⊕ ⊕ ⊛ Ⓔ
Fees: £25–35; Second visit: £20–30
Norwich NR3, Attleborough NR17,
Bury St Edmunds IP33
01603 660792

**Gillian Lawton RSHom**
⊕ O ⊕ ⊛ Ⓔ ❀
Fees: £25–35; Second visit: £20–30
Norwich NR3
01603 660792

**Tricia Stephenson RSHom**
⊕ O ⊕ ⊛ ∅ ❀
Fees: £36–45; Second visit: £20–30
Norwich NR2
01603 613228

**Sue Crump RSHom**
⊕ O ⊕ ⊕ Ⓔ
Fees: £25–35; Second visit: £20–30
Sedgeford PE36, Norwich NR3,
King's Lynn PE32
01485 570377

SUFFOLK

**Janet Cobill RSHom**
⊕ O ⊕ ⊛ ❀
Fees: £25–35; Second visit: <£20
Bungay NR35
01986 892846

**Lindsay Hickey RSHom**
⊕ ⊕ ⊛ ⊘ Ⓔ ❀
Fees: £25–35; Second visit: £20–30
Eye IP23
01379 870707

**Susan Saunders RSHom**
⊕ ⊕ ⊛ Ⓔ
Fees: £25–35; Second visit: £20–30
Eye IP23
01379 870707

**Maureen Wheeler RSHom**
O ⊛ Ⓔ ❀
Fees: £25–35; Second visit: <£20
Long Melford CO10
01787 378056

**John Carpmael RSHom**
⊕ O ⊛ Ⓔ
Fees: >£55; Second visit: £31–40
Woodbridge IP12
01394 389547

# Osteopathy

BEDFORDSHIRE

**Stephen Bass GOsC**
⊕ O ⊕ ⊛ Ⓔ ❀
Fees: £26–35; Second visit: £21–30
Bedford MK41
01234 308388

**Patricia M Bishop GOsC, BOA**
⊕ ⊛ ⊘ Ⓔ ❀
Fees: <£25; Second visit: £21–30
Bedford MK45
01525 712204

**Tessa Paget Daniels GOsC, BOA**
⊕ ⊕ ❀
Fees: <£25; Second visit: £21–30
Bedford MK45
01525 861281

**Kate Highstead GOsC**
⊕ ⊕ ⊕ ⊛ ❀
Fees: <£25; Second visit: £21–30
Bedford MK45
01525 841845

**Vicki Manners GOsC, BOA**
⊕ ⊕ ⊛ ❀
Fees: £26–35; Second visit: £21–30
Bedford MK40
01234 212788

**Joanne Pinny GOsC, BOA**
⊕ ⊕ ⊛
Fees: <£25; Second visit: £21–30
Bedford MK43
01234 823621

**Jason Pinny GOsC, BOA**
🔵
**Fees:** £26–35; Second visit: £21–30
Bedford MK43
01234 823621

**Julia Spivack GOsC, BOA**
○ ❀
**Fees:** £36–45; Second visit: £21–30
Bedford MK45
01525 719588

**Luisa Whitlock GOsC, BOA**
⊕ ⊕ ⊕ 🔵 ⊘ ❀
**Fees:** <£25; Second visit: £21–30
Bedford MK41
01234 353800

**Kevin Poynter GOsC**
○ 🔵
**Fees:** £26–35; Second visit: £21–30
Biggleswade SG18
01767 601879

**Sarah Fair GOsC, BOA**
⊕ 🔵 ❀
**Fees:** £26–35; Second visit: £21–30
Bromham MK43
01234 823621

**R D Bellamy GOsC, BOA**
⊕ 🔵 ❀
**Fees:** <£25; Second visit: £21–30
Dunstable LU5
01582 661199

**Jonathan Betser GOsC**
⊕ 🔵 ⊘
**Fees:** £26–35; Second visit: £21–30
Dunstable LU5
01582 608400

**Anne Johnson GOsC**
○ 🔵 ❀
**Fees:** <£25; Second visit: <£50
Dunstable LU6, Leighton Buzzard LU7
01525 221958

**Silva Schuldt GOsC, BOA**
⊕ 🔵 ⊘ Ⓔ ❀
**Fees:** £26–35; Second visit: £21–30
Flitwick MK45
01525 712204

**Glenn Lobo GOsC, BOA**
⊕ 🔵 Ⓔ ❀
**Fees:** £26–35; Second visit: £21–30
Luton LU1
0800 980 7151

**Richard Reilly GOsC, BOA**
🔵 ❀
**Fees:** <£25; Second visit: £21–30
Luton LU4
01582 560211

**Karen Robinson GOsC, BOA**
⊕ 🔵 ⊘ Ⓔ ❀
**Fees:** <£25; Second visit: £31–40
Shefford SG17
01462 811006

## CAMBRIDGESHIRE

**Marc Deora GOsC**
⊕ ○ ⊕ 🔵 Ⓔ
**Fees:** £26–35; Second visit: £21–30
Cambridge CB2
01223 242828

**Gaye Dixon GOsC, BOA**
⊕ 🔵 Ⓔ ❀
**Fees:** £26–35; Second visit: £21–30
Cambridge CB5
01223 277919

**Roger Giddings GOsC**
⊕ ⊕ 🔵 ❀
**Fees:** £26-35; Second visit: £21–30
Cambridge CB4
01223 237459

**Rebecca Mercer GOsC, BOA**
⊕ ○ ⊕ ⊕ 🔵 ❀
**Fees:** £26–35; Second visit: £21–30
Cambridge CB2
01223 315541

**Mojo Rathbone GOsC**
⊕ ⊕ ⊕ 🔵
**Fees:** £26-35; Second visit: £21–30
Cambridge CB2
01223 315541

**Philip Stockley GOsC, BOA**
⊕ ○ 🔵 ❀
**Fees:** £26-35; Second visit: £21–30
Cambridge CB1
01223 248233

# Osteopathy

**Neil Watson GOsC, BOA**
⊕ ⊕ ⊕ 🅝 ⊘ 🗲
**Fees:** <£25; Second visit: £21–30
Chatteris PE16
01354 694050

**Alexander Spence GOsC**
⊕ ⊕ ⊕ 🅝 ⓔ 🗲
**Fees:** £26-35; Second visit: £21–30
Ely CB7
01353 664476

**Nick Lunn GOsC, BOA**
⊕ Ⓞ ⊕ 🅝 ⓔ 🌑
**Fees:** £26–35; Second visit: £21–30
Haverhill CB9
01440 705020

**Garry Hares GOsC**
⊕ 🅝 🗲
**Fees:** £46-55; Second visit: £21–30
Huntingdon PE28
01487 830877

**Alison Kelly GOsC, BOA**
⊕ ⊕ 🅝
**Fees:** £26-35; Second visit: £21–30
Huntingdon PE29,London E17
01480 435554

**Alan Szmelskyj GOsC, BOA**
⊕ Ⓞ 🅝 🗲
**Fees:** £26-35; Second visit: £21–30
Huntingdon PE29
01480 435554

**Graham Thomas GOsC**
🅝 🗲
**Fees:** £26-35; Second visit: £21–30
Huntingdon PE27
01480 468921

**Benjamin Barker GOsC, BOA**
⊕ 🅝 🗲
**Fees:** <£25; Second visit: £21–30
Peterborough PE6
01778 347858

**David Cohen GOsC**
⊕ 🅝 🗲
**Fees:** £26-35; Second visit: £21–30
Peterborough PE6
01778 347858

**Phillip Hunt GOsC, BOA**
⊕ ⊕ 🅝 ⊘ 🗲
**Fees:** £26–35; Second visit: £31–40
Peterborough PE4
01733 770349

**David Longstaff GOsC**
⊕ 🅝 🗲
**Fees:** <£25; Second visit: £21–30
Peterborough PE1
01733 310978

**John Milborne GOsC**
⊕ Ⓞ 🅝 ⓔ 🗲
**Fees:** <£25; Second visit: £21–30
Peterborough PE8
01832 272527

**David A Hattersley GOsC, BOA,**
Ⓞ 🅝 🗲
**Fees:** <£25; Second visit: £31–40
Wisbech PE13
01945 700383

## ESSEX

**Graeme Stroud GOsC, BOA**
⊕ Ⓞ 🅝 🗲
**Fees:** £26-35; Second visit: £21–30
Basildon SS14
01268 287733

**James Dickason GOsC, BOA**
⊕ 🅝 ⊘ 🗲
**Fees:** £26–35; Second visit: £21–30
Braintree CM7
01376 322528

**Linda Aryaeenia GOsC, BOA**
⊕ ⊕ 🅝 🗲
**Fees:** <£25; Second visit: £21–30
Brentwood CM15
01277 212900

**Terry Rulten GOsC, BOA**
⊕ ⊕ 🅝 🗲
**Fees:** £26-35; Second visit: £21–30
Brentwood CM15
01277 848900

**Sean Wright GOsC**
⊕ 🅝 ⊘ 🗲
**Fees:** £26-35; Second visit: £21–30
Brentwood CM14
01277 224799

**Robin Woodleigh GOsC**
⊕ ⊕ ⊛ Ⓔ
Fees: £26–35; Second visit: £21–30
Buckhurst Hill IG9
020 8505 8353

**Francis Neil Bruce GOsC, BOA**
⊕ ⊕ ⊛ ❖
Fees: £26–35; Second visit: £31–40
Chelmsford CM17
01279 438444

**Tim Everett GOsC**
⊕ ⊛ ❖
Fees: <£25; Second visit: £21–30
Chelmsford CM2
01245 476677

**Anne Gibbons GOsC, BOA**
⊕ ⊕ ⊛ ⊘ Ⓔ ❖
Fees: £26-35; Second visit: £21–30
Chelmsford CM2
01245 283626

**Graham Hiscott GOsC, BOA**
⊕ O ⊛ ❖
Fees: <£25; Second visit: £21–30
Chelmsford CM3
01245 222804

**David Lindy GOsC, BOA**
O ⊕ ⊕ ⊛ ⊘ Ⓔ ❖
Fees: <£25; Second visit: £41–50
Chelmsford CM6
01371 872269

**Michael Maloney GOsC**
⊕ ⊛ ❖
Fees: <£25; Second visit: £21–30
Chelmsford CM2
01245 476677

**Gordon Service GOsC, BOA**
⊕ ⊛ ❖
Fees: <£25; Second visit: £21–30
Chelmsford CM3
01245 222804

**Robert Shanks GOsC, BOA**
⊕ O ⊛ ⊘ ❖
Fees: <£25; Second visit: £21–30
Chigwell IG7
020 8501 0937

**Lindsey Robinson GOsC, BOA**
⊕ ⊛ ❖
Fees: £26-35; Second visit: £21–30
Clacton-on-Sea CO15
01255 221651

**Colin Winer GOsC**
O ⊛ ⊘ ❖
Fees: <£25; Second visit: <£20
Clacton-on-Sea CO15
01255 421394

**Thorunn Bacon GOsC**
⊕ ⊕ ⊕ ⊛
Fees: £26-35; Second visit: £21–30
Coggeshall CO6
01376 562087

**Simon Bacon GOsC**
⊕ ⊛ ❖
Fees: £26-35; Second visit: £21–30
Colchester CO7
01206 825811

**Michael R Clarke GOsC**
⊕ ⊕ ⊛ ⊘ ❖
Fees: £26–35; Second visit: £21–30
Colchester CO2
01206 549325

**Karen Farrant GOsC, BOA**
⊕ ⊕ ⊛ ⊘ ❖
Fees: <£25; Second visit: £21–30
Colchester CO5
01206 385362

**Richard Kemp GOsC**
⊕ O ⊕ ⊛ ❖
Fees: £26-35; Second visit: £21–30
Colchester CD4P
01206 323427

**Michael Monk GOsC,**
O ⊛ ⊘ ❖
Fees: £46-55; Second visit: £31–40
Colchester CO6
01206 211370

**Susan Morrison GOsC, BOA**
O ⊘
Fees: <£25; Second visit: £21–30
Colchester CO7
01206 299027

# Osteopathy

**G J Sharp GOsC, BOA**
⊕ ⊕ ⦾ ⦿ ⦾ ⊘ Ⓔ ❈
Fees: £26–35; Second visit: £21–30
Colchester CO3
01206 769935

**Angus Hellier GOsC**
⊕ ⦿ ⦾ ⦿ ⊘ ❈
Fees: £26-35; Second visit: £21–30
Dunmow CM6
01371 875217

**Connie Mansueto GOsC**
⊕ ❈
Fees: £46-55; Second visit: £31–40
Epping CM16
01992 814620

**Kevin Roberts GOsC**
⦿ ⊘ ❈
Fees: £26-35; Second visit: £21–30
Epping CM16
01992 577606

**Peter Still GOsC, BOA**
⊕ ⦾ ⦿ ⊘ Ⓔ ❈
Fees: £26–35; Second visit: £21–30
Grays RM17
01375 396402

**Anita Watson GOsC**
⊕ ⦿ ⦿ ❈
Fees: £26–35; Second visit: £21–30
Grays RM16
01375 378608

**Lesley Kennedy GOsC**
⊕ ⊕ ⦾ ⦿ ❈
Fees: £26-35; Second visit: £21–30
Great Bentley CO7
01206 250890

**Jeremy Kenton GOsC, BOA**
⊕ ⊕ ⦿ ⊘ ❈
Fees: £46-55; Second visit: £21–30
Great Dunmow CM6
01371 876661

**Zoe Rumble GOsC**
⊕ ⦾ ❈
Fees: £36-45; Second visit: £21–30
Great Dunmow CM6
01371 875511

**Corina Breukel GOsC**
⊕ ⦿ Ⓔ ❈
Fees: £26-35; Second visit: £21–30
Halstead CO9
01787 476010

**Catherine Gawlinska GOsC**
⊕ ⦿ ⦿ ❈
Fees: £26-35; Second visit: £21–30
Harlow CM20
01279 410136

**Clive Kirby GOsC**
⊕ ⦾ ⦿ ❈
Fees: £26-35; Second visit: £21–30
Harlow CM17
07775 506807

**Keith Leeson GOsC, BOA**
⊕ ⦿ ⊕ ⦾ ⦿ ⊘ ❈
Fees: <£25; Second visit: £21–30
Hornchurch RM12
01708 472365

**Jonathan Shaw GOsC, BOA**
⊕ ⦾ ⦿ Ⓔ
Fees: £26–35; Second visit: £21–30
Loughton IG10
020 8508 7514

**Sara Mellor GOsC**
⊕ ⦿ ❈
Fees: £26-35; Second visit: £21–30
Maldon CM9
01621 856262

**Patrick Murphy GOsC**
⊕ ❈
Fees: <£25; Second visit: £21–30
Maldon CM9
01621 842750

**Wendy Saxby GOsC, BOA**
⊕ ⦿ ❈
Fees: £26-35; Second visit: £21–30
Maldon CM9
01621 852479

**Bill A J Wood GOsC, BOA**
⦿ ⦿ ❈
Fees: £36–45; Second visit: £21–30
Rayleigh SS6
01268 772212

**Richard C Holford GOsC, BOA**
✪ ⊛ ❖
**Fees:** <£25; Second visit: £21–30
Romford RM2
01708 740498

**Soraya Bish GOsC, BOA**
✪ ⊛ ❖
**Fees:** £26–35; Second visit: £21–30
Saffron Walden CB11
01799 524628

**Matthew Courtney-Jones GOsC**
✪ ⊛ ⊛ ⊘ ❖
**Fees:** £26–35; Second visit: £21–30
Saffron Walden CB11
01799 524628

**Anna Guthrie GOsC**
✪ ⊛ ⓔ ❖
**Fees:** £26–35; Second visit: £21–30
Southend-on-Sea SS7
01268 569639

**Anthony Larholt GOsC, BOA**
✪ ⊛ ⊛ ⊘ ❖
**Fees:** <£25; Second visit: £21–30
Southend-on-Sea SS1
01702 348221

**Silke Ukena-John GOsC, BOA**
○ ⊛ ⊘ ❖
**Fees:** £36–45; Second visit: £21–30
Southend-on-Sea SS7
01268 774249

**Matthew Voigts GOsC, BOA**
✪ ⊛ ❖
Southend-on-Sea SS1
01702 582485

**Daniel Moore GOsC**
✪ ⊛ ⊛ ❖
**Fees:** <£25; Second visit: £31–40
Stanford-le-Hope SS17
01375 361011

**Kim Tanner GOsC, BOA**
✪ ⊛ ⊛ ⊘ ❖
**Fees:** £26–35; Second visit: £21–30
Stanstead CM24
01279 815907

**Jacolin Sheaf GOsC, BOA**
✪ ⊛ ⊛ ⊘ ⓔ ❖
**Fees:** £26–35; Second visit: £21–30
Stansted CM24
01279 815907

**Bediz Akincioglu GOsC, BOA**
✪ ⊛ ⊘ ❖
**Fees:** £26–35; Second visit: <£20
Theydon Bois CM16
020 8591 2406

**Paul Masters GOsC**
✪ ❖
**Fees:** <£25; Second visit: <£20
Westcliff-on-Sea SS0
01702 346816

**Benjamin Calvert-Painter GOsC**
✪ ⊛ ⊘ ⓔ ❖
**Fees:** £26-35; Second visit: £21–30
Wickford SS11,Grays RM16
01268 477089

**Peter Jarvis GOsC**
✪ ⊛ ❖
**Fees:** £26–35; Second visit: £21–30
Witham CM8
01376 512188

**Justin Rata GOsC**
✪ ⊛ ❖
**Fees:** <£25; Second visit: £21–30
Witham CM8
01376 512188

## NORFOLK

**Kate Blanch GOsC**
✪ ⊕ ⊛ ⊛ ⊘
**Fees:** Second visit: £21–30
Attleborough NR17
01953 453166

**Anna Tonkin GOsC, BOA**
✪ ⊛ ⊛ ⓔ
**Fees:** £26–35; Second visit: £21–30
Diss IP22
01379 644407

**Isabel Latter GOsC, BOA**
✪ ⊛
**Fees:** <£25; Second visit: £21–30
Fakenham NR21
01328 856601

# Osteopathy

**Andrew Latter GOsC**
⊕ ⊕ ⊕ ⓃⒽⓈ ✿
**Fees:** <£25; Second visit: £21–30
Fakenham NR21
01328 856601

**Melvin A Jessup GOsC, BOA**
⊕ ⊕ ⓃⒽⓈ ✿
**Fees:** <£25; Second visit: £21–30
Great Yarmouth NR31
01493 443095

**Nicola Sturzaker GOsC**
⊕ ⓃⒽⓈ ✿
**Fees:** <£25; Second visit: £21–30
Great Yarmouth NR31
01493 414150

**Neil Fennel GOsC**
⊕ ⊕ ⓂⓌ Ⓔ ✿
**Fees:** <£25; Second visit: £21–30
King's Lynn PE30
01553 761484

**Averille Morgan GOsC**
Ⓞ ⓃⒽⓈ Ⓞ Ⓔ ✿
**Fees:** £26–35; Second visit: £21–30
King's Lynn PE31
01485 571559

**Caroline Bordoni GOsC**
Ⓞ ⓃⒽⓈ ✿
**Fees:** £26–35; Second visit: £21–30
Kings Lynn PE30
01553 769331

**Peggy Corney GOsC, BOA**
⊕ ⓃⒽⓈ Ⓞ
**Fees:** £36-45; Second visit: £21–30
Melton Constable NR24
01263 861184

**William Allchin GOsC, BOA**
⊕ ⓃⒽⓈ
**Fees:** <£25; Second visit: £41–50
Norwich NR3
07768 907756

**Anthony Ashford GOsC**
⊕ ⊕
**Fees:** £26–35; Second visit: £21–30
Norwich NR14
01508 570122

**Martin Booth GOsC**
⊕ ⊕ ⓃⒽⓈ ✿
**Fees:** <£25; Second visit: £21–30
Norwich NR3
01603 660792

**Charles Lim GOsC**
⊕ ⊕ ⓃⒽⓈ Ⓞ Ⓔ ✿
**Fees:** £26–35; Second visit: £21–30
Norwich NR1
01603 630226

**Cameron Reid GOsC**
⊕ ⊕ ⓃⒽⓈ Ⓞ ✿
**Fees:** <£25; Second visit: £21–30
Norwich NR19
01362 696079

**Helen Edwards GOsC**
⊕ Ⓞ ⓃⒽⓈ Ⓞ ✿
**Fees:** <£25
Thetford IP24
01892 750650

**Andrew Hamilton GOsC**
Ⓞ ⓃⒽⓈ Ⓞ ✿
**Fees:** <£25; Second visit: £21–30
Thetford IP24
01842 750650

---

**SUFFOLK**

**Miles James GOsC, BOA**
⊕ ⊕ ⓃⒽⓈ Ⓞ Ⓔ ✿
**Fees:** £26–35; Second visit: £21–30
Beccles NR34
01502 712505

**James S Miles GOsC, BOA**
⊕ ⊕ ⓃⒽⓈ ✿
**Fees:** <£25; Second visit: £21–30
Bungay NR35
01986 892846

**Jonathan Kettle GOsC, BOA**
⊕ ⓃⒽⓈ Ⓞ Ⓔ ✿
**Fees:** £26–35; Second visit: £21–30
Bury St Edmunds IP33
01284 769153

**Stephen Robinson GOsC, BOA**
Ⓞ ⓃⒽⓈ Ⓞ ✿
**Fees:** £26–35; Second visit: £21–30
Bury St Edmunds IP33
01284 760392

**Samantha Chapman GOsC, BOA**
Fees: <£25; Second visit: £21–30
Felixstowe IP11
01473 410708

**Tony Lutz GOsC**
Fees: £26–35; Second visit: £21–30
Halesworth IP19
01986 874618

**Owen Bull GOsC, BOA**
Fees: <£25; Second visit: £21–30
Ipswich IP4
01473 716340

**Beryl Churchman GOsC, BOA**
Fees: <£25; Second visit: £21–30
Ipswich IP1
01473 410708

**Adam Dallison GOsC**
Fees: £26–35; Second visit: £31–40
Ipswich IP1,New Malden KT3
01473 217592

**Andrew Gilmour GOsC, BOA**
Fees: £46–55; Second visit: £31–40
Ipswich IP1
01473 217592

**Amanda Green GOsC**
Fees: £26–35; Second visit: £31–40
Ipswich IP1
01473 217592

**John Steward GOsC, BOA**
Fees: £26–35; Second visit: £21–30
Ipswich IP1
01473 252378

**Stephen Francis Gold GOsC, BOA**
Fees: £26–35; Second visit: £21–30
Newmarket CB8
01638 667282

**Craig Cordiner GOsC**
Fees: £26–35; Second visit: £21–30
Stowmarket IP14
01449 613633

**Timothy Oxbrow GOsC, BOA**
Fees: £26–35; Second visit: £21–30
Stowmarket IP14
01449 613633

**Nicholas Salway GOsC**
Fees: £26–35; Second visit: £21–30
Stowmarket IP14
01449 613633

**Keith Brown GOsC**
Fees: £26–35; Second visit: £21–30
Sudbury CO10
01787 277523

**Phillip Tanswell GOsC, BOA**
Fees: £36–45; Second visit: £31–40
Sudbury CO10
01787 378320

**Jacky Wright GOsC, BOA**
Fees: <£25; Second visit: £21–30
Woodbridge IP12
01396 386540

# Chiropractic

## BEDFORDSHIRE

**Debbie Kibblewhite GCC, MCA**
O 🅝 ⊘
Fees: £36–45; Second visit: £21–30
Bedford MK40
01234 353273

**Eileen Naples GCC, BAAC, MCA**
O 🅝 ✤
Fees: £36–45; Second visit: £21–30
Leighton Buzzard LU7
01525 377384

**Graham Heale GCC, BCA**
⊕ 🅝 ⊘ Ⓔ ✤ 🅒
Fees: £36–45; Second visit: £21–30
Luton LU3
01582 579687

**Baiju A Khanchandanj GCC, BAAC**
⊕ ⊕ ⊕ 🅝
Fees: £36–45; Second visit: £21–30
Luton LU2
39 335 8428514

**Veronica Day GCC, MCA**
⊕ O 🅝 Ⓔ ✤
Fees: £36–45; Second visit: £21–30
Marston Moretaine MK43
01234 765174

## CAMBRIDGESHIRE

**Neil Broe GCC, BCA**
⊕ ⊕ 🅝 Ⓔ ✤
Fees: £26–35; Second visit: £21–30
Brampton PE28,
Peterborough PE8, Haverhill CB9
01480 436435

**Stuart White GCC, BCA**
⊕ ⊕ 🅝 ⊘ Ⓔ ✤
Fees: £36–45; Second visit: £21–30
Cambridge CB2
01223 355344

**Alison S J Edwards GCC, BCA**
⊕ ⊕ ⊕ 🅝 ⊘ Ⓔ ✤
Fees: £26–35; Second visit: £21–30
Huntingdon PE28
01480 417641

**Susan Kelley GCC, MCA**
O 🅝 ✤
Fees: £36–45; Second visit: £21–30
Peterborough PE28
01480 812179

**Kim Garnham GCC, BCA**
⊕ 🅝 ✤
Fees: £26–35; Second visit: £21–30
Peterborough PE1
01733 562638

**Charlotte Trip GCC, BCA**
⊕ 🅝 ⊘ ✤
Fees: £36–45; Second visit: £21–30
Peterborough PE1
01733 562638

**Victoria Emma Waller GCC, BCA**
⊕ ⊕ 🅝 ⊘
Fees: £36–45; Second visit: £21–30
Peterborough PE19
01480 473472

**Nicola Jennings GCC, MCA**
⊕ ⊕ 🅝 ✤
Fees: £36–45; Second visit: £21–30
Wisbech PE14, King's Lynn PE32
01945 880141

## ESSEX

**Sandokan Ayad GCC, BCA**
⊕ 🅝 ⊘ ✤
Fees: £36–45; Second visit: £21–30
Brentwood CM15, Ilford IG6,
London EC2M
01277 222221

**Suzanne Bober GCC, BCA**
⊕ 🅝 ⊘
Fees: <£25; Second visit: £21–30
Chelmsford CM1
01245 353078

**Brian Carter GCC, BCA**
⊕ O 🅝 ✤
Fees: £36–45; Second visit: £21–30
Chelmsford CM15
01277 222221

# Chiropractic

**Michele Hutchinson GCC, BCA**
Fees: <£25; Second visit: £21–30
Chelmsford CM7
01376 327474

**Ian Hutchinson GCC, BCA**
Fees: <£25; Second visit: £21–30
Braintree CM7
01376 327474

**David Owen MFHom**
Fees: <£25; Second visit: £21–30
Chelmsford CM1
01245 353078

**Robert Bateman GCC, BCA**
Fees: £26–35; Second visit: £21–30
Colchester CO2
01206 549809

**Ian Garrod GCC, BCA**
Fees: £26–35; Second visit: £21–30
Colchester CO2, Haverhill CB9
01206 549809

**Susan Goodwin GCC, BAAC**
Fees: £26–35; Second visit: <£20
Fordham CO6
01206 242534

**Sharon Lester GCC, BAAC**
Fees: £26–35; Second visit: £21–30
Harlow CM19
01279 838138

**Stuart Lawrence GCC, BCA**
Fees: <£25; Second visit: £21–30
Hockley SS5,Hockley SS5
01702 207017

**Pushka Deiana GCC, BCA**
Fees: £36–45; Second visit: £21–30
Ilford IG6
020 8500 1120

**Lyn Wilkinson GCC, BAAC, BCA**
Fees: £36–45; Second visit: £21–30
Illford GS1
020 8989 7707

**Joanne McCarey GCC, BCA**
Fees: £26–35; Second visit: £21–30
Saffron Walden CB11
07811 207142

**Lester Brayham GCC, BCA**
Fees: £26–35; Second visit: £21–30
Southend-on-Sea SS1
01702 342329

**Melanie Cutting GCC, BCA**
Fees: £26–35; Second visit: £21–30
Southend-on-Sea SS0
01702 430430

**Marcel Morelli GCC, BCA**
Fees: £26–35; Second visit: £21–30
Southend-on-Sea SS0
01702 430430

**Jennifer Stengler GCC, BCA**
Fees: £26–35; Second visit: £21–30
Southend-on-Sea SS1
01702 342329

**Rebecca Willard GCC, BCA**
Fees: £26–35; Second visit: £21–30
Southend-on-Sea SS11
01268 451663

**Mark Gurden GCC, BCA**
Fees: £36–45; Second visit: £21–30
Stansted CM24
01279 815336

**Frances Holt GCC, MCA**
Fees: £26–35; Second visit: £21–30
Thaxted CM6
01371 830433

# Chiropractic

**Arif O J Soomro GCC, BCA**
⊕ 🔵 ⊘ Ⓔ 🔵 🔵
**Fees:** £26–35; Second visit: £21–30
Westcliff-on-Sea SS0
01702 430430

## NORFOLK

**J A Rush GCC, BCA**
⊕ 🔵 ⊘ 🔵
**Fees:** £26–35; Second visit: £21–30
Diss IP22
01379 650020

**Sheila Lake GCC, MCA**
⊕ ⊕ 🔵 🔵
**Fees:** £36–45; Second visit: £21–30
King's Lynn PE32
01485 520123

**A J Norman GCC, BCA**
⊕ ⊕ 🔵 ⊘ Ⓔ 🔵 🔵
**Fees:** <£25; Second visit: £21–30
King's Lynn PE30
01553 772512

**Andrew Goddard GCC, BCA**
⊕ O 🔵 🔵
**Fees:** £26–35; Second visit: £21–30
Norwich NR7, Wymondham NR18
01603 414740

**Mark Owers GCC, MCA**
⊕ ⊕ 🔵 🔵
**Fees:** £26–35; Second visit: £21–30
Norwich NR2, Norwich NR11
01603 219264

## SUFFOLK

**Fiona M Jacobs GCC, BCA**
⊕ 🔵 ⊘ 🔵 🔵
**Fees:** £36–45; Second visit: £21–30
Ipswich IP33
01284 702155

**Rebecca Cowley GCC, MCA**
⊕ 🔵
**Fees:** £36–45; Second visit: £21–30
Ipswich IP13
01728 685960

**Peter J Miller GCC, BCA**
⊕ 🔵 Ⓔ 🔵 🔵
**Fees:** £26–35; Second visit: £21–30
Haverhill CB9, Colchester CO3,
Buntingford SG9
01440 705020

**Rachel Pick GCC, BCA**
⊕ 🔵 ⊘ 🔵 🔵
**Fees:** £26–35; Second visit: £21–30
Haverhill CB9
01440 705020

**Michael Bailey GCC, BCA**
⊕ ⊕ 🔵 🔵 🔵
**Fees:** £36–45; Second visit: £21–30
Ipswich IP22
01379 650020

**Kevin Correll GCC, BCA**
⊕ 🔵 Ⓔ 🔵 🔵
**Fees:** <£25; Second visit: <£20
Ipswich IP1
01473 463344

**Amada Hyde GCC, BCA**
⊕ 🔵 🔵
**Fees:** £26–35; Second visit: £21–30
Ipswich IP5
01473 624345

**Ray Martin GCC, BCA**
⊕ 🔵 ⊘ 🔵 🔵
**Fees:** £26–35; Second visit: £21–30
Ipswich IP5
01473 624345

**Paul Parolin GCC, BAAC**
⊕ ⊕ 🔵
**Fees:** £26–35; Second visit: £21–30
Ipswich IP12
01394 386079

**Richard Iveson GCC, BCA**
⊕ 🔵
**Fees:** £26–35; Second visit: £21–30
Newmarket CB8
01638 665858

**Anthony J Corrigan GCC, BCA**
⊕ 🔵 ⊘
**Fees:** £46–55; Second visit: £21–30
Sudbury CO10
01787 377300

## BEDFORDSHIRE

**J Cox MNIMH**
✦ ⊕ Ⓜ ⊘ ❋
**Fees:** £26–35; Second visit: £21–30
Ampthill MK45
01908 673933

**M Tassell MNIMH**
✦ ⊕ ⊕ ❋
Flitwick MK45
01525 712997

## CAMBRIDGESHIRE

**J Angus MNIMH**
O ⊕ ⊕ Ⓜ ❋
**Fees:** £26–35; Second visit: £21–30
Cambridge CB2
01223 315733

**A Davies MNIMH**
✦ O ⊕ Ⓜ ❋
**Fees:** £26–35; Second visit: <£20
Cambridge CB3
01223 264159

**Peter Jackson-Main AMH**
✦ Ⓜ ❋
**Fees:** £46–55; Second visit: £31–40
Cambridge CB1
01223 212744

**Vanessa Neville MNIMH**
✦ O ⊕ Ⓜ ❋
**Fees:** £26–35; Second visit: <£20
Cambridge CB11
07967 207326

**M Jilley MNIMH**
✦ ⊕ Ⓜ
**Fees:** £26–35; Second visit: <£20
Kings Lynn PE30
01485 540332

## ESSEX

**Katie Selves MNIMH**
✦ O ⊕ Ⓜ Ⓔ ❋
**Fees:** £26–35; Second visit: <£20
Braintree CM7, Saffron Walden CB10
,Halstead CO9
01376 339049

**Sherry Green MNIMH**
O Ⓜ ❋
**Fees:** <£25; Second visit: <£20
Essex CM3
01245 225928

**G Byde MNIMH**
O ❋
**Fees:** £26–35; Second visit: £21–30
Leigh-on-Sea SS9,Exeter EX4
01702 479578

## NORFOLK

**Julie Bruton-Seal AMH**
✦ O ⊕ Ⓜ ❋
**Fees:** £26–35; Second visit: £21–30
Norwich NR9
01603 507289

**Su Rayner AMH**
✦ O Ⓜ
**Fees:** £26–35; Second visit: <£20
Norwich NR15
01508 558135

**Jill Davies AMH**
✦
**Fees:** £26–35; Second visit: <£20
Pulham Market IP21
01379 608201

**Christine Herbert AMH**
✦ O ⊕ Ⓜ ❋
**Fees:** <£25; Second visit: <£20
Wymondham NR18
01953 603056

## SUFFOLK

**Joan M Atkinson AMH**
O Ⓜ ❋
Beccles NR34
01502 712779

**F Bevan MNIMH**
O Ⓜ
**Fees:** <£25; Second visit: <£20
Elmswell IP30
01359 241885

# Western Herbal Medicine

**Tobias Halbinger MNIMH**
**O**
Fees: £36–45; Second visit: £21–30
Ipswich IP27
01842 861124

**C J Wheeler MNIMH**
**⊕  ⊕  ✿**
Fees: £26–35; Second visit: <£20
Ipswich IP4
01473 788193

**Dorothy M Kitching AMH**
**⊕  O  ⊕  ⓦ**
Fees: £26–35; Second visit: <£20
Saxmundham IP17
01728 668633

**M Wade MNIMH**
**⊕  O  ⓔ  ✿**
Fees: £26–35; Second visit: <£20
Saxmundham IP17
01728 638504

**Nigel Wynn MNIMH**
**⊕  ⊕  ⓦ  ⓔ  ✿**
Fees: £26–35; Second visit: <£20
Woodbridge IP12,Colchester CO1
01394 380580

# Chinese Herbal Medicine

## BEDFORDSHIRE

**Jacqueline Arnold RCHM**
**O  ⊕**
Fees: <£25; Second visit: <£20
Stevenage SG5
01462 623533

## CAMBRIDGESHIRE

**Mark E Corcoran RCHM**
**⊕  O  ⊕  ⊕  ⓦ  ⊘  ✿**
Fees: <£25; Second visit: £21–30
Peterborough PE1
01733 315757

**Junsheng Wang RCHM**
**⊕  ⓦ  ✿**
Fees: £36–45; Second visit: £21–30
Peterborough PE1
01733 555899

## ESSEX

**S Koten MNIMH, RCHM**
**O  ✿**
Fees: £26–35; Second visit: £21–30
Upminster RM14
01708 223524

**Gillian Kelly RCHM**
**⊕  ⊕  ✿**
Fees: £36–45; Second visit: £21–30
Brentwood CM15
01277 260080

**Hong Van Trinh RCHM**
**⊕  O  ✿**
Fees: £36–45; Second visit: £21–30
Chelmsford CM1, Billericay CM12,
London SW3
01242 57085

**Jennifer Linstead RCHM**
**⊕  O  ⊕**
Fees: £26–35; Second visit: <£20
Clacton-on-Sea CO15
01255 221651

**Lei Zhou An RCHM**
**⊕  ⊕**
Fees: £36–45; Second visit: £41–50
Colchester CO1, London WC2H
01206 871122

**Robert Van't Hof RCHM**
**O  ⓦ  ⊘  ✿**
Fees: £26–35; Second visit: £21–30
Leigh-on-Sea SS9
01702 477588

**Anna Yang RCHM**
✛ ✿
Fees: £26–35; Second visit: £21–30
Leigh-on-Sea SS9
01702 482178

**Anh Nga Phan RCHM**
✛ ⬡
Fees: £26–35; Second visit: £21–30
Southend-on-Sea SS1,London
NW8,Loughton IG10
01702 390305

### NORFOLK

**Emma Farrant RCHM**
✛ ⬡ ⬤ ✿
Fees: £26–35; Second visit: <£20
Norwich NR2,London EC2A
01603 616126

**Timothy Gee RCHM**
O ✿
Fees: <£25; Second visit: <£20
Norwich NR7
01603 413272

**Naji Malak BAcC**
✛ ⬡ ✿
Fees: £26–35
Norwich NR2
01603 666546

# London

East London
East Central London
North London
North West London
South East London
South West London
West London
West Central London

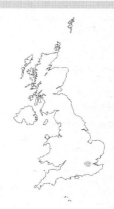

## Acupuncture

### LONDON (E)

**Maggie Bavington BAcC**
⊕ O ⊕ ⊕ ⊘ ❀ ⊕
Fees: £36–45; Second visit: £21–30
London (E) E17
020 8520 3315

**Alison Courtney BAcC**
⊕ ⊕ Ⓔ ❀ ⊕
Fees: £26–35; Second visit: £21–30
London (E) E8,London EC4
07790 264515

**Ollie Djurdjevic BAcC**
O ⊕ ⊕ ⊘ ❀ ⊕
Fees: £36–45; Second visit: £41–50
London (E) E2
020 8533 4745

**Victor N Foster BAcC**
⊕ ⊕ ⊕
Fees: £26–35; Second visit: £21–30
London (E) E17
020 8531 7188

**Josephine M Haworth BAcC**
⊕ O ⊕ ❀ ⊕
Fees: £26–35; Second visit: £21–30
London (E) E12
020 8989 7142

**Pippa Howell BAcC**
⊕ O ⊕ ❀ ⊕
Fees: £26–35; Second visit: £21–30
London (E) E17
020 8520 5268

**Sue Johnson BAcC**
O ⊕ ⊕ ❀ ⊕
Fees: £26–35; Second visit: £21–30
London (E) E5
020 8985 9326

**Steven Lindall BMAS,**
⊕ ⊘ ⊕
Fees: <£25; Second visit: £21–30
London (E) E17
020 8527 2563

**Robert Moore BAcC**
⊕ ⊕ ❀ ⊕
Fees: £36–45; Second visit: £31–40
London (E) E2
020 89816938

**Jagdish Pahwa BAcC, AACP**
⊕ ⊕ ⊕ ⊘ ❀ ⊕
Fees: £26–35; Second visit: £21–30
London (E) E7
020 8472 0170

# Acupuncture

**Peter Resteghini AACP**
⊕ ⊕ Ⓜ ⊘ ❀ ⊛
Fees: £36–45; Second visit: £31–40
London (E) E9
020 8510 7048

**Michael Theocharous BAcC**
⊕ Ⓞ ⊕ ⊘ ❀ ⊛
Fees: <£25; Second visit: £21–30
London (E) E4
020 8529 0815

**Mark Tittle BAcC**
⊕ ⊕ ⊕ ⊘ ❀ ⊛
Fees: £26–35; Second visit: £21–30
London (E) E18
020 8989 6848

**Snow Ruixue Wang BAcC**
Ⓞ ⊕ ⊛
Fees: £26–35; Second visit: £21–30
London (E) E14
020 7537 7165

## LONDON (EC)

**Ann Bradford BAcC**
⊕ ⊕ ⊘ ⊛
Fees: £36–45; Second visit: £31–40
London (EC) EC2
020 7729 8525

**Sarah Brawn BAcC**
⊕ Ⓞ ⊕ ❀ ⊛
Fees: £36–45; Second visit: £31–40
London (EC) EC1
020 7729 1912

**Louise Cole BAcC**
⊕ Ⓞ ⊕ ❀ ⊛
Fees: £26–35; Second visit: £21–30
London (EC) EC1
07989 950462

**Julie Gear AACP**
⊕ Ⓞ ⊛
Fees: £26–35; Second visit: £21–30
London (EC) EC4
020 7283 0108

**Huw Griffiths BAcC**
⊕ ⊕ ❀ ⊛
Fees: £36–45; Second visit: £41–50
London (EC) EC1
020 7336 0466

**Nicholas Masters RCHM**
⊕ ⊕ ⊕ Ⓜ ❀ ⊛
Fees: £36–45; Second visit: £31–40
London (EC) EC1
020 8981 4618

**Diane Wheatley BAcC**
⊕ ⊕ Ⓜ ❀ ⊛
Fees: >£55; Second visit: £31–40
London (EC) EC2
020 7628 3359

**Jane Wilson BAcC, AACP**
⊕ Ⓒ ❀ ⊛
Fees: £36–45; Second visit: £31–40
London (EC) EC2
020 7426 5129

## LONDON (N)

**Ghila Rodrik Bali BAcC**
Ⓞ ⊕ ⊘ ❀ ⊛
Fees: £26–35; Second visit: £31–40
London (N) N2
07767 272555

**P A Bartlett BAcC**
⊕ ⊕ ⊕ ⊘ ❀ ⊛
Fees: £26–35; Second visit: <£20
London (N) N5
020 7359 2609

**Karen Benson BMAS,**
⊕ ⊛
Fees: £26–35; Second visit: £31–40
London (N) N8
020 8340 7736

**David Berg BAcC**
⊕ Ⓞ ⊕ ❀ ⊛
Fees: £36–45; Second visit: £31–40
London (N) N16
020 7249 2990

**Andrew Carrington BAcC**
⊕ ⊕ ⊘ ❀ ⊛
Fees: £26–35; Second visit: £21–30
London (N) N20
020 8445 2660

**James Cattermole BAcC**
⊕ ⊕ ❀ ⊛
Fees: £26–35
London (N) N1
020 7354 8883

**Elizabeth Chang BAcC**
⊕ ⊕ ❄ ⊜
Fees: £26–35; Second visit: £21–30
London (N) N14
020 8886 5391

**Nadine Compernolle BAcC**
⊕ ⊕ ❄ ⊜
Fees: £26–35; Second visit: £31–40
London (N) N7
020 7281 1412

**Jo George BAcC**
⊕ ⊕ ❄ ⊜
Fees: £36–45; Second visit: £31–40
London (N) N6,London N6,
Muswell Hill N11
020 8348 5553

**Catherine Godley BAcC**
O ⊘ ❄ ⊜
Fees: £46–55; Second visit: £31–40
London (N) N12
020 8445 9057

**Shai Golan BAcC**
⊕ O ⊕ ⊕ ❄ ⊜
Fees: £36–45; Second visit: £31–40
London (N) N11
020 8361 5522

**Linda Gunn-Russell BAcC**
O ❄ ⊜
Fees: £36–45; Second visit: £31–40
London (N) N8
020 8348 1691

**Zadi Hasan BAcC**
⊕ ⊕ ⊕ ❄ ⊜
Fees: £46–55; Second visit: £31–40
London (N) N5
07939 247627

**Maeve Heavey BAcC**
⊕ ⊕ ⊕ ❄ ⊜
Fees: £36–45; Second visit: £31–40
London (N) N10,London N10,Waltham
Cross EN8
020 8808 0134

**Inga Heese BAcC**
⊕ ⊕ ❄ ⊜
Fees: £26–35; Second visit: £21–30
London (N) N21
020 8360 3485

**Christina Isaac BAcC**
⊕ O ⊜
Fees: £26–35; Second visit: £31–40
London (N) N11
020 8368 7926

**Oran Kivity BAcC**
⊕ O ⊕ ❄ ⊜
Fees: £36–45; Second visit: £31–40
London (N) N10
020 8365 3545

**Caroline Kunzler AACP**
⊕ ⊕ ⊜
Fees: £26–35; Second visit: £31–40
London (N) N14
020 8440 3629

**Poh Gek Lim BAcC**
O ⊕ Ⓔ ❄ ⊜
Fees: £26–35; Second visit: £21–30
London (N) N8, London N22
020 8881 9494

**K H Liu BAcC**
O ⊜
Fees: <£25
London (N) N8
020 8340 9625

**Stephen Lock BAcC**
O ❄ ⊜
Fees: £36–45; Second visit: £31–40
London (N) N19
020 7281 2324

**Wendy Longworth AACP, BAcC**
O ⊘ ⊜
Fees: £26–35; Second visit: £21–30
London (N) N2
020 8883 5888

**David Lurie BAcC**
⊕ ⊕ ⊘ ❄ ⊜
Fees: £46–55; Second visit: £31–40
London (N) N19
020 7281 5869

**Angela Mansfield BAcC**
O ❄ ⊜
Fees: £26–35; Second visit: £21–30
London (N) N16
020 8806 3018

# Acupuncture

**Daniel Maxwell BAcC**
⊕ ⊕ ⊕ ⊕ ⊘ ✿ ⊕
**Fees:** £36–45; Second visit: £21–30
London (N) N8
07946 390212

**Christina McCausland BAcC**
⊕ O ⊕ ⊕ ✿ ⊕
**Fees:** £36–45; Second visit: £31–40
London (N) N16
020 7249 2768

**Jan McCorquodale BAcC**
⊕ ⊕ ✿ ⊕
**Fees:** £36–45; Second visit: £31–40
London (N) N19
020 7687 1125

**Cinzia Scorzon BAcC**
⊕ O ⊕ ⊕ ⊘ ✿ ⊕
**Fees:** £46–55; Second visit: £31–40
London (N) N1,London EC1V
020 7935 7848

**Sara Mokone BAcC, AACP**
⊕ ⊕ ✿ ⊕
**Fees:** £36–45; Second visit: £31–40
London (N) N15
020 8809 1626

**Samir Mostafa BAcC**
O ⊕ ✿ ⊕
**Fees:** £36–45
London (N) N3
07901 590197

**David Nesbitt AACP**
⊕ ⊕ ✿ ⊕
**Fees:** £26–35; Second visit: £21–30
London (N) N20
020 8361 8681

**Gillian Price BAcC**
⊕ O ⊕ ✿ ⊕
**Fees:** £36–45; Second visit: £31–40
London (N) N16
020 7249 2990

**Nama Ryu BAcC**
⊕ ⊕ ✿ ⊕
**Fees:** £26–35; Second visit: £21–30
London (N) N19
020 7272 6888

**Aki Sasaki BAcC**
⊕ O ⊕ ⊕ ✿ ⊕
**Fees:** £26–35; Second visit: £21–30
London (N) N12
07958 280994

**Jinal Shah BAcC**
⊕ ⊕ ⊕ ✿ ⊕
**Fees:** £26–35; Second visit: £21–30
London (N) N14
020 8368 3150

**Dilip Shah BMAS,**
⊘ ✿ ⊕
**Fees:** <£25; Second visit: <£20
London (N) N14
020 88864035

**Yana Stajno BAcC**
⊕ ⊕ ✿ ⊕
**Fees:** £46–55; Second visit: £31–40
London (N) N19
020 7281 5869

**Bianca Stroll BAcC**
⊕ O ⊕ ⊕ ✿ ⊕
**Fees:** £36–45; Second visit: £31–40
London (N) N19,London W8,London N8
020 7263 6737

**Okamoto Takeshi BAcC**
O ✿ ⊕
**Fees:** £26–35; Second visit: £31–40
London (N) N12
020 8446 2877

**Martin P S Underwood BAcC**
O ⊘ ✿ ⊕
**Fees:** £36–45; Second visit: £31–40
London (N) N19
020 7607 5265

**Trina Ward BAcC**
⊕ ⊕ ⊕ © ✿ ⊕
**Fees:** £26–35; Second visit: £31–40
London (N) N5,London NW5
020 7226 1143

# Acupuncture

## LONDON (NW)

**Silvio Andrade BAcC**
Fees: £46–55; Second visit: £31–40
London (NW) NW1
07957 325399

**Helen Barnett BAcC**
Fees: £26–35; Second visit: £21–30
London (NW) NW5
020 7485 6477

**Phillip Beach BAcC**
Fees: £36–45; Second visit: £31–40
London (NW) NW3
020 7794 1140

**Shelagh Brady BAcC**
Fees: £26–35; Second visit: £21–30
London (NW) NW6
0207 3723215

**Simon Canney BAcC**
Fees: £36–45; Second visit: £31–40
London (NW) NW3
020 7482 0443

**Tamar Dhiri BAcC**
Fees: >£55; Second visit: >£50
London (NW) NW8
0766 903 6286

**Gloria Else BAcC**
Fees: £36–45; Second visit: £31–40
London (NW) NW3
07968 282142

**Marian Fixler BAcC**
Fees: £36–45; Second visit: £31–40
London (NW) NW6
020 7419 1211

**Joseph Goodman BAcC**
Fees: £46–55; Second visit: £41–50
London (NW) NW4
020 8202 6242

**Alan J Grant BMAS,**
Fees: £26–35; Second visit: £21–30
London (NW) NW11,Enfield EN2
020 8351 0790

**Gideon Hajioff BAcC**
Fees: £36–45; Second visit: £31–40
London (NW) NW4
07958 282123

**Ruth Hajioff BAcC**
Fees: £46–55; Second visit: £31–40
London (NW) NW3
020 8731 7030

**C Hector BAcC**
Fees: £26–35; Second visit: £21–30
London (NW) NW6
020 8960 1801

**Barbara Hezelgrave BAcC**
Fees: £46–55; Second visit: £31–40
London (NW) NW3
020 7485 8150

**Stephen Kriss BAcC**
Fees: £26–35; Second visit: £31–40
London (NW) NW11
01923 858162

**Ana Maria Lavin-Parot BAcC**
Fees: >£55; Second visit: £41–50
London (NW) NW8
020 7722 3939

**Anne Lewthwaite BAcC**
Fees: >£55; Second visit: £31–40
London (NW) NW3
020 7267 9995

**Kezheng Liang BAcC**
Fees: £26–35; Second visit: £21–30
London (NW) NW1
020 7383 4575

# Acupuncture

**Neil Munro BAcC**
⊕ ⊕ ✿ ⊛
**Fees:** £26–35; Second visit: £21–30
London (N) NW2
020 7281 8585

**Solveig Nielsen-Brown BAcC**
O ⊕ ✿ ⊛
**Fees:** £46–55; Second visit: £31–40
London (NW) NW8
020 7722 3939

**Janine Norris BAcC**
⊕ ✿ ⊛
**Fees:** £36–45; Second visit: £31–40
London (NW) NW3
020 7483 3568

**Helen Robertson BAcC**
⊕ ⊕ ✿ ⊛
**Fees:** £36–45; Second visit: £31–40
London (NW) NW3
020 7483 2345

**Eve Rogans BAcC**
O ⊕ ⊛
**Fees:** £26–35; Second visit: £21–30
London (NW) NW5
020 7813 8708

**Nguyen Tinh Thong BAcC**
⊕ ⊕ ⊕ ⓦ Ⓔ ⊛
**Fees:** >£55
London (NW) NW8
020 7586 6543

**Clare Walter BAcC**
✿ ⊛
**Fees:** £36–45; Second visit: £31–40
London (NW) NW6
020 8459 2188

**Judi Wilson BAcC**
✿ ⊛
**Fees:** £36–45; Second visit: £21–30
London (NW) NW6
020 7402 8746

**Robert W Zagar BAcC**
⊕ ⊘ ✿ ⊛
**Fees:** £36–45; Second visit: £31–40
London (NW) NW5
020 7482 3293

## LONDON (SE)

**Sylvia Beattie BAcC**
⊕ ⊕ ⓦ ⊛
**Fees:** >£55; Second visit: £31–40
London (SE) SE1
020 7928 8333

**Lydia Coles BAcC**
⊕ ⓦ ✿ ⊛
**Fees:** >£55; Second visit: £31–40
London (SE) SE1
020 8980 3819

**Giles Davies BAcC**
⊕ O ⊕ ✿ ⊛
**Fees:** £36–45; Second visit: £21–30
London (SE) SE22
020 8516 0769

**Jennifer Hobbs BAcC**
⊕ ⊕ ✿
**Fees:** £36–45; Second visit: £31–40
London (SE) SE1
07761 902907

**Charles John BAcC**
✿ ⊛
**Fees:** £46–55
London (SE) SE23
020 8291 7457

**Anastasios Lambridis AACP**
⊕ ⊕ ⊘ ⊛
**Fees:** £36–45; Second visit: £21–30
London (SE) SE1
020 7328 7314

**Mary Lenihan BAcC**
⊕ ⊕ ⓦ ✿ ⊛
**Fees:** £36–45; Second visit: £21–30
London (SE) SE22
020 8299 2152

**Elizabeth McAulay BAcC**
⊕ ⊕ ⓦ ✿ ⊛
**Fees:** £36–45; Second visit: £31–40
London (SE) SE18
020 8854 8787

**Gail Newton BAcC**
⊕ O ⊕ ✿ ⊛
**Fees:** £36–45; Second visit: £31–40
London (SE) SE25
07889 485915

**Fionnula Orrom BAcC**
O ⊕ ✿ ⊕
Fees: £46–55; Second visit: £31–40
London (SE) SE14,London NW1
020 7652 2572

**Fatma Ozerk BAcC**
⊕ ⊕ ⊕
Fees: £46–55; Second visit: £31–40
London (SE) SE5
020 7346 3572

**Malcolm Reeve BAcC**
⊕ ⊕ ⊕ ⊕ ✿ ⊕
Fees: £36–45; Second visit: £31–40
London (SE) SE3
020 8692 0628

**Richard Royds BAcC**
⊕ ⊕ € ✿ ⊕
Fees: >£55
London (SE) SE1
020 7928 8333

**Aruna Sahni BAcC**
⊕ ⊕ € ✿ ⊕
London (SE) SE1
020 7928 8333

**Clarence D Thenuwara BAcC, BMAS,**
O ⊘ ✿ ⊕
Fees: £26–35; Second visit: £21–30
London (SE) SE9
020 8859 7941

**Lorna Withers BAcC**
⊕ O ⊕ ✿ ⊕
Fees: £36–45; Second visit: £21–30
London (SE) SE23
020 8291 1713

**Christopher Woodward BAcC**
⊕ ⊕ ⊕ ✿ ⊕
Fees: >£55; Second visit: £41–50
London (SE) SE1
0207 9288333

**Anthony Yardley-Jones BMAS,**
⊕ O ⊕ ⊘ ⊕
Fees: £26–35; Second visit: £21–30
London (SE) SE1
020 7407 3100

## LONDON (SW)

**Ala Al Hussaini BMAS**
⊕ ⊕ ⊕ ⊘ ✿ ⊕
Fees: £26–35; Second visit: £21–30
London (SW) SW5
020 7460 8915

**Martin J Barry BAcC**
⊕ ⊕ ✿
Fees: £36–45; Second visit: £31–40
London (SW) SW18
020 8875 1101

**Barbara Barrymore BAcC**
⊕ ⊕ ✿ ⊕
Fees: >£55; Second visit: £31–40
London (SW) SW7
020 7835 0400

**James Bentley BAcC**
⊕ ✿ ⊕
Fees: <£25; Second visit: £21–30
London (SW) SW7
07989 973121

**Balbir S Bhogal BAcC**
⊕ O ⊕ ⊘ ✿ ⊕
Fees: £26–35; Second visit: £31–40
London (SW) SW4
020 7627 8890

**Ronald Bishop BAcC**
⊕ ⊕ ⊘
Fees: £36–45; Second visit: £31–40
London (SW) SW1
020 7834 6229

**Dolores Lola Boix BAcC**
⊕ O ⊕ ⊕ ⊕ € ✿ ⊕
Fees: £26–35; Second visit: £31–40
London (SW) SW, London SE22,
London SW9
020 7326 4568

**Karen Byrne BAcC**
⊕ O ⊕ ⊕ ⊕
Fees: >£55; Second visit: >£50
London (SW) SW7
020 7589 6414

**Amadis Cammell BAcC**
⊕ ⊕ ⊕ ⊕ ⊘ ✿ ⊕
Fees: £26–35; Second visit: £31–40
London (SW) SW17
020 8671 4224

# Acupuncture

**Emma Cannon BAcC**
⊕ ⊕ ⊕ ⊕ ⊘ ⊕
Fees: £36–45; Second visit: £31–40
London (SW) SW18
020 88771877

**Bridget A Cassey BAcC**
O ✿ ⊕
Fees: £36–45; Second visit: £31–40
London (SW) SW11
020 7738 9149

**Cecil Chen BAcC**
⊕ ⊘ ⊕
Fees: £46–55; Second visit: £31–40
London (SW) SW1
020 7834 1012

**Craig Coman BAcC**
⊕ ⊕ ✿ ⊕
Fees: £26–35; Second visit: £21–30
London (SW) SW10
020 7352 3074

**Philip J Davies BAcC**
⊕ ⊕ ⊕ ✿ ⊕
Fees: >£55; Second visit: £41–50
London (SW) SW1
07956 665933

**Julia Davis BAcC**
O ✿ ⊕
Fees: £46–55; Second visit: £31–40
London (SW) SW17
020 86720455

**Roisin Golding BAcC**
⊕ O ⊕ ⊘ ✿ ⊕
Fees: £46–55; Second visit: £31–40
London (SW) SW1
020 7978 8009

**Robert Graham BAcC**
O ✿ ⊕
Fees: £26–35; Second visit: £21–30
London (SW) SW19
020 8946 5424

**Mina Haeri BAcC**
⊕ ⊕ ⊕
Fees: >£55; Second visit: £31–40
London (SW) SW11
020 7228 0309

**N A Hamami BMAS,**
⊕ ⊕ ⊕ ⊘ ✿ ⊕
Fees: £26–35; Second visit: £21–30
London (SW) SW5,London W6
020 7460 2000

**Nick Johnson BAcC**
⊕ ⊕ ⊕ ⊘ ✿ ⊕
Fees: £26–35; Second visit: £31–40
London (SW) SW4
020 7720 8817

**Anna Kiff BAcC**
⊕ ⊕ ⊕
Fees: £26–35; Second visit: £31–40
London (SW) SW4
020 7627 8890

**Tabitha Anne Laksimi BAcC**
⊕ ⊕ ✿ ⊕
Fees: £36–45; Second visit: £31–40
London (SW) SW2
020 8674 3850

**Angela Lapadula BAcC**
⊕ O ⊕ ✿ ⊕
Fees: £36–45; Second visit: £21–30
London (SW) SW4
020 7622 9079

**Christopher Latter BAcC**
O ⊘ ✿ ⊕
Fees: >£55; Second visit: >£50
London (SW) SW8
020 7735 6325

**Tom Lawrence BAcC**
⊕ O ⊕ ✿ ⊕
Fees: £36–45; Second visit: £31–40
London (SW) SW11
07887 682291

**Mark Leopold BAcC**
⊕ ⊕ ⊕ ✿ ⊕
Fees: £26–35; Second visit: £31–40
London (SW) SW15
020 8789 5848

**Siop Lim-Cooper BAcC**
O ⊕ ⊕ ⊕ ✿ ⊕
Fees: £26–35
London (SW) SW15
020 8789 2548

**Alex Maas BAcC**
Fees: £36–45; Second visit: £21–30
London (SW) SW1
020 7730 9977

**Vicky Maljanovska BAcC**
Fees: £36–45; Second visit: £31–40
London (SW) SW13
07957 210971

**Yvette Masure BAcC**
Fees: >£55; Second visit: £41–50
London (SW) SW1
020 7730 9977

**Anne Mather BAcC**
Fees: £36–45; Second visit: £21–30
London (SW) SW18
020 8874 5810

**Victoria Neill AACP**
Fees: £26–35
London (SW) SW18
020 8874 2895

**Jonathan Orchard BAcC**
Fees: £26–35; Second visit: £21–30
London (SW) SW20
020 8946 2331

**Purnima Patel BAcC**
Fees: <£25; Second visit: £21–30
London (SW) SW16
020 8679 4081

**Pom Pearson-Enz BAcC**
Fees: >£55; Second visit: £41–50
London (SW) SW1
020 7798 8685

**James Pinkney BAcC, AACP**
Fees: £36–45; Second visit: £31–40
London (SW) SW4
020 8673 6820

**John Pudduck BAcC**
Fees: £26–35; Second visit: £21–30
London (SW) SW16,Wells BA5,East
Grinstead RH19
020 8769 7409

**Fiona Ratti BAcC**
Fees: £36–45; Second visit: £31–40
London (SW) SW11
020 7350 1600

**Sally J Roberts AACP**
Fees: £26–35; Second visit: £31–40
London (SW) SW17
020 8682 1800

**Sylvia Schroer BAcC**
Fees: >£55; Second visit: £41–50
London (SW) SW1
020 7590 8000

**Lesley Spencer BAcC**
Fees: £26–35
London (SW) SW6
020 7736 7813

**Adrian Stoddart BAcC**
Fees: £36–45; Second visit: £31–40
London (SW) SW18
020 8874 4125

**Daniel Tapsell BAcC**
Fees: £26–35; Second visit: £31–40
London (SW) SW1
020 8981 4006

**Geoffrey Van Klaveren AACP**
Fees: £26–35; Second visit: £31–40
London (SW) SW19
020 8879 3608

**Penelope Wall BAcC**
Fees: £36–45; Second visit: £31–40
London (SW) SW9
020 7274 9252

# Acupuncture

**Elizabeth S Ward BAcC,**
O ⊕
**Fees:** £36–45; Second visit: £31–40
London (SW) SW18
020 8874 4938

**Petra Werth BAcC**
O ✿ ⊕
**Fees:** £36–45; Second visit: £31–40
London (SW) SW19
020 8540 6062

## LONDON (W)

**Keith J Ashton BAcC**
⊕ O ⊕ ⊕ ✿ ⊕
**Fees:** >£55; Second visit: £41–50
London (W) W1
020 8348 7151

**Yogini Rawal BAcC**
⊕ ✿ ⊕
**Fees:** £26–35; Second visit: £21–30
London (W) W1
07931 884682

**Rebecca Avern BAcC**
⊕ ⊕ ✿ ⊕
**Fees:** >£55; Second visit: £41–50
London (W) W1
020 7731 5329

**Aliza Baron-Cohen BAcC**
⊕ ⊕ NHS ✿ ⊕
**Fees:** £26–35; Second visit: £21–30
London (W) W10
020 8969 3331

**Simon Berkowitz BAcC**
⊕ O ⊕ ✿ ⊕
**Fees:** £36–45; Second visit: £31–40
London (W) W11
020 7727 4544

**Bai-Shu Bian BAcC, BMAS**
⊕ ✿ ⊕
**Fees:** £26–35; Second visit: £21–30
London (W) W2
020 7792 8626

**Kim Chan BAcC**
⊕ ⊕ ✿ ⊕
**Fees:** £36–45; Second visit: £31–40
London (W) W5
020 8847 4887

**Ross Chellew BAcC**
⊕ ⊕ Ⓔ ✿ ⊕
**Fees:** £26–35; Second visit: £21–30
London (W) W10
020 8969 3331

**Stefan Chmelik BAcC**
⊕ O ⊕ ✿ ⊕
**Fees:** >£55; Second visit: £31–40
London (W) W8
020 7221 4602

**Sarah Collison BAcC**
⊕ ⊕ ✿ ⊕
**Fees:** £46–55; Second visit: £31–40
London (W) W10
020 8960 0846

**Linda Coviello BAcC**
O ✿
London (W) W7
020 8566 4478

**Abid Dar BAcC**
⊕ ⊕ ✿ ⊕
**Fees:** £36–45; Second visit: £31–40
London (W) W4
020 8742 7701

**Cheryll Davies BAcC**
O ⊕
**Fees:** £36–45; Second visit: £31–40
London (W) W8
020 7937 4968

**Arnold Desser BAcC**
⊕ ⊕ NHS ⊘ ⊕
**Fees:** £46–55; Second visit: £41–50
London (W) W1
020 7383 4410

**Selwyn Dexter BMAS,**
⊕ ⊕ ⊘ ✿ ⊕
**Fees:** £26–35; Second visit: £21–30
London (W) W9
020 7624 2504

**Guru Dharam Khalsa BAcC**
⊕ ⊕ NHS ✿ ⊕
**Fees:** >£55; Second visit: £41–50
London (W) W1
07958 928252

### Suzanne G Harper BAcC
Fees: £46–55; Second visit: £41–50
London (W) W1
020 7224 3387

### Susan Horrocks BAcC
Fees: £26–35; Second visit: £31–40
London (W) W1
020 7935 7585

### Virginie Host AACP
Fees: £36–45; Second visit: £31–40
London (W) W1
020 7405 1996

### Mark Kane BAcC
Fees: >£55; Second visit: >£50
London (W) W1
020 7486 9588

### Song Ke BAcC
Fees: £46–55; Second visit: £31–40
London (W) W1
020 7467 8300

### Steve Kippax BAcC
Fees: >£55; Second visit: £31–40
London (W) W1
020 7439 7332

### Dve N Ledermann BMAS,
Fees: £26–35; Second visit: £21–30
London (W) W1
020 7935 8774

### Patrick Magovern BMAS,
Fees: £46–55; Second visit: £31–40
London (W) W1
020 7486 1096

### Naji Malak BAcC
Fees: £36–45; Second visit: £31–40
London (W) W13
020 7734 6263

### Bryan Melville BAcC
Fees: £36–45; Second visit: £31–40
London (W) W10
020 7602 4330

### Uberlinda Munoz BAcC
Fees: £36–45; Second visit: £31–40
London (W) W11
020 8208 1309

### R Newman Turner GOsC, BOA
Fees: >£55; Second visit: £41–50
London (W) W1,Letchworth SG6
020 7436 1446

### Samara Reid BAcC
Fees: £46–55; Second visit: £41–50
London (W) W1
0207 6310156

### Erica Salisbury BAcC, AACP
Fees: £46–55; Second visit: £31–40
London (W) W1
020 7262 1490

### Stella Simpson BAcC
Fees: £36–45; Second visit: £31–40
London (W) W6
07973 684908

### Georgina Stourton BAcC
Fees: £26–35; Second visit: £21–30
London (W) W6
07970 499292

### Anna Szabolcsi BMAS,
Fees: £46–55; Second visit: £31–40
London (W) W1
020 7935 9795

### Virginia Tacey BAcC
Fees: £26–35; Second visit: £21–30
London (W) W11
020 8640 3301

# Acupuncture

### Garry Trainer BAcC
⊕ O ✿
**Fees:** >£55; Second visit: £41–50
London (W) W1
020 7224 1750

### A Treharne BAcC
⊕ O ⊕ ✿ ⊕
**Fees:** >£55; Second visit: >£50
London (W) W1G
020 7935 7835

### Rose Uniacke BAcC
O ⊘ ✿ ⊕
**Fees:** £36–45; Second visit: £31–40
London (W) W4
020 8994 2098

### Rosario Varela BAcC
O ✿ ⊕
**Fees:** £46–55; Second visit: £31–40
London (W) W10
020 8964 3156

### Trevor A Wing BAcC
⊕ ⊕ ⊕ ⊕ ⊕
**Fees:** >£55; Second visit: >£50
London (W) W1
07796 958228

### Alan Wysman BAcC
O ⊕ ✿ ⊕
**Fees:** <£25; Second visit: £21–30
London (W) W1
020 7636 3139

## LONDON (WC)

### David Braime BAcC
⊕ ⊕ ✿ ⊕
**Fees:** £36–45; Second visit: £21–30
London (WC) WC2
020 8723 3725

### Si Tu Xing Chang BAcC
⊕ ⊕ ⊕ ✿ ⊕
**Fees:** £36–45; Second visit: £31–40
London (WC) WC2, London W9,
Amersham HP7
020 7379 7662

### Simeen Khoylou BAcC
⊕ ⊕ ✿ ⊕
**Fees:** £36–45; Second visit: £31–40
London (WC) WC2
020 7379 1312

### Gerad Kite BAcC
⊕ O ⊕ ⊕
**Fees:** >£55; Second visit: >£50
London (WC) WC2
020 7379 7662

### Brit Muhleisen BAcC
O ⊕ ⊘ ✿ ⊕
**Fees:** £36–45
London (WC) WC1
020 7405 9689

### Reiko Oshima-Barclay MNIMH
⊕
London (W) WC2
07946 651742

### Ena Poon BAcC
⊕ ⊕ ✿ ⊕
London (WC) WC1
020 7833 2143

### Joska Ramelow BAcC
⊕ O ⊕ ✿ ⊕
**Fees:** £36–45; Second visit: £31–40
London (WC) WC2
020 7379 7662

### John Renshaw BAcC
⊕ O ⊕ ⊕ ⊕ ✿ ⊕
**Fees:** £36–45; Second visit: £41–50
London (WC) WC2
020 7379 1312

### Dominique Joire BAcC
⊕ ⊕ ⊕ ⊕ ✿
**Fees:** >£55; Second visit: £31–40
London (SW) SW6
07957 222219

## LONDON (E)

**Ganesh C Dutt MFHom**
⊕ Ⓔ
Fees: £25–35; Second visit: <£20
London (E) E14
020 7515 5525

**Kathleen Moore RSHom**
⊕ O ⓃⒽⓈ Ⓔ ✿
Fees: £25–35; Second visit: £20–30
London (E) E11
020 8989 7194

**Lesley Murphy RSHom**
⊕ O ⊕ ⓃⒽⓈ Ⓔ ✿
Fees: £36–45; Second visit: £31–40
London (E) E1
020 7790 8421

**Vivienne Patchett RSHom**
⊕ O ⊕ ⓃⒽⓈ Ⓔ ✿
Fees: £36–45; Second visit: £31–40
London (E) E17
020 8520 5268

**Anita Wicks RSHom**
⊕ O ⊕ ⊕ ⓃⒽⓈ Ⓔ ✿
Fees: £46–55; Second visit: £31–40
London (E) E17,London N4
020 8527 5570

## LONDON (N)

**Grazyna Baran RSHom**
⊕ O ✿
Fees: >£55; Second visit: £31–40
London (N) N8
020 8340 1307

**Richard Bocock RSHom**
O ⓃⒽⓈ Ⓔ ✿
Fees: >£55; Second visit: £31–40
London (N) N1,London E1
020 7226 8705

**Cathryn Brooks RSHom**
⊕ O ⊕ ⓃⒽⓈ Ⓔ ✿
Fees: £46–55; Second visit: £31–40
London (N) N12
020 83469385

**Peter Crockett RSHom**
⊕ ⓃⒽⓈ ⊘
Fees: £36–45; Second visit: £41–50
London (N) N7
020 7700 4234

**Hilary Fairclough RSHom**
⊕ O ⊕ Ⓔ ✿
Fees: £46–55; Second visit: £31–40
London (N) N7
020 7607 3613

**Wendy Glaze RSHom**
⊕ O ⊕ ⓃⒽⓈ Ⓔ ✿
Fees: £46–55; Second visit: £31–40
London (N) N17
020 8801 9356

**Lesley Gregerson RSHom**
⊕ O ⊕ ⓃⒽⓈ Ⓔ
Fees: >£55; Second visit: £41–50
London (N) N21
020 8360 8757

**Jane Harter RSHom**
O ⓃⒽⓈ Ⓔ ✿
Fees: >£55; Second visit: £31–40
London (N) N2
020 8365 2564

**Lynne Howard RSHom**
⊕ O ⊕ ⓃⒽⓈ ✿
Fees: >£55; Second visit: £31–40
London (N) N1,London W8,Buckhurst
Hill IG9
020 7254 7621

**Marie McShea RSHom**
⊕ O ⊕ ⓃⒽⓈ Ⓔ ✿
Fees: £46–55; Second visit: £31–40
London (N) N16
020 7254 8494

**Lindsay Nash RSHom**
O ⓃⒽⓈ Ⓔ ✿
Fees: >£55; Second visit: £31–40
London (N) N11,Nottingham NG7
020 8888 1252

**Jan Perivolas RSHom**
O ⓃⒽⓈ Ⓔ ✿
Fees: £36–45; Second visit: £31–40
London (N) N8
020 8348 1091

# Homeopathy

**Meg Portal RSHom**
● ⊕ ⊕ ⓝ ⓔ ✦
Fees: £36–45
London (N) N7
020 72542867

**Louise Salmon RSHom**
● ⊕ ⊕ ⓝ ⓔ ✦
Fees: £46–55; Second visit: £31–40
London (N) N10
0208 444 8489

**Sharon White RSHom**
● ○ ⊕ ⓝ ⓔ ✦
Fees: £46–55; Second visit: £31–40
London (N) N16
020 7249 2990

**Jane Wood RSHom**
● ⓝ ⓔ
Fees: >£55; Second visit: £31–40
London (N) N3
020 8346 2939

**Susan Young RSHom**
○ ⓝ ⓔ ✦
Fees: £36–45; Second visit: £31–40
London (N) N16
020 7502 0383

## LONDON (NW)

**Elizabeth Adalian RSHom**
● ○ ⊕ ⓝ ⓔ
Fees: £46–55; Second visit: £31–40
London (NW) NW5
0207 4823293

**Michael Bridger RSHom**
○ ⓝ ⓔ
Fees: >£55; Second visit: £41–50
London (NW) NW6
020 7624 8650

**Janet Cokeliss RSHom**
○ ✦
Fees: >£55; Second visit: £31–40
London (NW) NW6
020 8968 0433

**Jayne L M Donegan MFHom**
○ ⓝ ⊘ ⓔ ✦
Fees: >£55; Second visit: >£50
London (NW) NW4
020 8632 1634

**Sara Eames MFHom**
○ ⓝ ⊘ ✦
Fees: >£55; Second visit: £31–40
London (NW) NW6
020 8830 0549

**Felicity Fine RSHom**
● ⊕ ⊕ ⓝ ⓔ ✦
Fees: >£55; Second visit: £41–50
London (NW) NW3
020 7431 9394

**Annie Friedmann RSHom**
● ○ ⓝ ⓔ ✦
Fees: >£55; Second visit: £41–50
London (NW) NW2
020 8452 2946

**Moira Houston MFHom**
● ⊕ ⊕ ⓔ ✦
Fees: >£55; Second visit: £41–50
London (NW) NW2,Letchworth SG6
020 8450 3304

**Margaret Johnson RSHom**
● ○ ⊕ ⊕ ⓝ ✦
Fees: £46–55; Second visit: £31–40
London (NW) NW3,Sheffield
S21,Rotherham S60
020 7916 1866

**Cassandra Marks Lorius RSHom**
● ○ ⊕ ⓔ ✦
Fees: £46–55; Second visit: £31–40
London (NW) NW5
020 7485 9362

**David Mundy RSHom**
● ⊕ ⓝ ✦
Fees: >£55; Second visit: £41–50
London (NW) NW1
020 7388 8030

**Jane Parkin RSHom**
● ⊕ ⓝ ⊘ ⓔ ✦
Fees: >£55; Second visit: £31–40
London (NW) NW5
020 7609 2069

**Rachel Roberts RSHom**
○ ⊕ ⊕ ⓝ ⊘ ⓔ ✦
Fees: £46–55; Second visit: £31–40
London (NW) NW6
020 7794 6256

## Gordon Sambidge RSHom

Fees: £46–55; Second visit: £41–50
London (NW) NW8
020 7483 1288

## Caroline Schuck RSHom

Fees: >£55; Second visit: £41–50
London (NW) NW3
020 77221924

## Michelle Shine RSHom

Fees: >£55; Second visit: £41–50
London (NW) NW7
020 8959 8855

## Francis Treuherz RSHom

Fees: >£55; Second visit: £31–40
London (NW) NW2, London W1
020 8450 6564

## Vicki Turmaine RSHom

Fees: £25–35; Second visit: £20–30
London (NW) NW2
020 8907 0062

## Frances Turner RSHom

Fees: £36–45; Second visit: £20–30
London (NW) NW3
020 7916 2983

## Joseph Zarfaty RSHom

Fees: £46–55; Second visit: £20–30
London (NW) NW11
020 7722 4098

## LONDON (SE)

## Pippa Bow RSHom

Fees: £36–45; Second visit: £20–30
London (SE) SE15
020 76396112

## Marita Byrne RSHom

Fees: £46–55; Second visit: £20–30
London (SE) SE22
020 8693 6867

## Maureen Chapple RSHom

Fees: £36–45; Second visit: £20–30
London (SE) SE12, Southampton
SO45, London SE10
020 8297 8887

## Roger Dyson RSHom

Fees: £36–45; Second visit: £20–30
London (SE) SE26
020 8659 5001

## Carol Lewis RSHom

Fees: £36–45; Second visit: £20–30
London (SE) SE18, London E15
020 8855 9266

## Linda Razzell RSHom

Fees: £46–55; Second visit: £20–30
London (SE) SE10
020 8691 5408

## Elizabeth Sawyer RSHom

Fees: £46–55; Second visit: £31–40
London (SE) SE6, London SE12
020 8698 1809

## Linda Shannon RSHom

Fees: >£55; Second visit: £31–40
London (SE) SE22
01305 824996

## Jacqueline Taylor RSHom

Fees: £36–45; Second visit: £20–30
London (SE) SE3, London SE14,
London N21
020 82935380

## Judith Watson RSHom

Fees: £36–45; Second visit: £20–30
London (SE) SE15
07971 224635

## Elizabeth Whitehead RSHom

Fees: £36–45; Second visit: £20–30
London (SE) SE21
020 84882027

# Homeopathy

**Anne Wynne-Simmons MFHom**
O 🔵 ⊘ ❋
Fees: >£55; Second visit: £31–40
London (SE) SE10
020 8694 2320

## LONDON (SW)

**Melissa Assilem RSHom**
⊕ O ⊕ 🔵
Fees: >£55; Second visit: £41–50
London (SW) SW4
020 7720 2267

**Penelope Barnard RSHom**
O 🔵 ❋
Fees: £36–45; Second visit: £20–30
London (SW) SW16
020 8769 1930

**Jacqueline Becker RSHom**
⊕ ⊕ ⊕ 🔵 Ⓔ
Fees: £36–45; Second visit: £20–30
London (SW) SW4
0207 627 8890

**Elizabeth Bevan-Jones RSHom**
⊕ O ⊕ 🔵 Ⓔ ❋
Fees: £36–45; Second visit: £31–40
London (SW) SW17,London SW19
020 8540 0486

**Inez Claus RSHom**
O 🔵 Ⓔ ❋
Fees: £25–35; Second visit: £20–30
London (SW) SW16
020 8769 0141

**John Cummiing RSHom**
O 🔵
Fees: >£55; Second visit: £31–40
London (SW) SW11
020 7924 2955

**Ilana Snyder Dannheisser RSHom**
⊕ O ⊕ 🔵 Ⓔ
Fees: £46–55; Second visit: £31–40
London (SW) SW17
020 8682 1800

**Christine De Groot RSHom**
⊕ O 🔵 Ⓔ ❋
Fees: £46–55; Second visit: £31–40
London (SW) SW16
020 8677 6212

**Penelope Edwards RSHom**
⊕ O ⊕ 🔵 Ⓔ ❋
Fees: £46–55; Second visit: £31–40
London (SW) SW15
020 87885761

**Sylvia Ennis RSHom**
O 🔵 Ⓔ ❋
Fees: £25–35; Second visit: £20–30
London (SW) SW16
020 8677 3497

**Catherine Frazer RSHom**
O 🔵 ❋
Fees: £46–55; Second visit: £31–40
London (SW) SW10
020 7351 5398

**Barbara Geraghty RSHom**
⊕ O 🔵 Ⓔ ❋
Fees: £46–55; Second visit: £31–40
London (SW) SW19
020 8946 4950

**Christina Grayson MFHom**
⊕ ⊘ ❋
Fees: >£55; Second visit: £41–50
London (SW) SW14
020 88763901

**Christina Head RSHom**
⊕ ⊕ 🔵 Ⓔ ❋
Fees: >£55; Second visit: £31–40
London (SW) SW11
020 7978 4519

**Charles Innes MFHom**
⊕ ⊕ ⊕ 🔵
Fees: >£55; Second visit: >£50
London (SW) SW7
020 7589 6414

**Clare Lincoln RSHom**
⊕ ⊕ 🔵 ❋
Fees: £46–55; Second visit: £31–40
London (SW) SW15
020 89462650

**Kieran Linnane RSHom**
⊕ Ⓔ ❋
Fees: >£55; Second visit: >£50
London (SW) SW15
020 8870 1808

# Homeopathy

**Diane Margolis RSHom**
⊕ ⊕ 🌐 ℰ ✿
**Fees:** >£55; Second visit: £31–40
London (SW) SW11
020 7978 4519

**Adriana Marian RSHom**
⊕ ⊕ 🌐 ℰ ✿
**Fees:** >£55; Second visit: £31–40
London (SW) SW17
020 8672 5253

**Barbara McIntosh RSHom**
🌐 ℰ ✿
**Fees:** £46–55; Second visit: £20–30
London (SW) SW2
020 8671 0061

**Claudia Rice RSHom**
⊕ ⊕ 🌐 ∅ ✿
**Fees:** £46–55; Second visit: £20–30
London (SW) SW4,Crawley RH10
020 7627 8890

**Fran Sinclair Taylor RSHom**
⊕ O ℰ
**Fees:** >£55; Second visit: £31–40
London (SW) SW17,London SW14
020 8672 5253

**Charles Wansbrough RSHom**
⊕ ⊕ 🌐 ℰ ✿
**Fees:** >£55; Second visit: >£50
London (SW) SW15
020 8870 1808

## LONDON (W)

**Helen Austerberry RSHom**
O 🌐 ℰ ✿
**Fees:** £46–55; Second visit: £20–30
London (W) W2, London SE22
020 7792 2844

**Frances Beer-Jones RSHom**
⊕ O ⊕ 🌐 ✿
**Fees:** £46–55; Second visit: £31–40
London (W) W5
0208 579 4323

**Erroll Bowyer RSHom**
⊕ ⊕ 🌐 ℰ ✿
**Fees:** >£55; Second visit: £31–40
London (W) W6
020 8741 9264

**Mr Cannell MFHom**
⊕ 🌐 ∅ ✿
**Fees:** >£55
London (W) W1,St Albans AL2
020 7580 5489

**Rose Chisholm RSHom**
⊕ O ⊕ ℰ
**Fees:** £46–55; Second visit: £31–40
London (W) W6
020 8992 4445

**David Curtin MFHom**
⊕ ⊕ ⊕ 🌐 ∅ ✿
**Fees:** >£55; Second visit: >£50
London (W) W1
020 7224 5111

**Alice Greene FFHom,**
⊕ ⊕ 🌐 ∅ ℰ
**Fees:** >£55; Second visit: >£50
London (W) W1
020 7580 4188

**Paul Hughes RSHom**
O 🌐 ℰ ✿
**Fees:** £36–45; Second visit: £20–30
London (W) W12
020 8749 3472

**Brian Kaplan MFHom**
⊕ ⊕ ⊕ ∅ ℰ ✿
**Fees:** >£55; Second visit: >£50
London (W) W1
020 7487 3416

**Anne Macalpine-Leny RSHom**
⊕ ⊕ ⊕ ℰ
**Fees:** £46–55; Second visit: £20–30
London (W) W14
020 7371 3458

**Annette Middleton RSHom**
⊕ O ⊕ 🌐 ℰ ✿
**Fees:** >£55; Second visit: >£50
London (W) W8,London SW11
020 7221 4602

**David Peters MFHom**
⊕ ⊕ ∅ ℰ
**Fees:** >£55; Second visit: £41–50
London (W) W1, London W1
020 7486 6664

# Homeopathy

**David Ratsey FFHom,**
◉ ⊘
**Fees:** >£55; Second visit: >£50
London (W) W1
020 7589 2776

**Penny Rushton RSHom**
✪ ⊕ ⊕ ◉ Ⓔ
**Fees:** >£55; Second visit: >£50
London (W) W1
020 7631 0604

**Liz Salter RSHom**
✪ ⊕ ◉ Ⓔ ✿
**Fees:** >£55; Second visit: £31–40
London (W) W12, London NW5,
Ingatestone CM4
07976 368052

**Jodi Sher RSHom**
✪ O ⊕ ◉ ⊘ ✿
**Fees:** >£55; Second visit: £41–50
London (W) W8, London SW5
020 72212266

**Imogen Spencer RSHom**
✪ ⊕ ◉ Ⓔ ✿
**Fees:** £36–45; Second visit: £20–30
London (W) W6
020 8741 9264

**Kathryn Tomlinson RSHom**
O Ⓔ
**Fees:** £46–55; Second visit: £20–30
London (W) W13
020 8840 2468

**Nigel Williamson RSHom**
✪ ⊕ ◉ Ⓔ
**Fees:** £46–55; Second visit: £41–50
London (W) W11, London NW2
020 7229 0014

**Veda Young RSHom**
✪ O ⊕ ◉ ⊘ Ⓔ ✿
**Fees:** £46–55; Second visit: £31–40
London (W) W12
020 8749 6523

## LONDON (WC)

**Ann Bowden MFHom**
⊕ ◉ ⊘
London (WC) WC1
020 7837 8833

**Peter Fisher FFHom,**
◉ ⊘
**Fees:** >£55; Second visit: £41–50
London (WC) WC1
020 7837 8833

**Marysia Kratimenos MFHom**
⊕ ⊕ ◉ ⊘
**Fees:** >£55; Second visit: >£50
London (WC) WC1
07654 241340

**Helmut Roniger MFHom**
◉ ⊘
**Fees:** >£55; Second visit: >£50
London (WC) WC1, London
WC1,Tunbridge Wells TN1
020 7837 8833

**Andrea Wiessner MFHom**
◉ ⊘
London (WC) WC1
020 7837 8833

# Osteopathy

## LONDON (E)

**Anthony Agius GOsC**
◉ ✿
**Fees:** £26–35; Second visit: £21–30
London (E) E4
020 85296677

**Alison Brown GOsC, BOA**
O ◉ Ⓔ ✿
**Fees:** £26–35; Second visit: £21–30
London (E) E6
020 8470 8678

### Iain Chapman GOsC, BOA
⊕ 🌐 ❄
Fees: £26–35; Second visit: £31–40
London (E) E17
020 8521 7888

### Simon Curtis GOsC, BOA
O 🌐 ❄
Fees: <£25; Second visit: £21–30
London (E) E1
020 7265 8262

### Robert Davies GOsC, BOA
⊕ 🌐
Fees: £26–35; Second visit: £21–30
London (E) E6, Billericay CM12
07761 965620

### Feriedoun Eftekhari GOsC, BOA
⊕ 🌐 ❄
Fees: <£25; Second visit: £31–40
London (E) E18
020 8989 7569

### Daryl Herbert GOsC
⊕ ⊕ ⊕ 🌐 ⊘ Ⓔ ❄
Fees: £26–35; Second visit: £21–30
London (E) E4
020 8524 1505

### Bhavesh Joshi GOsC, BOA
O ⊕ ⊘ ❄
Fees: £26–35; Second visit: £21–30
London (E) E15
020 8522 1414

### Penelope Kelly GOsC, BOA
O 🌐 ❄
Fees: £26–35; Second visit: £21–30
London (E) E10
020 8558 6841

### James Last GOsC
⊕ 🌐 ⊘ ❄
Fees: £36–45; Second visit: £21–30
London (E) E2
020 7739 8009

### John Mallinder GOsC
⊕ ⊕ 🌐 Ⓔ ❄
Fees: £26–35; Second visit: £21–30
London (E) E2
020 8981 6938

### Bridgit McKay GOsC
⊕ ⊕ 🌐 ❄
Fees: £26–35; Second visit: £21–30
London (E) E10
85566902

### Stephen Moore GOsC, BOA
⊕ 🌐 ❄
Fees: <£25; Second visit: £21–30
London (E) E1
020 7426 0622

### Patricia Row GOsC, BOA
O 🌐 ❄
Fees: £26–35; Second visit: £21–30
London (E) E5
020 8985 2355

### Stephen Sandler GOsC, BOA
⊕ ⊕ ⊕ 🌐 ⊘ Ⓔ ❄
Fees: £26–35; Second visit: £21–30
London (E) E4
020 8529 0815

### Claire Saxby GOsC, BOA
⊕ ⊕ Ⓔ ❄
Fees: £26–35; Second visit: £21–30
London (E) E2
020 8981 6938

### Natalie Seager GOsC, BOA
⊕ ⊕ ⊕ 🌐 ⊘ ❄
Fees: <£25; Second visit: £21–30
London(E), London N10
020 8883 6079

### Amanda Thomas GOsC
⊕ ⊕ ⊕ 🌐 ⊘ ❄
Fees: £26–35; Second visit: £21–30
London (E) E18
020 8532 2922

### Kitty Valentine GOsC
⊕ O ⊕ 🌐 ❄
London (E) E17
020 8527 6276

## LONDON (EC)

### Thomas-Wai Fan GOsC, BOA
⊕ ⊕ ⊕ Ⓔ
Fees: £36–45; Second visit: £31–40
London (EC) EC4
020 7353 5678

# Osteopathy

**Fiona Greer GOsC**
Fees: £36–45; Second visit: £21–30
London (EC) EC1
020 72788070

**Torben Hersborg GOsC, BOA**
Fees: £26–35; Second visit: £31–40
London (EC) EC1
020 7729 1912

**Anthony Kanutin GOsC**
Fees: £36–45; Second visit: £41–50
London (EC) EC3
020 7626 2020

**Yuri Korvatko GOsC**
Fees: £36–45; Second visit: £31–40
London (EC) EC3
020 7680 5000

**Holly Makin GOsC, BOA**
Fees: £36–45; Second visit: £31–40
London (EC) EC2
020 7729 8525

**Michael Vassiliou GOsC, BOA**
Fees: £36–45; Second visit: £31–40
London (EC) EC4
020 7283 9797

**Joyce Vetterlein GOsC**
Fees: £36–45; Second visit: £41–50
London (EC) EC2
020 7729 8525

## LONDON (N)

**Ana Bennett GOsC**
Fees: £26–35; Second visit: £21–30
London (N) N19
020 7272 6695

**Pamla Bowmaker GOsC, BOA**
Fees: £26–35; Second visit: £21–30
London (N) N6
020 7281 0841

**Jane S Brannan GOsC, BOA**
Fees: <£25; Second visit: £21–30
London (N) N8
020 8340 6832

**Kevin Brownhill GOsC**
Fees: £26–35; Second visit: £21–30
London (N) N8
020 8347 9990

**Stephen Choy GOsC, BOA**
Fees: £26–35; Second visit: £21–30
London (N) N1
020 7354 2314

**Geoffrey Clark GOsC, BOA**
Fees: £26–35; Second visit: <£20
London (N) N10
020 8883 2130

**Penelope Conway GOsC, BOA**
Fees: £26–35; Second visit: £21–30
London (N) N21
020 8882 0026

**Caroline Ellwood GOsC**
Fees: £36–45; Second visit: £31–40
London (N) N1
020 7837 3451

**Hussein Eshref GOsC**
Fees: £26–35; Second visit: £31–40
London (N) N1
020 7226 0011

**Jeremy Feilder GOsC, BOA**
Fees: £36–45; Second visit: £21–30
London (N) N2
020 8365 2841

**Carole Finch GOsC**
Fees: £46–55; Second visit: £41–50
London (N) N5
020 7704 1002

### John Fudge GOsC, BOA
Fees: <£25; Second visit: £21–30
London (N) N4
020 7226 1193

### Jimmy Georgious GOsC, BOA
Fees: £36–45; Second visit: £21–30
London (N) N12
020 8445 5439

### Nigel Graham GOsC, BOA
Fees: <£25; Second visit: £21–30
London (N) N12
020 8445 3344

### Sibyl Grundberg GOsC, BOA
Fees: £36–45; Second visit: £31–40
London (N) N4
020 8341 2904

### Andrew Harwich GOsC
Fees: £36–45
London (N) N1
020 7833 3748

### Michael Hunt GOsC
Fees: £26–35; Second visit: £31–40
London (N) N21
020 8360 3485

### Michael Kern GOsC
Fees: <£25; Second visit: £21–30
London (N) N3
020 8349 0297

### Adam Lancaster GOsC, BOA
Fees: £26–35; Second visit: £21–30
London (N) N3
020 3930 5840

### Eyal Lederman PhD GOsC
Fees: £36–45; Second visit: £31–40
London (N) N19
020 7263 8551

### Antony Marsh GOsC
Fees: £26–35; Second visit: £21–30
London (N) N8
020 8348 7432

### Dennis G Michael GOsC, BOA
Fees: £46–55; Second visit: £21–30
London (N) N3
020 8343 3423

### Helen Morton GOsC
Fees: £26–35; Second visit: £21–30
London (N) N11
020 7226 0011

### Savash Mustafa GOsC
Fees: £26–35; Second visit: £21–30
London (N) N1
020 8889 1200

### Simeon Niel-Asher GOsC
Fees: >£55; Second visit: £41–50
London (N) N6
020 8347 6160

### Brian O'Flynn GOsC, BOA
Fees: £36–45; Second visit: £31–40
London (N) N8
020 8347 8300

### Sue Palfreyman GOsC, BOA
Fees: £36–45; Second visit: £21–30
London (N) N8
020 8348 3600

### Sonal Patel GOsC
Fees: £36–45; Second visit: £21–30
London (N) N10
020 8444 8212

### Anthony Perdikis GOsC, BOA
Fees: £26–35; Second visit: £21–30
London (N) N10
020 8444 1920

# Osteopathy

**Steven Pratsides GOsC**
✚ ◯ ⓝ ⊘ Ⓔ ✿
**Fees:** £36–45; Second visit: £31–40
London (N) N14
020 8882 3666

**Anette Schreiber GOsC**
✚ ◯ Ⓔ ✿
**Fees:** £36–45; Second visit: £31–40
London (N) N16
020 7485 8034

**Paul Strange GOsC, BOA**
◯ ⊕ ⓝ ⊘ ✿
**Fees:** £26–35; Second visit: £21–30
London (N) N4
020 8800 3094

**Stella Strong GOsC, BOA**
◯ ⊕ ✿
**Fees:** £36–45; Second visit: £31–40
London (N) N1
020 7226 8499

**Garnett B Symonds GOsC**
✚ ⓝ ✿
**Fees:** £36–45; Second visit: £31–40
London (N) N12
020 8361 2293

**Jeanette Thomson GOsC, BOA**
✚ ⊕ ⓝ ⊘ ✿
**Fees:** £26–35; Second visit: £31–40
London (N) N8
020 8340 1518

**Simon Thurgood GOsC**
✚ ⊕ ⓝ ⊘ Ⓔ ✿
**Fees:** £36–45; Second visit: £21–30
London (N) N13
020 8886 9977

**T Togelong GOsC, BOA**
◯ ⓝ ⊘
**Fees:** <£25; Second visit: £21–30
London (N) N3
020 8346 4869

**Lance Turvey GOsC**
✚ ◯ ⓝ ✿
**Fees:** <£25; Second visit: £21–30
London (N) N8
020 8347 9990

**Martin Underwood GOsC**
◯ ⓝ ✿
**Fees:** £36–45; Second visit: £31–40
London (N) N19
020 7607 5265

**Hedwig Verdonk GOsC**
◯ ✿
**Fees:** £26–35; Second visit: £31–40
London (N) N7
020 7609 8973

**M Vizinczey-Lambert GOsC**
✚ ⓝ ⊘ ✿
**Fees:** <£25; Second visit: £21–30
London (N) N6
07957 228430

**O Joy Wardell GOsC**
◯
**Fees:** £26–35; Second visit: £21–30
London (N) N3
020 8346 6715

**Leonard Wardell GOsC, BOA**
◯
**Fees:** £26–35; Second visit: £21–30
London (N) N3
020 8346 6715

**Sarah Whitehead GOsC, BOA**
✚ ⓝ Ⓔ ✿
**Fees:** £36–45; Second visit: £31–40
London (N) N1
020 7226 7027

**Elsworth Wray GOsC**
✚ ⊕ ⓝ ✿
**Fees:** £26–35; Second visit: £21–30
London (N) N21
07956 826546

## LONDON (NW)

**Alistair Blank GOsC, BOA**
✚ ⊕ ⊕ ⓝ Ⓔ ✿
**Fees:** £36–45; Second visit: £31–40
London (NW) NW1
020 7722 8890

**Gavin Burt GOsC, BOA**
✚ ⊕ ✿
**Fees:** £26–35; Second visit: £31–40
London (NW) NW5
020 7485 9362

**Anthony Charlaff GOsC**
✚ ⊕ 🅝 🅔 ❄
Fees: £26–35; Second visit: £31–40
London (NW) NW5
020 7485 9362

**Laura David GOsC, BOA**
✚ 🅝 ❄
Fees: £26–35; Second visit: £21–30
London (NW) NW5
020 7209 3243

**Isabelle De Reyher GOsC**
✚ 🅝 ⊘ ❄
Fees: >£55; Second visit: >£50
London (NW) NW1
020 7267 8847

**Andrew Doody GOsC**
✚ ⊕ 🅝 ⊘ ❄
Fees: <£25; Second visit: £21–30
London (NW) NW3
07957 430126

**Jadwiga Iga Downing GOsC, BOA**
O 🅝 🅔 ❄
Fees: £36–45; Second visit: £21–30
London (NW) NW6
020 7624 3987

**Dominic G Eglinton GOsC, BOA**
✚ ⊕ 🅝 ❄
Fees: <£25; Second visit: £21–30
London (NW) NW7
020 8959 1123

**Sebastien Escure GOsC, BOA**
✚ ⊕ 🅝 ⊘ ❄
Fees: £26–35; Second visit: £21–30
London (NW) NW4
020 8201 5555

**Lee Freed GOsC, BOA**
✚ ⊕ 🅝 ❄
Fees: £26–35; Second visit: £31–40
London (NW) NW4
020 8202 7543

**Alex Fugallo GOsC, BOA**
✚ O ⊕ ❄
Fees: <£25; Second visit: >£50
London (NW) NW6
020 7209 5889

**Philip Godfrey GOsC**
✚ O 🅝 ❄
Fees: £36–45; Second visit: £21–30
London (NW) NW4
020 8203 8977

**Guy Gold GOsC**
✚ ⊕ 🅝 ❄
Fees: £36–45; Second visit: £31–40
London (NW) NW3
07957 652182

**Joseph Goodman GOsC**
O ⊕ 🅝
Fees: £46–55; Second visit: £41–50
London (NW) NW4
020 8202 6242

**Morwenna Gough GOsC**
✚ ⊕ ⊕ 🅝
Fees: £36–45; Second visit: £31–40
London (NW) NW2
020 8452 9063

**Daniel Graham GOsC, BOA**
O ⊕ ❄
Fees: £26–35; Second visit: £21–30
London (NW) NW1
07810 498676

**Nesli Harris GOsC, BOA**
🅝
Fees: <£25; Second visit: £21–30
London (NW) NW11
07710 214368

**J Headifen GOsC, BOA**
✚ ⊕ 🅝
Fees: <£25; Second visit: £21–30
London (NW) NW5
020 7485 9362

**Timothy D H John GOsC, BOA**
✚ ⊕ 🅝
Fees: >£55; Second visit: £41–50
London (NW) NW7,London W1
020 8959 1123

**Brian Joseph GOsC**
✚ ⊕ 🅝 ⊘ ❄
Fees: £46–55; Second visit: £31–40
London (NW) NW11
020 8458 2586

# Osteopathy

**E F Keeling GOsC, BOA**
⊕ O ⓝⓗⓢ
Fees: <£25; Second visit: £21–30
London (NW) NW3
020 7435 1740

**Ronald Klein GOsC**
⊕ ⊕ ⓝⓗⓢ ⊘ ✿
Fees: <£25; Second visit: £21–30
London (NW) NW1
020 7267 0110

**Jane Langer GOsC**
O ⓝⓗⓢ
Fees: £26–35; Second visit: £31–40
London (NW) NW7
020 8959 5435

**Anthony Longaretti GOsC**
O ⓝⓗⓢ ✿
Fees: £36–45; Second visit: £21–30
London (NW) NW6
020 7328 7269

**Alexander Lubel GOsC, BOA**
⊕ ⓝⓗⓢ ✿
Fees: £26–35; Second visit: £21–30
London (NW) NW2
020 8450 8854

**Josephine Manton GOsC**
⊕ ⓝⓗⓢ ⊘ ✿
Fees: £26–35; Second visit: £21–30
London (NW) NW5
020 7267 6445

**Robert McLoughlin GOsC, BOA**
⊕ ⓝⓗⓢ ✿
Fees: <£25; Second visit: £21–30
London (NW) NW3
07956 185123

**Lyndsay Mudford GOsC, BOA**
⊕ ⊕ ⓝⓗⓢ
Fees: <£25; Second visit: £21–30
London (NW) NW11
020 8458 2586

**Lazarus Nono GOsC, BOA**
⊕ ⓝⓗⓢ ✿
Fees: £26–35; Second visit: £21–30
London (NW) NW10
020 8450 8688

**Robi Persad GOsC, BOA**
O ⊕ ⓝⓗⓢ ✿
Fees: £26–35; Second visit: £21–30
London (NW) NW5
020 7209 3243

**Martin Pidd GOsC, BOA**
O ⓝⓗⓢ ⊘ Ⓔ ✿
Fees: £36–45; Second visit: £21–30
London (NW) NW11
020 8455 2675

**Stephen Pirie GOsC**
⊕ ⓝⓗⓢ ✿
Fees: £46–55; Second visit: £41–50
London (NW) NW1
020 7935 3207

**David J Powers GOsC, BOA**
⊕ ⊕ ⓝⓗⓢ Ⓔ ✿
Fees: £26–35; Second visit: £21–30
London (NW) NW4
020 8959 0823

**Giulia Quintarelli GOsC, BOA**
⊕ ⊘
Fees: >£55; Second visit: >£50
London (NW) NW1
020 7267 8847

**Berwyn Rutherford GOsC**
O ⓝⓗⓢ ⊘ ✿
Fees: £36–45; Second visit: £31–40
London (NW) NW3
020 7435 4753

**Bronwyn Stevens GOsC, BOA**
⊕ O ⓝⓗⓢ ⊘ ✿
Fees: £36–45; Second visit: £31–40
London (NW) NW3
020 7485 8787

**Grania Stewart-Smith GOsC, BOA**
⊕ ⓝⓗⓢ ⊘ Ⓔ
Fees: £46–55; Second visit: >£50
London (NW) NW8
020 7286 2615

**Thomas Zacharia GOsC, BOA**
⊕ ⓝⓗⓢ ⊘ ✿ ⊜
Fees: £46–55; Second visit: £31–40
London (NW) NW4
020 8202 1140

## Osteopathy

**Lubna Zaidi GOsC**
🟢 ⭕ 🔵 🔵 ⊘ 🔵
**Fees:** £36–45; Second visit: £31–40
London (NW) NW6
07761 83494

### LONDON (SE)

**Michael Adams GOsC**
🟢 🔵 🔵 🔵
**Fees:** £26–35; Second visit: £21–30
London (SE) SE9
020 8294 1113

**David Annett GOsC, BOA**
🟢 🔵 ⊘ 🔵
**Fees:** <£25; Second visit: £31–40
London (SE) SE19
020 8771 9050

**Christina Ashton GOsC**
🟢 ⭕ 🔵 🔵 ⊘ Ⓔ 🔵
**Fees:** £36–45; Second visit: £21–30
London (SE) SE23
020 8291 3905

**Remi Baudriboc GOsC, BOA**
🟢 ⊕ 🔵 🔵
**Fees:** <£25; Second visit: £31–40
London (SE) SE22
020 8299 9798

**Charlotte Bucknill GOsC**
⭕ 🔵
**Fees:** £26–35; Second visit: £21–30
London (SE) SE24
020 7733 8555

**Kevan Bumstead GOsC, BOA**
🟢 🔵 ⊘ Ⓔ 🔵
**Fees:** £26–35; Second visit: £21–30
London (SE) SE13
020 8852 5577

**F D Campbell GOsC, BOA**
🟢 🔵 ⊘ 🔵
**Fees:** £26–35; Second visit: £21–30
London (SE) SE19
020 8771 9050

**Gemma Colbert GOsC, BOA**
🟢 🔵 ⊘ 🔵
**Fees:** £26–35; Second visit: £21–30
London (SE) SE13
020 8852 5577

**Dan Delap GOsC, BOA**
⭕ 🔵 ⊘
**Fees:** £36–45; Second visit: £21–30
London (SE) SE10
020 8692 2831

**Neil Fennel GOsC**
🟢 ⭕ 🔵 🔵 ⊘ Ⓔ 🔵
**Fees:** <£25; Second visit: £21–30
London (SE) SE4
020 8691 1051

**Amberin Fur GOsC, BOA**
🟢 🔵 🔵 🔵
**Fees:** <£25; Second visit: £21–30
London (SE) SE22
020 8299 9798

**Elaine Gregory GOsC, BOA**
🟢 🔵 🔵 Ⓔ 🔵
**Fees:** £26–35; Second visit: £21–30
London (SE) SE22
020 8693 5515

**Donald Kean GOsC, BOA**
🟢 ⭕ 🔵 🔵 Ⓔ 🔵
**Fees:** £36–45; Second visit: £21–30
London (SE) SE10
020 8691 5408

**Donald J Kean GOsC, BOA**
🟢 ⭕ 🔵 Ⓔ 🔵
**Fees:** £36–45; Second visit: £21–30
London (SE) SE3
020 8853 2275

**Robin Kirk GOsC, BOA**
🟢 ⊕ 🔵 🔵
**Fees:** £36–45; Second visit: £31–40
London (SE) SE1
020 7378 0850

**Pierre Andre LaRouch GOsC, BOA**
🟢 🔵 🔵 ⊘ 🔵
**Fees:** <£25; Second visit: £21–30
London (SE) SE3
020 8853 0800

**Julie Lewis GOsC**
🟢 🔵 🔵 🔵
**Fees:** £26–35; Second visit: £21–30
London (SE) SE3
020 8852 1706

# Osteopathy

**Cyprian Londt GOsC, BOA**
⊕ ⊕ ⊕ ⊛ Ⓔ ❈
**Fees:** <£25; Second visit: £21–30
London (SE) SE15
020 7701 2535

**Alexander Low GOsC**
⊕ ⊛ ⊘ ❈
**Fees:** £26–35; Second visit: £21–30
London (SE) SE4
020 8694 2714

**Neil Lunt GOsC, BOA**
⊕ O ⊕ ⊛ Ⓔ ❈
**Fees:** £26–35; Second visit: £21–30
London (SE) SE23
020 8699 3156

**Joanna Mitchell GOsC**
⊕ ⊛
**Fees:** £26–35; Second visit: £21–30
London (SE) SE4
020 8773 4122

**Nikki Moss GOsC, BOA**
⊕ ⊕ ⊛
**Fees:** <£25; Second visit: £21–30
London (SE) SE12
020 8297 8887

**Margaret Ohuche GOsC, BOA**
O ⊕ ⊛ ⊘ ❈
**Fees:** £26–35; Second visit: £21–30
London (SE) SE20
020 8778 9468

**Kate-Emma Osazuwa GOsC**
⊕ ⊕ ❈
**Fees:** £26–35; Second visit: £21–30
London (SE) SE19
020 8653 5646

**Ross Payn GOsC, BOA**
⊕ ⊛ ❈
**Fees:** £26–35; Second visit: £21–30
London (SE) SE4
020 8694 2714

**Carol Plumridge GOsC**
⊕ ⊕ ⊛ ❈
**Fees:** £36–45; Second visit: £21–30
London (SE) SE10
020 8691 5408

**Trevor Reeves GOsC**
⊕ ❈
**Fees:** £26–35; Second visit: £21–30
London (SE) SE11
020 8387 8132

**Thomas Sheehan GOsC**
⊕ ⊛ ❈
**Fees:** £26–35; Second visit: £21–30
London (SE) SE5
020 7737 8007

**Fabiano Da Silva GOsC, BOA**
⊕ ⊕ ⊛ ❈
**Fees:** <£25; Second visit: £21–30
London(SE) SE5
07956 257980

**Romeo Stafford GOsC**
⊕ O ⊕ ⊛ ❈
**Fees:** £36–45; Second visit: £21–30
London (SE) SE22
020 82490159

**Catherine Varnon GOsC, BOA**
⊕ ⊕ ⊛ ⊘ ❈
**Fees:** £26–35; Second visit: £21–30
London (SE) SE1
020 7378 0850

**Charlotte Webb GOsC, BOA**
O ⊕ ⊛ ❈
**Fees:** £36–45; Second visit: £21–30
London (SE) SE3, Rotherhithe SE16
020 8318 9123

**Carol B Williams GOsC, BOA**
⊕ O ⊕ ⊛ ❈
**Fees:** £36–45; Second visit: £21–30
London (SE) SE10
020 8691 5408

**K Fan Yau GOsC**
⊕ ⊕ ⊛ ❈
**Fees:** <£25; Second visit: £21–30
London (SE) SE1
07973 769077

## LONDON (SW)

**Adam Beaumont GOsC**
⊕ O ⊕ ⊛ ⊘ ❈
**Fees:** <£25; Second visit: £21–30
London (SW) SW15
020 8788 1991

**Stephen Beaver & Associates
GOsC, BOA**
● ● ●
Fees: £36–45; Second visit: £31–40
London (SW) SW19
020 8543 3673

**Ronald Bishop GOsC**
● ● ● ●
Fees: £36–45; Second visit: £31–40
London (SW) SW1
020 7834 1012

**Jo Bowyer GOsC**
● ● ● ● ●
Fees: <£25; Second visit: £21–30
London (SW) SW4
020 7627 0291

**Deryck Breinburg GOsC, BOA**
● ● ● ● ● ●
Fees: £26–35; Second visit: £21–30
London (SW) SW4
020 76274901

**Helena Bridge GOsC**
● ● ●
Fees: £36–45; Second visit: £31–40
London (SW) SW15
020 8788 5761

**Ashling Casey GOsC, BOA**
● ● ● ●
London (SW) SW11
020 7350 1600

**R Chapman GOsC, BOA**
● ● ● ● ● ●
Fees: £26–35; Second visit: £31–40
London (SW) SW1
020 7834 0861

**Kieran G Chhabra GOsC**
● ● ● ●
Fees: <£25; Second visit: £21–30
London (SW) SW19
020 8545 0965

**Alan Coles GOsC**
● ● ● ● ●
Fees: <£25; Second visit: £21–30
London (SW) SW5
07802 826109

**Andrew Cotton GOsC**
● ● ●
Fees: <£25; Second visit: £21–30
London (SW) SW6
020 7384 1851

**Melinda Cotton GOsC**
● ● ● ●
Fees: <£25; Second visit: £21–30
London (SW) SW6
020 7384 1851

**Michael Cummings GOsC, BOA**
● ● ●
Fees: £26–35; Second visit: £21–30
London (SW) SW15
020 8788 1991

**James Dodd GOsC, BOA**
● ● ● ● ●
Fees: <£25; Second visit: £21–30
London (SW) SW18
020 8946 5681

**Beatrice Duchier GOsC, BOA**
● ● ●
Fees: £36–45; Second visit: £31–40
London (SW) SW19
020 8542 8596

**Oluyinka Fabusuyi GOsC, BOA**
● ● ●
Fees: <£25; Second visit: £21–30
London (SW) SW2
020 8674 5883

**Daniel Fenocchi GOsC**
● ● ●
Fees: £26–35; Second visit: £31–40
London (SW) SW19
020 8947 1555

**Daren Fletcher GOsC**
● ● ●
Fees: £36–45; Second visit: £31–40
London (SW) SW1
020 7828 6888

**Viraj Gopaul GOsC, BOA**
● ● ● ● ●
Fees: £36–45; Second visit: £31–40
London (SW) SW15
020 8255 6255

# Osteopathy

**Fiona Hamilton GOsC, BOA**
⊕ ⊛ ✿
Fees: £26–35; Second visit: £21–30
London (SW) SW20
020 8946 3898

**Marcia M Harewood GOsC, BOA**
⊕ ⊛ ✿
Fees: £36–45; Second visit: £31–40
London (SW) SW11
020 7498 9966

**Penelope J Haslam GOsC, BOA**
◯ ⊕ ⊛ Ⓔ ✿
Fees: £46–55; Second visit: £41–50
London (SW) SW6
020 7736 2013

**George Hughes GOsC**
⊕ ◯ ⊕ ⊛ ✿
Fees: £36–45; Second visit: £31–40
London (SW) SW1
020 7834 6229

**Stephen Humphreys GOsC**
⊕ ⊕ ⊛ Ⓔ ✿
Fees: £36–45; Second visit: £31–40
London (SW) SW1
020 7834 3149

**David Isherwood GOsC, BOA**
◯ ⊛ Ⓔ ✿
Fees: £36–45; Second visit: £31–40
London (SW) SW11
020 7228 6336

**Vispi Jamooji GOsC, BOA**
⊕ ⊕ ⊕ ⊛ ⊘ ✿
Fees: £26–35; Second visit: £21–30
London (SW) SW20
020 8946 2331

**Emyr Jones GOsC**
◯ ⊛ ✿
Fees: £36–45; Second visit: £21–30
London (SW) SW19
020 8540 5543

**Charles Lankester GOsC, BOA**
⊕ ⊕ ⊛ ✿
Fees: £26–35; Second visit: £21–30
London (SW) SW18
020 8870 8761

**Philippa Last GOsC, BOA**
⊕ ⊕ ⊛ ⊘ ✿ ⊕
Fees: £26–35; Second visit: £21–30
London (SW) SW1
020 8746 5736

**Liv Lowrie GOsC**
⊕ ⊕ ⊛ ⊘ Ⓔ ✿
Fees: £36–45; Second visit: £31–40
London (SW) SW1
020 7245 6372

**Colin Mahon GOsC**
⊕ ⊛ ⊘ ✿
Fees: £36–45
London (SW) SW15
020 8789 3881

**Naval Mair GOsC, BOA**
⊕ ⊛ ⊘ ✿
Fees: £36–45; Second visit: £31–40
London (SW) SW11
020 77389199

**Leo Meyer GOsC, BOA**
⊕ ⊕ ⊕ ⊛ ✿
Fees: £36–45; Second visit: £31–40
London (SW) SW10
07958 491244

**Khalid Mahmood Mughal GOsC, BOA**
⊕ ◯ ⊕ ⊛ ⊘ ✿
Fees: £36–45; Second visit: £31–40
London (SW) SW5
020 7373 4102

**Maggie Murray GOsC**
⊕ ⊛ ⊘
Fees: <£25; Second visit: £21–30
London (SW) SW20
020 8543 8297

**Jean-Marie Noiret GOsC**
◯ ⊛ ⊘ ✿
Fees: £36–45; Second visit: £31–40
London (SW) SW11
020 7738 9354

**Salome Olivia GOsC, BOA**
⊕ ⊕ ⊕ ⊛ ✿
Fees: £26–35; Second visit: £31–40
London (SW) SW16
020 8679 5900

**Brent Osborn-Smith GOsC, BOA**
Fees: >£55; Second visit: £41–50
London (SW) SW1
020 7228 9995

**Sue Philbey GOsC, BOA**
Fees: <£25; Second visit: £21–30
London (SW) SW18
020 8870 7345

**Suzanne Pinsker GOsC, BOA**
Fees: £26–35; Second visit: £31–40
London (SW) SW10
020 7352 9385

**Emma Poole GOsC**
Fees: £26–35; Second visit: £21–30
London (SW) SW18
020 8870 0822

**Farrah Pradhan GOsC, BOA**
Fees: <£25; Second visit: £21–30
London (SW) SW3

**John Prescott GOsC, BOA**
Fees: £36–45; Second visit: £31–40
London (SW) SW15
020 8780 2727

**David Propert GOsC**
Fees: £46–55; Second visit: £31–40
London (SW) SW1
020 7798 8685

**Karen Robertson GOsC, BOA**
Fees: £26–35; Second visit: >£50
London (SW) SW19
020 8946 6103

**Michael Robinson GOsC**
Fees: <£25; Second visit: <£20
London (SW) SW15
020 8788 0723

**Frederic Roscop GOsC**
Fees: £36–45; Second visit: £31–40
London (SW) SW3
07941 796268

**Simone Ross GOsC**
Fees: >£55; Second visit: >£50
London (SW) SW1
020 7235 8300

**David Rowland GOsC**
Fees: £36–45; Second visit: £31–40
London (SW) SW19
020 8946 6103

**Matthew Schrock GOsC, BOA**
Fees: >£55; Second visit: >£50
London (SW) SW7, Woking GU21
020 7589 6414

**Ajay Shah GOsC, BOA**
Fees: £26–35; Second visit: £21–30
London (SW) SW12
020 8767 3834

**Peter Simpson GOsC, BOA**
Fees: £26–35; Second visit: £21–30
London (SW) SW2
020 8674 7554

**Nicolas Snelling GOsC**
Fees: £36–45; Second visit: £31–40
London (SW) SW13
020 8876 9897

**Piers Spencer GOsC**
Fees: £36–45; Second visit: £21–30
London (SW) SW1
020 7730 5171

**Richard Stimson GOsC**
Fees: £26–35; Second visit: £21–30
London (SW) SW16
020 8677 0486

# Osteopathy

**Martin Stokes And Associates**
**GOsC, BOA**
⊕ 🔵 ✿
**Fees:** £26–35; Second visit: £21–30
London (SW) SW4
07930 324827

**Maxine Hamilton Stubber GOsC**
⊕ ⊕ ⊘ ©
**Fees:** £46–55; Second visit: £41–50
London (SW) SW1
020 7730 7928

**John Telford GOsC, BOA**
○ 🔵 ✿
**Fees:** £36–45; Second visit: £31–40
London (SW) SW20
0181 947 5827

**Steven Vogel GOsC, BOA**
○ ⊕ 🔵 ⊘ ✿
**Fees:** <£25; Second visit: £31–40
London (SW) SW9
020 8674 5883

**Philip Von Hauenschild GOsC**
⊕ ○ 🔵 ✿
**Fees:** £26–35; Second visit: £31–40
London (SW) SW10
020 7376 7649

**Philip Waldman GOsC**
⊕ ⊕ 🔵 ✿
**Fees:** £26–35; Second visit: £31–40
London (SW) SW10
020 7352 3074

**Didier Wart GOsC**
⊕ 🔵 ✿
**Fees:** £46–55; Second visit: £41–50
London (SW) SW7
020 7591 3847

**Claire Webster GOsC**
⊕ ⊕ 🔵 ⊘ ✿
**Fees:** £26–35; Second visit: £21–30
London (SW) SW1, Maldon CM9
020 8746 5736

**Caroline Wells GOsC**
⊕ 🔵 ✿
**Fees:** £26–35; Second visit: £21–30
London (SW) SW13
020 8878 8998

**Krystyna Zielinski GOsC, BOA**
○ 🔵 ✿
**Fees:** £36–45; Second visit: £21–30
London (SW) SW19
020 8542 8596

## LONDON (W)

**Antonia Adeniji GOsC**
⊕ ⊕ © ✿
**Fees:** £36–45; Second visit: £21–30
London (W) W12
020 8749 3792

**Tracey Aird GOsC, BOA**
⊕ 🔵 © ✿
**Fees:** £36–45; Second visit: £21–30
London (W) W1
020 7486 6160

**Peter Bartlett GOsC**
⊕ ○ ⊕ ⊕ 🔵 ✿ 🔵
**Fees:** £46–55; Second visit: £41–50
London (W) W1, Reading RG10
020 7935 2030

**Robert Chaffe GOsC**
⊕ ⊕ 🔵 ⊘ ✿
**Fees:** £36–45; Second visit: £31–40
London (W) W1
0207 499 3555

**Leon Chaitow GOsC, BOA**
⊕ ⊕ 🔵
**Fees:** >£55; Second visit: £41–50
London (W) W1
020 7486 6664

**Maria Clarke GOsC**
⊕ ⊕ 🔵 ✿
**Fees:** £46–55; Second visit: >£50
London (W) W1
020 7436 7010

**Juliette Cole GOsC, BOA**
⊕ ⊕ 🔵 ⊘ ✿
**Fees:** £36–45; Second visit: £31–40
London (W) W1
020 7935 8505

**Nina Constandinou GOsC, BOA**
⊕ 🔵 ✿
**Fees:** £46–55; Second visit: £41–50
London (W) W2
020 7221 3557

**Simon Cooke GOsC, BOA**
⊕ ⊕ ⊛ ⊛
**Fees:** <£25; Second visit: £21–30
London (W) W1
07979 862816

**Philippa Cossens GOsC**
⊕ O
**Fees:** <£25; Second visit: £21–30
London (W) W1
020 7486 6160

**Marcus Davis GOsC, BOA**
⊕ ⊕ ⊕ ⊛ ⊘ ⊛
**Fees:** <£25; Second visit: £21–30
London (W) W1
07957 637666

**Tajinder K Deoora GOsC**
⊕ O ⊕ ⊕ ⊛ ⊛
**Fees:** >£55; Second visit: £41–50
London (W) W1
0207 4874568

**Gary Derrick GOsC**
⊕ O ⊕ ⊕ © ⊛
**Fees:** >£55; Second visit: >£50
London (W) W1
020 76369595

**John Durkan GOsC**
⊕ ⊕ ⊕ ⊛ ⊘ ⊛ ⊛
**Fees:** >£55; Second visit: >£50
London (W) W1
07880 746077

**Martyn Edwards GOsC**
⊕ O ⊕ ⊛ ⊛
**Fees:** £26–35; Second visit: £21–30
London (W) W2
020 7229 8144

**Lissie Evans GOsC, BOA**
⊕ O ⊕ ⊛ ⊛
**Fees:** <£25; Second visit: £21–30
London (W) W10
020 8960 0846

**Mary Evers GOsC, BOA**
⊕ O ⊛ © ⊛
**Fees:** £36–45; Second visit: £31–40
London (W) W9
020 7289 4705

**Sholeh Fadami GOsC, BOA**
⊕ ⊛ ⊘ ⊛
**Fees:** <£25; Second visit: £31–40
London(W) W13
020 8998 8873

**Robin Fairman GOsC, BOA**
⊕ ⊛ ⊛
**Fees:** £36–45; Second visit: £31–40
London (W) W3
020 8743 5140

**Susan Farwell GOsC**
O ⊛ ⊘
**Fees:** <£25; Second visit: £21–30
London (W) W3
020 8993 1994

**Andrew Ferguson GOsC, BOA**
⊕ ⊛ ⊛
**Fees:** >£55; Second visit: >£50
London (W) W11
020 7937 2298

**Michael Francis GOsC, BOA**
⊕ ⊕ ⊕ ⊛ ⊛
**Fees:** £26–35; Second visit: £21–30
London (W) W12
020 8749 3792

**Celia Frank GOsC, BOA**
⊕ ⊛ © ⊛
**Fees:** £36–45; Second visit: £31–40
London (W) W12
020 8749 0581

**G Gajadharsingh GOsC**
⊕ O ⊕ ⊛ ⊘ ⊛
**Fees:** <£25; Second visit: £21–30
London (W) W1
020 7487 4204

**Jeremy Gilbey GOsC**
⊕ ⊕ ⊛
**Fees:** £46–55; Second visit: £41–50
London (W) W2
020 7221 3557

**Alison Grant GOsC, BOA**
⊘
**Fees:** £26–35; Second visit: £21–30
London (W) W3
020 89923372

# Osteopathy

### Ashley Gregory GOsC, BOA
❖
**Fees:** £26–35; Second visit: £21–30
London (W) W6
020 8741 4640

### Suzanne Harper GOsC
⊕ O ⊕ ⊕ ⊕ ❖
**Fees:** £46–55; Second visit: £41–50
London (W) W1
020 7224 3387

### Alexandra L Havard GOsC
⊕ O ⊕ ⊕ ❖
**Fees:** £26–35; Second visit: £21–30
London (W) W6
020 7610 5459

### Amos Heller GOsC, BOA,
⊕ ⊕ ⊕
**Fees:** <£25; Second visit: £21–30
London (W) W2
020 7221 3557

### Iqbal A Hussein GOsC
⊕ ⊕ ⊕ ⊘ ❖
**Fees:** >£55; Second visit: >£50
London (W) W1
020 7486 1920

### Alison Judah GOsC, BOA
⊕ ⊕ ❖
**Fees:** £36–45; Second visit: £31–40
London (W) W5
07956 287776

### Mark Kane GOsC
⊕ ⊕ ⊘ ❖
**Fees:** >£55; Second visit: >£50
London (W) W1
020 7486 9588

### Victoria Kent GOsC
⊕ ⊕ ⊘ ⓔ ❖
**Fees:** >£55; Second visit: >£50
London (W) W1
020 7486 9588

### Robin Kiashek GOsC
⊕ ⊕ ⊕ ⊕ ❖
**Fees:** £36–45; Second visit: £31–40
London (W) W1
74376383

### Corinne Kirby GOsC, BOA
⊕ ⊕
**Fees:** £26–35; Second visit: £21–30
London (W) W2,London E4
020 8524 1505

### David J Knight GOsC, BOA
⊕ ⓔ ⊕ ❖
**Fees:** £36–45; Second visit: £21–30
London (W) W1T
07931 501257

### Jenny Lalau-Keraly GOsC
⊕ ⊕ ⊕ ❖
**Fees:** £36–45; Second visit: £31–40
London (W) W2
020 7229 8144

### Gerald Lamb GOsC
⊕ ⊕ ⊕
**Fees:** >£55; Second visit: £41–50
London (W) W1
020 7486 2875

### Jonathan Le Bon GOsC
⊕ ⊕ ⊕ ⊕ ❖
**Fees:** >£55; Second visit: £41–50
London (W) W1
020 7724 2464

### Christine Lister GOsC, BOA
O ⊕ ❖
**Fees:** £36–45; Second visit: £21–30
London (W) W7
020 8567 4044

### Julie Lyons GOsC, BOA
⊕ ⊕ ❖
**Fees:** <£25; Second visit: £21–30
London (W) W11
0207 2298 666

### Luciana Magalotti GOsC
⊕ ⊕ ⓔ
**Fees:** £46–55; Second visit: £41–50
London (W) W1
020 7435 4620

### Marie-Louise Mahieu GOsC
O ⊘ ❖
**Fees:** £46–55; Second visit: £41–50
London (W) W8
020 7584 3424

**Lorna McGrigor GOsC, BOA**
**Fees:** >£55; Second visit: >£50
London (W) W1
020 7262 1437

**David Melrose GOsC**
**Fees:** >£55; Second visit: >£50
London (W) W1
020 7487 5926

**Stephen Moore GOsC, BOA**
**Fees:** £36–45; Second visit: £31–40
London (W) W1
020 7499 3444

**Jonathan Nunn GOsC, BOA**
**Fees:** £46–55; Second visit: £41–50
London (W) W1
07976 278053

**Amanda O'Connor GOsC**
**Fees:** £26–35; Second visit: £21–30
London (W) W5
07956 444385

**Lucinda Palmer GOsC**
**Fees:** £26–35; Second visit: £21–30
London (W) W10
020 89641811

**Sohini Patel GOsC, BOA**
**Fees:** >£55; Second visit: >£50
London (W) W1
07866 227901

**Martin Pendry GOsC, BOA**
**Fees:** <£25; Second visit: £31–40
London (W) W11
07973 287273

**Nedialka Penner GOsC, BOA**
**Fees:** >£55; Second visit: £21–30
London (W) W3
020 8992 7252

**C Petter GOsC**
**Fees:** <£25; Second visit: £31–40
London (W) W1
0207631056

**Sandra Price GOsC**
London (W) W1
020 7935 0023

**Sharon Quilter GOsC**
**Fees:** <£25; Second visit: £31–40
London (W) W1

**Shakeela Rashid GOsC, BOA**
**Fees:** £36–45; Second visit: £21–30
London (W) W3
020 8992 3190

**Thomas Remaud GOsC, BOA**
**Fees:** £36–45; Second visit: £41–50
London (W) W11
020 7727 6827

**Laurent Reynolds GOsC**
**Fees:** £36–45
London (W) W2
020 7467 0544

**Erica Salisbury GOsC, BOA**
**Fees:** £46–55; Second visit: £31–40
London (W) W1
020 7262 1490

**Ida Scheibelhoffer GOsC, BOA**
**Fees:** <£25; Second visit: £21–30
London (W) W1
020 7437 6383

**Max Secchi GOsC**
**Fees:** <£25; Second visit: £21–30
London (W) W11
020 7937 2298

# Osteopathy

**Barbara A Sherringham GOsC, BOA**
➊ ⓝ ✿
Fees: <£25; Second visit: £21–30
London (W) W1
020 7724 2329

**Guru Singh GOsC**
➊ ⓖ ⓝ ⓔ ✿
Fees: £26–35; Second visit: £21–30
London (W) W8
020 7221 4602

**Michael J G Skipwith GOsC**
➊ ⓝ ⊘ ✿
Fees: <£25; Second visit: £21–30
London (W) W1
020 7486 2875

**Ashley Stafford GOsC, BOA**
➊ ⓖ ⓝ ✿
Fees: £36–45; Second visit: £31–40
London (W) W12
020 8749 3792

**Richard Stubbs GOsC, BOA**
➊ ⭕ ⓖ ⓝ ⊘
Fees: >£55; Second visit: £41–50
London (W) W1
020 7262 3022

**David Tatton GOsC, BOA**
➊ ⓖ ⓝ ⓔ ✿
Fees: £36–45; Second visit: £31–40
London (W) W12
020 8749 0581

**Sarah Towers GOsC**
➊ ⓖ ⓝ
Fees: <£25; Second visit: £31–40
London (W) W3
020 8752 0902

**Kenneth Underhill GOsC, BOA**
⭕ ⊕ ⓖ ⓝ ✿
Fees: £36–45; Second visit: £31–40
London (W) W1
020 7402 4430

**Carol Vile GOsC**
⭕ ✿
Fees: £26–35; Second visit: £21–30
London (W) W13
020 8991 8141

**Vasiliki Vlachonis GOsC**
➊ ⊕ ⓖ ⓝ ⊘ ✿
Fees: >£55; Second visit: >£50
London (W) W1
020 7224 5111

**Sarah Weldon GOsC**
➊ ⓝ ✿
Fees: <£25; Second visit: £21–30
London (W) W8
020 7937 4333

**Julia Williams GOsC**
➊ ⓖ ⓝ ✿
Fees: £26–35; Second visit: £31–40
London (W) W4
07966 243459

**Danny Williams GOsC, BOA**
➊ ⊕ ⓖ ⊘
Fees: £46–55; Second visit: £41–50
London (W) W1
020 7439 7332

**James Wilson GOsC**
➊ ⓝ ⊘ ✿
Fees: £26–35; Second visit: £21–30
London (W) W1U
020 7535 5619

**Kristian Joseph Wood GOsC**
➊ ⓝ ✿
Fees: £36–45; Second visit: £31–40
London (W) W12
020 8749 7449

**Frank Ying GOsC, BOA**
➊ ⓝ ⊘ ⓔ ✿
Fees: £46–55; Second visit: £41–50
London (W) W2
0207 2217077

## LONDON (WC)

**Iain Chapman GOsC, BOA**
➊ ⓖ ⓝ ✿
Fees: £26–35; Second visit: £31–40
London (WC) WC2
020 7836 3646

**Simon Freedman GOsC**
➊ ⓝ ✿
Fees: <£25; Second visit: £21–30
London (WC) WC2
020 7379 5531

# Osteopathy

**Tim Hanwell GOsC**
⊕ ⊕ ⊛
**Fees:** £26–35; Second visit: £21–30
London (WC) WC2
020 7955 7016

**Helen Harris GOsC, BOA**
⊕ ⊕ ⊛ ✿
**Fees:** £26–35; Second visit: £21–30
London (WC) WC1
020 7343 1710

**Brit Muhleisen GOsC**
O ⊕ ⊛ ⊘ ✿
**Fees:** <£25; Second visit: £21–30
London (WC) WC1
020 7405 9689

**Harry Phillips GOsC**
O ⊛ ✿
**Fees:** <£25; Second visit: £31–40
London (WC) WC2
020 7836 4007

**Ian Schofield GOsC, BOA**
⊕ ⊛ ✿
**Fees:** £26–35; Second visit: £31–40
London (WC) WC2
07778 636363

**Andreas Syrimis GOsC, BOA**
⊕ ⊕ ⊛ ⊘ ⓔ
**Fees:** £26–35; Second visit: £31–40
London (WC) WC1
020 7813 7546

# Chiropractic

### LONDON (EC)

**John C Adam GCC, BCA**
⊕ ⊕ ⊛ ✿
**Fees:** £46–55; Second visit: £31–40
London (EC) EC2
020 7638 4330

**Richard Hollis GCC, BCA**
⊕ ⊛ ⊘
**Fees:** £46–55; Second visit: £31–40
London (EC) EC2
020 7638 4330

### LONDON (N)

**Jane Griffiths GCC, MCA**
O ✿
**Fees:** £36–45; Second visit: £31–40
Finchley N3
020 8371 0522

**Hemi Patel GCC, BCA**
⊕ ⊛ ⊘ ✿
**Fees:** £36–45; Second visit: £21–30
London (N) N21
020 8360 0204

**Rosie Priest GCC, BAAC**
⊕ O ⊛
**Fees:** £26–35; Second visit: £21–30
London (N) N11
020 8361 0865

**Olaf Silins GCC, BCA**
⊕ ⊕ ⊛ ✿
**Fees:** £36–45; Second visit: £21–30
London (N) N12
020 8446 7575

### LONDON (NW)

**Kay McCarroll GCC, MCA**
⊕ ⊕ ✿
**Fees:** £46–55; Second visit: £31–40
London (NW) NW4
020 8202 9747

**George Rogerson GCC, MCA**
⊕ O ⊕ ✿
**Fees:** £36–45; Second visit: £31–40
London (NW) NW10, London NW4
020 8459 2903

**Thomas Zacharia GCC, BCA**
⊕ ⊛ ⊘ ✿ ⓔ
Fees: Second visit: >£50
London (NW) NW4
020 8202 1140

# Chiropractic

## LONDON (SE)

### Daniel Cheung GCC, BCA
⊕ ⊕ ❖ ⊕
Fees: £36–45; Second visit: £21–30
London (SE) SE25
020 8771 2070

### Jean-Baptist Garrone GCC, BCA
⊕ ⊕ ❖
Fees: £36–45; Second visit: £21–30
London (SE) SE3
020 8463 0607

### Daniel Harvey GCC, BAAC
⊕ ⊕ ❖
Fees: £26–35; Second visit: £21–30
London (SE) SE22
020 8693 1115

### Jagdish S Patel GCC, BCA
⊕ ⊕ ❖
Fees: <£25
London (SE) SE25
020 8653 0831

### Jen Sanders GCC, MCA
⊕ ○ ⊕ ❖
Fees: £36–45; Second visit: £21–30;
Second visit: £31–40
London (SE) SE20
020 8659 8897

## LONDON (SW)

### Adrian Audsley GCC, MCA
⊕ ○ ⊕ ⊕ ⊘ € ❖
Fees: £36–45; Second visit: £21–30
London (SW) SW12
020 86732201

### Dominic Cheetham GCC, BCA
⊕ ⊕ ⊕ ⊘ €
Fees: >£55; Second visit: £41–50
London (SW) SW1
020 7730 3031

### Julian Keel GCC, BCA
⊕ ❖
Fees: £36–45; Second visit: £21–30
London (SW) SW13,Reading RG1
020 8282 1661

### Andrew Kerklaan GCC, BCA
⊕ ⊕ ⊕ ⊕ € ❖
Fees: >£55; Second visit: £41–50
London (SW) SW1
020 7730 3031

### Anthony Kerrigan GCC, BCA
⊕ ⊕ ⊕ ❖
Fees: £26–35; Second visit: £21–30
London (SW) SW20
020 8241 2515

### Ida Norgaard GCC, BCA
⊕ ⊕ ⊕ ⊘ ❖
Fees: >£55; Second visit: £31–40
London (SW) SW7
020 7591 1929

### Anne Rampacher GCC, BCA
⊕ ⊕ ⊕
Fees: £46–55; Second visit: £21–30
London (SW) SW6
020 7731 3737

### Matthew James Stears GCC, BCA
⊕ ⊕ ⊘ ❖
Fees: £36–45; Second visit: £21–30
London (SW) SW20
020 8543 1144

### Robert Van Schalkwyk GCC, BCA
⊕ ❖ ⊕
Fees: £46–55; Second visit: £21–30
London (SW) SW6
0207 731 3737

### Stephanie Wright GCC, BCA
⊕ ⊕ ⊕ ⊘ ❖
Fees: £46–55; Second visit: £31–40
London (SW) SW3
020 7881 5800

## LONDON (W)

### Neil Austin GCC, BCA
⊕ ⊕ ⊘
Fees: £36–45; Second visit: £21–30
London (W) W1
020 7 935 8117

### Christopher Berlingieri GCC, BCA
⊕ ⊕ ⊕ ⊘ € ⊕
Fees: >£55; Second visit: £41–50
London (W) W8,London W1
020 7937 8978

# Chiropractic

**Robert Brydges GCC, BCA**
⊕ ⓝ ⊘ ⓔ ✿
**Fees:** £46–55; Second visit: £31–40
London (W) W8, London SW15
020 7937 4988

**Michael Durtnall GCC, BCA**
⊕ ⓝ ⓔ ⓖ
**Fees:** >£55; Second visit: £41–50
London (W) W8,London W1
020 7937 8978

**Stephen Hughes GCC, BCA**
⊕ ⓝ ⊘
**Fees:** £36–45; Second visit: £21–30
London (W) W6
020 8563 2608

**Johan Jeronimus GCC, BCA**
⊕ ⓝ ⊘ ✿
**Fees:** £36–45; Second visit: £21–30
London (W) W13
020 8566 3757

**Caragh Pittam GCC, BCA**
⊕ O ⊕ ⊕ ⓝ ⓔ ✿
**Fees:** £46–55; Second visit: £21–30;
Second visit: £31–40
London (W) W6, London W1,London W5
020 8741 3556

**Roger Reid GCC, BCA**
⊕ ⊕ ⓝ ⊘ ⓖ
**Fees:** £36–45; Second visit: £31–40
London (W) W2
0207 706 7003

**Alan Reid GCC, BCA**
⊕ ⊕ ⓝ ⊘ ✿ ⓖ
**Fees:** £36–45; Second visit: £31–40
London (W) W2
020 7706 7003

**Aarti Shah GCC, MCA**
⊕ O ⊕ ⓝ ✿
**Fees:** >£55; Second visit: £31–40
London W8,Stevenage SG2
020 7221 4602

**Jason Sykes GCC, BCA**
⊕ O ⊕ ⓝ ⊘
**Fees:** £46–55; Second visit: £21–30
London (W) W4
020 8994 2527

## LONDON (WC)

**Mike Piercey GCC, BAAC, MCA**
⊕ ⊕ ⊕ ⓝ ✿
**Fees:** £36–45; Second visit: £31–40
London (W) WC2
020 7379 7662

# Western Herbal Medicine

## LONDON (E)

**F Abdullah MNIMH**
⊕ ⓝ
**Fees:** £26–35; Second visit: £21–30
London (E) E4
020 8923 0892

**Sue Eldin MNIMH**
O ⊕ ⓝ ⊘ ⓔ ✿
**Fees:** £36–45; Second visit: £21–30
London (E) E1
020 7481 9376

**J Elphinstone MNIMH**
⊕ O ⊕ ⓝ
**Fees:** £26–35; Second visit: <£20
London (E) E11
020 8989 9761

**George R Foster IRCH**
⊕ ⊕ ⊘
**Fees:** £26–35; Second visit: £21–30
London (E) E17
020 8531 7188

**W Hoyland MNIMH**
⊕ O ✿
**Fees:** £36–45; Second visit: £21–30
London (E) E5
020 8806 0909

**N Hunt MNIMH**
O ⓝ ✿
**Fees:** £26–35; Second visit: £21–30
London (E) E2
020 7729 3099

# Western Herbal Medicine

**A Knowles MNIMH**
⊕ O ⊕ Ⓔ ✿
Fees: £26–35; Second visit: <£20
London (E) E1,Northampton
NN6,London NW6
020 8981 6938

**F M Mazurka MNIMH**
O ✿
Fees: £26–35; Second visit: £21–30
London (E) E5
020 8533 7674

**A M McDermott MNIMH**
⊕ O ⊕ �désᵒ ⊘ ✿
Fees: £36–45; Second visit: £21–30
London (E) E11
020 8341 7425

**S F Robbins MNIMH**
⊕ O ⊕ ⓦ ✿
Fees: £26–35; Second visit: <£20
London (E) E5
020 8806 0997

## LONDON (EC)

**R Standeven MNIMH**
⊕ ⊕ ⊕
Fees: >£55; Second visit: £31–40
London (EC) EC3
020 7283 8908

## LONDON (N)

**H Brice-Ytsma MNIMH**
ⓦ
Fees: <£25; Second visit: <£20
London (N) N19
020 8411 4411

**S Burns MNIMH**
⊕ O ⊕ ✿
Fees: £36–45; Second visit: £31–40
London (N) N1
020 8883 9773

**J Griffiths MNIMH**
O ⓦ ✿
Fees: £36–45; Second visit: £21–30
London (N) N3
020 8371 0522

**E M Holly MNIMH**
⊕ O ⊕ ⊕ ⓦ ⊘ ✿
Fees: £26–35; Second visit: £21–30
London (N) N8
020 8347 5674

**M Logue MNIMH**
⊕ ⊕ ✿
Fees: £26–35; Second visit: £21–30
London (N) N13
020 8882 3957

**Deanna Millard AMH**
O ⓦ ✿
Fees: £36–45
London (N) N16
020 7503 4672

**S H Mitchell MNIMH**
O ✿
Fees: £26–35; Second visit: £21–30
London (N) N5, Hailsham BN27
020 7690 6785

**Christine Poster IRCH**
⊕ ⓦ ✿
Fees: £36–45; Second visit: £21–30
London (N) N20
020 8446 4031

**Krishna Ramamurthy MNIMH**
⊕ O ⊕ ⊕ ✿
Fees: £26–35; Second visit: £21–30
London (N) N15
020 8808 7744

**Julia Russell AMH**
⊕ ⊕ ⓦ
Fees: £36–45; Second visit: <£20
London (N) N6
020 8348 5553

**C L Stedman MNIMH**
⊕ ⓦ ⊘ ✿
Fees: £26–35; Second visit: <£20
London (N) N9
020 8805 8180

## LONDON (NW)

**S Goddard MNIMH**
⊕ ⓦ ⊘ ✿
Fees: <£25; Second visit: <£20
London (NW) NW1
020 7916 9861

**Ruth Hajioff MNIMH**
⊕ O ⊕ ❀
Fees: £46–55; Second visit: £21–30
London (NW) NW3
020 8731 7030

**M Hayward MNIMH**
⊕ ❀
Fees: £26–35; Second visit: £21–30
London (NW) NW6
07960 241897

**Christopher Hedley MNIMH**
London (NW) NW1
020 7722 6261

**G Most MNIMH**
ⓔ
London (NW) NW3
020 7431 4292

**A Pavier MNIMH**
⊕ ⊕ ❀
Fees: £26–35; Second visit: £21–30
London (NW) NW1
020 7689 0768

**S F Robbins MNIMH**
⊕ O ⊕ ⊕ ⊛ ⊘ ❀
Fees: £46–55; Second visit: £20–30
London (NW) NW1
020 8806 0997

**E Waters MNIMH**
⊕ ⊕
Fees: £26–35; Second visit: £21–30
London (NW) NW3
020 7431 0651

## LONDON (SE)

**P J Appleton MNIMH**
⊕ O ⊕ ⊕ ⊛ ❀
Fees: <£25; Second visit: <£20
London (SE) SE15
020 7732 8980

**S Hamer MNIMH**
⊕ O ⊕ ⓔ ❀
Fees: £26–35; Second visit: £21–30
London (SE) SE12, London SE22
020 8297 8887

**Marilena Hettema MNIMH**
⊕ ⊕ ❀
Fees: £26–35; Second visit: £21–30
London (SE) SE1
020 7720 8817

**P Hoyte MNIMH**
O ❀
Fees: £26–35; Second visit: £21–30
London (SE) SE23
020 8291 3198

## LONDON (SW)

**Jessica Adams MNIMH**
O ❀
Fees: £26–35; Second visit: <£20
London (SW) SW2
020 8674 5201

**Peter Bradbury MNIMH**
O ⊛
Fees: >£55; Second visit: £41–50
London (SW) SW1
020 7834 3579

**J C Dare MNIMH**
O ⓔ ❀
Fees: £36–45; Second visit: £31–40
London (SW) SW14, Kent
020 8878 7579

**Kosara Petrovic MNIMH**
⊕ ⊛
Fees: £26–35; Second visit: <£20
London (SW) SW15
020 8876 1188

**S F Robbins MNIMH**
⊕ O ⊕ ⊛ ⊘ ❀
Fees: £46–55
London (SW) SW4
020 7720 8817

**A Williams MNIMH**
O ⊛ ⊘ ❀
Fees: £26–35; Second visit: <£20
London (SW) SW8
020 7587 1710

**N Woodward MNIMH**
⊕ ⓔ ❀
Fees: £26–35; Second visit: £21–30
London (SW) SW11
07989 968349

# Western Herbal Medicine

## LONDON (W)

### J Beaton MNIMH
✛ O ⊕ ⊘ ❈
Fees: £36–45; Second visit: £21–30
London (W) W6
020 8741 3556

### Ellie Holly MNIMH
✛ ⊕ ⊘ ❈
Fees: £36–45; Second visit: £31–40
London (W) W8, London N8
0845 1219001

### S Kippax MNIMH
✛ ⊕ ⊕ ⓝ ⊘ ❈
Fees: >£55; Second visit: £31–40
London (W) W1
020 7439 7332

### M A Mendoza MNIMH
✛ O ⊕ ⓝ ⊘
Fees: £26–35; Second visit: <£20
London (W) W1
020 7911 5041

### K M Watson Mnimh MNIMH
O ⊕ ❈
Fees: £36–45; Second visit: £21–30
London (W) W2
020 7792 8188

### D J Norden MNIMH
✛ O ⊕ ⓝ ❈
Fees: £26–35; Second visit: £21–30
London (W) W4
020 8995 5988

## LONDON (WC)

### A Syrimis MNIMH
✛ ⊕ ⊕ ⓝ ⊘
Fees: £26–35; Second visit: £21–30
London (WC) WC1
020 7813 7546

# Chinese Herbal Medicine

## LONDON (E)

### Stefan Chmelik RCHM
✛ ⊕ ⓝ ❈
Fees: >£55; Second visit: £31–40
London (E) E1
020 7247 0204

### Yan Huang RCHM
✛ ⓝ ❈
Fees: <£25; Second visit: <£20
London (E) E2
020 7729 5100

## LONDON (EC)

### Ann Bradford RCHM
✛ ⊕ ⊘
Fees: £26–35; Second visit: £21–30
London (EC) EC2
020 7729 8525

## LONDON (N)

### Kim Wells RCHM
✛ ⊕ ⓝ ❈
Fees: £26–35; Second visit: £21–30
London (N) N8, Stroud GL5
020 8340 1518

### James Cattermole RCHM
✛ ⊕ ❈
Fees: £26–35; Second visit: £31–40
London (N) N1
020 7354 8883

### Elizabeth Chang RCHM
✛ ⓝ ⊘ ❈
Fees: <£25; Second visit: <£20
London (N) N14, London N12,
London N13
020 8886 5391

**Nadine Compernolle RCHM**
➌ ⊕ ❋
**Fees:** £36–45; Second visit: £31–40
London (N) N7
020 7281 1412

**Shai Golan RCHM**
➌ O ⊕ ⊕ ⓝ ❋
**Fees:** £36–45; Second visit: £31–40
London (N) N11
020 8361 5522

**Linda Gunn-Russell RCHM**
O ⓔ ❋
**Fees:** £36–45; Second visit: £31–40
London (N) N8
020 8348 1691

**Veronica Howard RCHM**
➌ O ⊕ ❋
**Fees:** £26–35; Second visit: £21–30
London (N) N4

**Laurens Holve RCHM**
➌ ⊕ ❋
**Fees:** £26–35; Second visit: <£20
London (N) N6
020 7681 9127

**Dany Lee-Hepple RCHM**
➌ ⊕ ❋
**Fees:** £36–45; Second visit: £31–40
London (N) N7
020 7700 3897

**David Lurie RCHM**
➌ ⊕ ⓝ ⊘ ❋
**Fees:** £26–35; Second visit: £21–30
London (N) N19
020 7281 5869

**Neil Munro RCHM**
➌ ⊕ ❋
**Fees:** £26–35; Second visit: £21–30
London (N) N7
07941 339811

**Nama Ryu RCHM**
**Fees:** £26–35; Second visit: £21–30
London (N) N19
020 7272 6888

**Aki Sasaki RCHM**
➌ O ⊕ ⊕ ❋
**Fees:** £26–35; Second visit: <£20
London (N) N12
07958 280994

**Trina Ward RCHM**
➌ ⊕ ⊕ ⓝ ⓔ ❋
**Fees:** £26–35; Second visit: £31–40
London (N) N5
020 7226 1143

**Hong Yang RCHM**
⊕ ⊕ ⓝ ❋
**Fees:** £26–35; Second visit: £21–30
London (N) N11
020 8556 8843

---

## LONDON (NW)

**Rosalind Beeton RCHM**
O ⓝ ❋
**Fees:** £46–55; Second visit: £21–30
London (NW) NW11
020 8455 6184

**B LINHARES MNIMH, RCHM**
➌ O ⊕
**Fees:** £36–45; Second visit: £31–40
London (NW) NW5, London NW11
020 7485 9362

**Ana Maria Lavin-Parot RCHM**
➌ ⊕ ⓝ ⊘ ❋
**Fees:** >£55; Second visit: £21–30
London (NW) NW8
020 7722 3939

**Helen Robertson RCHM**
➌ ⊕ ⓝ ⓔ ❋
**Fees:** £36–45
London (NW) NW3
020 74832345

**Eve Rogans RCHM**
O
**Fees:** £26–35; Second visit: £21–30
London (NW) NW5
020 7813 3708

# Chinese Herbal Medicine

**Lin Jun Wen RCHM**
⊕ ❀
**Fees:** <£25; Second visit: <£20
London (NW) NW3, London NW1,
London NW11
020 7722 9808

**Fang Liang Xue RCHM**
⊕ ⬤ ❀
**Fees:** <£25; Second visit: <£20
London (NW) NW9
020 8206 2848

**Vincent Wei S Yu RCHM**
⊕ ❀
**Fees:** <£25
London (NW) NW6
020 73722184

## LONDON (SE)

**Lesley Brew RCHM**
⊕ ❀
**Fees:** £36–45; Second visit: £31–40
London (SE) SE18
020 8854 8787

**Nancy Joan Holroyde-Downing RCHM**
⊕ ⊕ ⬤ ⊘ ❀
**Fees:** >£55; Second visit: £31–40
London (SE) SE1
020 7928 8333

**Hui Lan Lin RCHM**
⊕ ⊕ ⬤ Ⓔ ❀
London (SE) SE17
020 8518 7338

**Gail Newton RCHM**
⊕ ⊕ ❀
**Fees:** £36–45; Second visit: £31–40
London (SE) SE25
020 8676 8418

**Aruna Sahni RCHM**
⊕ ⊕ ⊘ Ⓔ ❀
London (SE) SE1
020 86924148

**Mark Tittle RCHM**
⊕ ⊕ ⊕ ⊘ ❀
**Fees:** £26–35; Second visit: £21–30
London (SE) SE9, London E18 London
SE13
0208 8576000

## LONDON (SW)

**Simon Leung K Cheung RCHM**
⊕ O ⊕ ⬤ ⊘ ❀
**Fees:** £36–45; Second visit: £31–40
London (SW) SW6, Cobham KT11,
London SW18
020 7367557

**Lim Cooper RCHM**
O ⊕ ⬤ ❀
**Fees:** <£25; Second visit: <£20
London (SW) SW15
020 8789 2548

**Steve Heydt RCHM**
⊕ ⊕ ⊕ ⬤ ❀
London (SW) SW18

**Nick Johnson RCHM**
⊕ ⊕ ⬤ ❀
**Fees:** £26–35; Second visit: <£20
London (SW) SW4
020 7720 8817

**Simon Lau RCHM**
⊕
**Fees:** £26–35; Second visit: <£20
London (SW) SW19
020 7581 1118

**Mark Leopold RCHM**
⊕ ⊕ ❀
**Fees:** £26–35; Second visit: £31–40
London (SW) SW18
020 8789 5848

**S Lim-Cooper RCHM**
O ⊕ ⬤
**Fees:** <£25; Second visit: <£20
London (SW) SW15
020 8789 2548

**Xia Liu RCHM**
⊕ ⬤ ❀
**Fees:** <£25; Second visit: <£20
London (SW) SW15
020 8780 1112

**Sylvia Schroer RCHM**
🜨 ⊕ 🜨 🌑 🍀
**Fees:** £36–45; Second visit: £21–30
London (SW) SW1
020 7590 8000

**John Tindall RCHM**
🜨 🜨 🌑 🍀
**Fees:** >£55; Second visit: £31–40
London (SW) SW4
020 7622 9079

**Yong Jun Zheng RCHM**
🜨 🜨 🍀
**Fees:** £26–35; Second visit: £21–30
London (SW) SW7, London SW18
020 7244 9550

## LONDON (W)

**Susan Astbury RCHM**
🜨 🜨
**Fees:** >£55; Second visit: £31–40
London (W) W8
0207 2212266

**Linda Coviello RCHM**
O Ⓔ 🍀
London (W) W7
020 8566 4478

**Atsuko Cowley RCHM**
🜨 🜨 🍀
**Fees:** £46–55; Second visit: £31–40
London (W) W6
020 8741 9264

**Abid Dar RCHM**
🜨 🜨
**Fees:** £36–45; Second visit: £31–40
London (W) W4
020 8747 4946

**Catherine Gatacre RCHM**
O 🌑 Ⓔ
London (W) W12
020 8743 8984

**Guru Dharam S Khalsa RCHM**
🜨 ⊕ 🜨 🌑 🍀
**Fees:** £36–45; Second visit: £21–30
London (W) W1
07958 928252

**Stephen Kippax MNIMH, RCHM**
🜨 ⊕ 🜨 🌑 🍀
**Fees:** >£55; Second visit: £41–50
London (W) W1
020 7439 7332

**Tai Long RCHM**
🜨 🜨 🌑 ⊘ Ⓔ 🍀
**Fees:** £46–55; Second visit: £41–50
London (W) W11
0207 2213899

**Solveig Nielsen-Brown RCHM**
🜨 O 🜨 ⊘ 🍀
**Fees:** £36–45; Second visit: £31–40
London (W) W13
020 8567 8849

**Friedrich Staebler RCHM,**
🜨 O ⊘ 🍀
**Fees:** >£55; Second visit: £31–40
London (W) W11, London N7
020 7221 2479

**Georgina Stourton RCHM**
O 🍀
**Fees:** £26–35; Second visit: £21–30
London (W) W6 9
07970 499292

**Sharon Subner RCHM**
🜨 🜨 🌑 ⊘ 🍀
**Fees:** >£55; Second visit: >£50
London (W) W5 3
020 7792 5623

**Alan Treharne RCHM**
🜨 O 🜨 🍀
**Fees:** >£55; Second visit: >£50
London (W) W1G
020 7935 7835

**Jining Zhang RCHM**
🍀
London (W) W3 9
020 8993 6253

## LONDON (WC)

**Simeen Khoylou RCHM**
🜨 🜨 🌑 🍀
**Fees:** <£25; Second visit: <£20
London (WC) WC2H
0207 379 1312

# Chinese Herbal Medicine

**John Renshaw RCHM**
⊕ ⊕ ⊕ ⊛ ✦
Fees: £36–45; Second visit: £31–40
London (WC) WC2H
020 7379 1312

**Xing Chang Situ RCHM**
⊕ ⊕ ✦
Fees: £26–35; Second visit: £21–30
London (WC) WC2H,London
W9,Amersham HP7
020 7379 7662

**Hong Sun RCHM**
⊕ ⊕ ⊛ ⊘ ✦
Fees: <£25
London (WC) WC2H
020 7287 1086

# Ayurvedic Medicine

## LONDON (N)

**Seema R Datta AMAUK**
○ ✦
Fees: <£25; Second visit: <£20
London (N) N8 9
020 8340 0759

## LONDON (NW)

**Mauroof M Athique AMAUK**
⊕ ○ ⊕ ⊛ ⊘ ✦
Fees: £26–35; Second visit: £31–40
London (NW) NW8
020 7722 3939

**Rekhaben Depala AMAUK**
⊕ ○
Fees: £46–55; Second visit: £21–30
London (NW) NW4
020 8931 2642

## LONDON (SE)

**Amarshi Gohel AMAUK**
⊕ ○ ⊛ ✦
Fees: £26–35; Second visit: <£20
London (SE) SE21
020 8761 5252

## LONDON (SW)

**N Sathiyamoorthy AMAUK**
⊕ ⊛ ✦
Fees: £36–45; Second visit: £31–40
London (SW) SW17
020 8682 3876

**Alvi Kaushal AMAUK**
⊕ ⊕ ✦
Fees: £26–35; Second visit: <£20
Wimbledon SW19
020 8543 6826

## LONDON (W)

**Shantha Godagama AMAUK**
⊕ ⊕ ⊕ ⊛ ⊘ ✦
Fees: £26–35; Second visit: £21–30
London (W) W1N
020 7631 0156

# Greater London

North East (Enfield to Barking & Dagenham)
North West (Uxbridge to Barnet)
South East (Bexley to Croydon)
South West (Sutton to Hounslow)

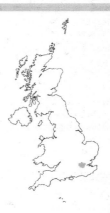

## Acupuncture

### NORTH EAST

**Daniela Matal BAcC**
⊕ ⊕ ✿ ⊜
Fees: £26–35
Dagenham RM8
020 8599 2628

**Jacqueline Fraser RCHM**
⊕ ⊕ ✿ ⊜
Fees: £26–35; Second visit: £21–30
Enfield EN2,London W4
020 8366 2300

**C Wu BAcC**
⊕ ∅ ✿ ⊜
Fees: £26–35; Second visit: £21–30
Ilford IG3
020 8598 8880

**Professor Ye Zhang BAcC**
⊕ O ⓃⒽⓈ ✿ ⊜
Fees: <£25; Second visit: £21–30
Romford RM1
01708 764909

### NORTH WEST

**Adam Leighton BAcC**
⊕ ⊕ ⊕ ✿ ⊜
Fees: £46–55; Second visit: £31–40
Barnet EN5
020 8441 0231

**Revana Swales BAcC**
O ∅ Ⓔ ✿ ⊜
Fees: £26–35; Second visit: £31–40
Barnet EN5
020 8449 0211

**Ling Wang BAcC**
⊕ ⓃⒽⓈ ✿ ⊜
Fees: £26–35; Second visit: £31–40
Barnet EN5,Gloucester GL1
020 8441 6478

**Muthuccumaru Kaneshanathan BAcC, AACP**
⊕ ⓃⒽⓈ ∅ ⊜
Fees: £26–35
Edgware HA8
020 89589820

# Acupuncture

**Rita Kalagate Vel'kalagow BAcC**
⊕ ⊘ ❀ ⓣ
**Fees:** £46–55; Second visit: £21–30
Greenford UB6
020 8991 2088

**Shipra Amin BAcC**
⊕ ⊘ ❀
**Fees:** £26–35; Second visit: £21–30
Harrow HA2
020 8868 4146

**Woeng Choong Gee RCHM**
⊕ ⓜ ⊘ ❀ ⓣ
**Fees:** £26–35; Second visit: £21–30
Harrow HA1
020 8863 1699

**Anna Colmer BAcC**
⊕ ⊕ ⊕ ❀ ⓣ
**Fees:** £46–55; Second visit: £31–40
Harrow HA3
020 8563 8133

**Qian Feng Huang BAcC**
⊕ ⓔ ❀ ⓣ
**Fees:** £26–35; Second visit: £21–30
Harrow HA2
020 8429 3535

**Anand Marshall BAcC**
⊕ ⊕ ⊕ ❀ ⓣ
**Fees:** £26–35; Second visit: £21–30
Harrow HA2
020 8861 4280

**Indira Patel BAcC**
⊕
**Fees:** £26–35; Second visit: £21–30
Harrow HA3
020 8907 6542

**Minerva O P Singh BAcC**
⊕ ❀ ⓣ
**Fees:** £26–35; Second visit: £21–30
Harrow HA1
020 8861 1839

**Y Zhou BAcC**
⊕ ⊘ ❀
**Fees:** <£25; Second visit: <£20
Harrow HA1
020 8930 9236

**J Thoeye BAcC**
⊕ ⊕ ⊕ ⊕ ⊘ ⓔ ❀ ⓣ
**Fees:** £36–45; Second visit: £31–40
Harrow on the Hill HA2, London W4,
Harrow HA1
020 8423 1570

**Surendrakumar Patel BAcC**
⊕ ⊕ ⓣ
**Fees:** £26–35; Second visit: £21–30
Hayes UB3
020 8561 0819

**Maher Succar BAcC**
⊕ ⊕ ⊕ ⊕ ❀ ⓣ
**Fees:** £36–45; Second visit: £41–50
Hayes UB3
020 8450 2292

**J S Bansal BAcC**
⊕ ⊕ ⓣ
**Fees:** £26–35; Second visit: £31–40
Northwood HA6
07973 667213

**Davinder Sohal BAcC**
⊕ ⊕ ⊕ ⓜ ❀ ⓣ
**Fees:** £26–35; Second visit: £21–30
Southall UB1
020 8843 0666

**N N V O'Sullivan BAcC, BMAS,**
⊕ ❀ ⓣ
**Fees:** £36–45; Second visit: £21–30
Stanmore HA7
020 8954 1333

**Margaret Romer AACP**
⊕ ⊘ ❀ ⓣ
**Fees:** £36–45; Second visit: £31–40
Stanmore HA7
07050 038954

**Juliette Ros BMAS,**
⊕ ⊘ ❀ ⓣ
**Fees:** £26–35; Second visit: £21–30
Stanmore HA7
020 8954 1851

**Beverley De Valois BAcC**
⊕ ⊕ ❀ ⓣ
**Fees:** £26–35; Second visit: £21–30
Uxbridge UB8
01895 231772

**Yizhen Jia BAcC**

⊕ ⊕ ⊕ ❀ ⊕
Fees: £36–45; Second visit: £21–30;
Second visit: £31–40
Uxbridge UB10,London EC2A
01895 230519

**Melanie Pottle BAcC**

⊕ ⊕ ⊕ ❀ ⊕
Fees: £36–45; Second visit: £31–40
Wembley HA0
020 8904 3212

**Yong Chai Siow BAcC**

O ⊕ ❀ ⊕
Fees: £26–35; Second visit: £21–30
Wembley HA9
020 89049388

## SOUTH EAST

**Emma Chambers AACP**

O ⊘ ⊕
Fees: £36–45; Second visit: £21–30
Beckenham BR3
020 8466 6911

**Rao Kadambari BAcC, BMAS,**

⊕ ❀ ⊕
Fees: <£25; Second visit: <£20
Beckenham BR3,London SW11,London SW17
020 8658 5627

**Jonathan Sourcott BAcC**

⊕ ⊕ ❀ ⊕
Fees: £36–45; Second visit: £21–30
Beckenham BR3,London SE16
020 8402 7265

**Ilkay Zihni Chirali BAcC**

O ❀ ⊕
Fees: £26–35; Second visit: £21–30
Bexleyheath DA6
020 8306 6736

**Denise Callaghan BAcC**

⊕ ❀ ⊕
Fees: £26–35; Second visit: £21–30
Bromley BR1
020 8313 0510

**Craig Minto BAcC**

⊕ O ⊕ ❀ ⊕
Fees: £26–35; Second visit: £21–30
Bromley BR1
020 8464 2544

**Terry Simou BAcC**

⊕ ⊕ ❀ ⊕
Fees: £36–45; Second visit: £21–30
Bromley BR1
020 8313 1577

**Baifang Zhu BAcC**

⊕ ⊕ ❀ ⊕
Fees: £26–35; Second visit: £21–30
Bromley BR1,Beckenham BR3
020 8290 4688

**Tosca Zuidyk BAcC**

Fees: £36–45; Second visit: £21–30
Bromley BR2
020 8467 9001

**Gillian Allsop BAcC**

⊕ O ⊕ ⊕
Fees: £36–45; Second visit: £21–30
Chislehurst BR7
020 8295 0893

**Clare Stenner AACP**

⊕ ⊕ ❀ ⊕
Fees: £36–45; Second visit: £31–40
Coulsdon CR5
020 8660 8070

**Anthony Booker BAcC**

⊕ ⊕ ❀ ⊕
Fees: £26–35; Second visit: £21–30
Dartford DA2
07966 474722

**Robyn Selby AACP**

⊕ ⊕ ⊘ ❀ ⊕
Fees: £26–35; Second visit: £31–40
Orpington BR6
01689 852483

**Lifei Zhang BAcC**

⊕ ⊕ ❀ ⊕
Fees: <£25; Second visit: <£20
Purley CR8
020 8763 1119

# Acupuncture

**Sally Dixon BAcC**

**Fees:** £36–45; Second visit: £21–30
Sidcup DA14,Crawley RH10
020 8302 2624

**David Wilson BAcC**

Denham UB9
01895 834213

## SOUTH WEST

**Po Chi-Kin BAcC**

**Fees:** £26–35
Carshalton SM5
020 8646 7697

**Peter Warwick BAcC**

**Fees:** £36–45; Second visit: £21–30
Carshalton SM5
020 8647 4135

**Steven J Ash BAcC**

**Fees:** >£55; Second visit: £41–50;
Second visit: >£50
Effingham KT24,Cranleigh GU6
01483 281428

**Po-Yee Wong BAcC**

**Fees:** £46–55; Second visit: £31–40
Feltham TW14
020 8890 8008

**Barrie Stone BAcC**

**Fees:** £36–45; Second visit: £31–40
Kingston Upon Thames KT2
020 8549 7401

**Won-Kyu Kim BAcC**

**Fees:** £26–35; Second visit: £21–30
New Malden KT3
020 8949 3888

**Ute Wilde BAcC**

**Fees:** £26–35; Second visit: £21–30
New Malden KT3
020 89490557

**Pamela R Davis BAcC**

**Fees:** £26–35; Second visit: £31–40
Sunbury-on-Thames TW16
01932 785815

**Stephanie Mills BAcC**

**Fees:** £36–45; Second visit: £21–30
Surbiton KT5
020 8399 3215

**Alicia Grant BAcC, AACP**

**Fees:** £36–45; Second visit: £31–40
Sutton SM2
020 8770 0018

**Toon Min BAcC**

**Fees:** £26–35; Second visit: £21–30
Sutton SM2
020 8661 6168

**Aideen O'Sullivan BAcC**

**Fees:** £36–45; Second visit: £31–40
Sutton SM1
020 8642 2307

**David Penwarden BAcC**

**Fees:** £26–35; Second visit: £21–30
Sutton SM2
020 8642 6639

**P A Brougham BMAS,**

**Fees:** £26–35; Second visit: £21–30
Teddington TW11,Sutton SM1
020 8943 2424

**Greg Dorn BAcC**

**Fees:** £46–55; Second visit: £31–40
Twickenham TW1,Hampton
TW12,Teddington TW11
020 8941 0966

**Richard Wegrzyk BAcC**

**Fees:** £26–35; Second visit: £21–30
Twickenham TW1
07973 184427

## Acupuncture

**David Campbell BAMS**
⊕ ⓦ ⊘ ✿
**Fees:** £26–35; Second visit: £21–30
Croydon CR0
020 8656 9573

## Homeopathy

### NORTH EAST

**Lesley Isaacson RSHom**
O ⓔ ✿
**Fees:** >£55; Second visit: £41–50
Ruislip HA4
01895 639942

### NORTH WEST

**Sally Ann Hutcheson RSHom**
⊕ O ⊕ ⓦ ⓔ ✿
**Fees:** >£55; Second visit: £31–40
Barnet EN5
020 8446 7935

**Glenda Fraser RSHom**
O ⓦ ⓔ ✿
**Fees:** >£55; Second visit: £31–40
Harrow HA2
020 8423 3071

**Jane Gathercole RSHom**
O ⓦ ⓔ ✿
**Fees:** £46–55; Second visit: £31–40
Harrow HA1
020 8621 0931

**Mina Mehta RSHom**
⊕ O ⓦ ⓔ ✿
**Fees:** £46–55; Second visit: £20–30
Northwood HA6
01923 822750

**Jyoti Pathak RSHom**
O ⓦ ✿
**Fees:** >£55; Second visit: £31–40
Wembley HA9
020 8904 8049

### SOUTH EAST

**Patricia Macrae RSHom**
⊕ O ⊕ ⓦ ⓔ
**Fees:** £36–45; Second visit: £20–30
Beckenham BR3, Bromley BR2, London SE12
020 8289 2378

**Moira Ruth RSHom**
⊕ O ⓦ ✿
**Fees:** >£55; Second visit: £31–40
Beckenham BR3, Orpington BR6
020 86909375

**Janice Micallef RSHom**
O ⓦ ✿
**Fees:** >£55; Second visit: £31–40
Bexley DA5
01322 558334

**Linda Peacock RSHom**
⊕ O ⊕ ⓦ ⓔ ✿
**Fees:** £46–55; Second visit: £20–30
Bromley BR1, Caterham CR3
020 8325 9503

**Ingrid Daniels RSHom**
⊕ O ⊕ ⓦ ⓔ ✿
**Fees:** £46–55; Second visit: £31–40
Carshalton SM5, South Croydon CR2
020 83956550

**Poonam Sharma MFHom**
⊕ ⓦ ⊘
**Fees:** >£55; Second visit: £31–40
Chislehurst BR7
07956 827160

**Tom Meeneghan RSHom**
⊕ O ⓦ ⓔ ✿
**Fees:** £25–35; Second visit: £20–30
Croydon CR0
020 8688 7588

# Homeopathy

### Sandra Baker RSHom
⊕ ◐ ⊕ ⊚ ⓔ ❁
**Fees:** £36–45; Second visit: £20–30
Orpington BR6,Gillingham
01689 898787

### Pat Bromley RSHom
⊕ ⊕ ⊚ ⓔ ❁
**Fees:** £36–45; Second visit: £20–30
West Wickham BR4
020 8776 1525

### Paul Burnett RSHom
⊕ ⊕ ⊚ ❁
**Fees:** £36–45; Second visit: £20–30
West Wickham BR4
020 87762536

### Marian Byham RSHom
⊕ ◐ ⊕ ⊚ ⊘ ⓔ ❁
**Fees:** £36–45; Second visit: £20–30
West Wickham BR4
020 8776 1525

## SOUTH WEST

### Brenda McBride RSHom
◐ ⊚ ❁
**Fees:** £46–55; Second visit: £31–40
Cheam SM2
020 8786 8812

### Frances Penwarden RSHom
⊕ ⊕ ⊚ ⓔ ❁
**Fees:** £36–45; Second visit: £20–30
Cheam SM2
020 8642 6639

### Jacqueline Olesker RSHom
◐ ⊚ ⓔ ❁
**Fees:** £36–45; Second visit: £20–30
Feltham TW13
020 8707 1784

### Christine Collins RSHom
⊕ ◐ ⊚
**Fees:** £36–45; Second visit: £31–40
Hampton TW12,Slough SL1
020 8941 2016

### Doy Dalling RSHom
⊕ ◐ ⊕ ⊚ ⓔ ❁
**Fees:** £46–55; Second visit: £31–40
Hampton TW12,Richmond
TW9,Ashford TW15
020 8979 0497

### Meike Lawrence RSHom
⊕ ◐ ❁
**Fees:** £36–45; Second visit: £20–30
Kingston KT2
020 8541 1319

### Kerry Larkman RSHom
⊕ ◐ ⊕ ⊚ ⓔ ❁
**Fees:** >£55; Second visit: £20–30
Long Ditton KT6
020 8398 0263

### Justin W Blake-James MFHom
⊕ ◐ ⊕ ⊚ ⊘ ⓔ ❁
**Fees:** >£55; Second visit: £41–50
Richmond TW9,Cambridge
CB4,Sudbury CO10
020 8940 2802

### Annie Gould RSHom
◐ ⊚ ⊘ ❁
**Fees:** £46–55; Second visit: £31–40
Richmond TW9
020 8404 7636

### Stephne Monaghan RSHom
◐ ⊚ ⓔ
**Fees:** £46–55; Second visit: £20–30
Richmond TW10
020 8948 4702

### Annette Gamblin RSHom
⊕ ⊕ ⊚ ⓔ ❁
**Fees:** >£55; Second visit: £31–40
Surbiton KT6
020 8399 2772

### Sylvia Neubacher RSHom
⊕ ◐ ⊕ ⊚ ⓔ ❁
**Fees:** £46–55; Second visit: £31–40
Surbiton KT6
020 8941 4334

### Erica Gustavsson RSHom
◐ ⊕ ⊕ ⊚ ⓔ ❁
**Fees:** £36–45; Second visit: £20–30
Teddington TW11
020 8977 6140

# Homeopathy

**Anne Hetherton RSHom**
⊕ O ⊕ ⦿ ❀
**Fees:** >£55; Second visit: £41–50
Teddington TW11,
35a Welbeck Street W1M
020 8977 7530

**David Weiss RSHom**
O ⦿ ❀
**Fees:** £36–45; Second visit: £20–30
Teddington TW11
020 8943 9573

**Cathy Bland RSHom**
⊕ ⊕ € ❀
**Fees:** £36–45; Second visit: £31–40
Twickenham TW1,Isleworth TW7
020 8891 5762

**Christina Isis RSHom**
⊕ O ⊕ ⦿ € ❀
**Fees:** £36–45; Second visit: £20–30
Twickenham TW2
020 8408 1746

**Roger Sharpley RSHom**
⊕ ⊕ ⊕ ⦿ ❀
**Fees:** £36–45; Second visit: £31–40
Twickenham TW2
020 8898 1952

**Carolyn Festa RSHom**
O ⦿ € ❀
**Fees:** >£55; Second visit: £20–30
Walton-on-Thames KT12
01932 252899

# Osteopathy

### NORTH EAST

**Lindsey Howley GOsC, BOA**
⊕ ⦿ ❀
**Fees:** £26–35; Second visit: £21–30
Barking IG11
020 8591 2406

**John Yeboah GOsC, BOA**
⊕ ⊕ ❀
**Fees:** £26–35; Second visit: £21–30
Enfield EN1
020 8482 1112

**Andria Marchant GOsC, BOA**
O ⦿ ❀
**Fees:** <£25; Second visit: £21–30
Enfield EN2
020 8367 4054

**Elizabeth Bagley GOsC, BOA**
O ⦿ ❀
**Fees:** £26–35; Second visit: £21–30
Hornchurch RM12
01708 621119

**Colin Crowder GOsC, BOA**
O ⦿ ⊘ ❀
**Fees:** <£25; Second visit: £21–30
Ilford IG1
020 8554 3849

**George Foster GOsC, BOA**
⊕ O ⦿ ❀
**Fees:** £26–35; Second visit: £21–30
Ilford IG4
020 8550 2552

**Jonathan Friend GOsC**
⊕ ⦿ ❀
**Fees:** £26–35; Second visit: £21–30
Ilford IG4
020 8550 0982

**John Kirkwood GOsC, BOA**
⊕ ⊕ ⦿ ⊘ ❀
**Fees:** <£25; Second visit: £21–30
Rainham RM13
01708 551771

**Louise Alexander GOsC, BOA**
⊕ ⦿ ❀
**Fees:** £26–35; Second visit: <£20
Romford RM1
01708 762441

**Emma Chippendale GOsC, BOA**
⊕ ⦿ ❀
**Fees:** <£25; Second visit: £41–50
Romford RM1
01708 762441

# Osteopathy

### Daraius Cooper GOsC
✚ O Ⓔ ❖
**Fees:** £26–35; Second visit: £21–30
Romford RM1
01708 762441

### Colin I Dove GOsC
✚ ⊕ ⊘
**Fees:** <£25; Second visit: £21–30
Romford RM1
01708 762441

### Roy Knightbridge GOsC
✚ ⓝ ⊘ ❖
**Fees:** <£25; Second visit: £21–30
Romford RM1
01708 762441

### David Langford GOsC
✚ O ⊕ ⓝ ❖
**Fees:** £26–35; Second visit: £21–30
Romford RM16
01375 382308

### Jeffrey Grumball GOsC
✚ ⓝ ❖
**Fees:** £26–35; Second visit: £21–30
Upminster RM14
01708 227888

### Lorne Gutteridge GOsC, BOA
ⓝ ❖
**Fees:** £26–35; Second visit: £21–30
Upminster RM14
01708 227786

### Christopher Thomas GOsC
✚ ⓝ
**Fees:** £26–35; Second visit: £21–30
Upminster RM14
01708 227888

## NORTHWEST

### Marcus Webb GOsC, BOA
✚ ⊕ ⓝ ❖
**Fees:** £26–35; Second visit: £21–30
Barnet EN4
020 8441 8352

### Melvyn Eyres GOsC
✚ O ⓝ ❖
**Fees:** £36–45; Second visit: £31–40
Barnet EN5
020 8449 3746

### Hilary Hubbers GOsC, BOA
O ⓝ ❖
**Fees:** <£25; Second visit: £41–50
Edgware HA8
020 8952 2197

### Sophie King GOsC, BOA
✚ ⊕ ⓝ ⊘ ❖
**Fees:** £26–35; Second visit: £21–30
Edgware HA8
020 8905 4427

### Davinder Sohal GOsC
✚ ⊕ ⊕ ⓝ ⊘ ❖
**Fees:** £26–35; Second visit: £21–30
Edgware HA8
020 8732 6210

### Caroline Weber GOsC
O ⊘
**Fees:** £26–35; Second visit: £31–40
Edgware HA8
020 8958 1948

### Annika Adodra GOsC,
⊕ ⊕ ⓝ ❖
**Fees:** £26–35; Second visit: £21–30
Greenford UB6
020 8575 8058

### Emma Shanahan GOsC
✚ ⓝ ❖
**Fees:** £26–35; Second visit: £21–30
Harrow HA1
020 8427 8811

### Jan Thoeye GOsC
✚ ⊕ ⓝ ⊘ ❖
**Fees:** £36–45; Second visit: £31–40
Harrow HA1
020 8861 1221

### Shipra Amin GOsC
O Ⓔ ❖
**Fees:** £26–35; Second visit: £21–30
Harrow HA2
020 8868 4146

### Khalid Mughal GOsC, BOA
✚ O ⊕ ⓝ ⊘ ❖
**Fees:** £36–45; Second visit: £31–40
Harrow HA2
020 8864 5615

**Ian Bird GOsC**
O · ⬤

**Fees:** £36–45; Second visit: £21–30
Harrow HA3
020 8954 4394

**Jayant Joshi GOsC**
O · ⬤ · ⬤

**Fees:** £26–35; Second visit: £21–30
Harrow HA3
020 8907 1660

**Tony Vogel GOsC**
⬤ · ⬤ · ⬤ · ⬤

**Fees:** £26–35; Second visit: £21–30
Ickenham UB10
01895 631945

**Jonathan McSwiney GOsC**
⬤ · ⬤ · ⬤

**Fees:** £26–35; Second visit: £21–30
Northolt UB5
020 8841 5611

**Aileen A Fenn GOsC, BOA**
O · ⬤ · ⬤ · ⬤

**Fees:** <£25; Second visit: £21–30
Northwood HA6
01923 827756

**Jeremy Gilbey GOsC**
⬤ · ⬤ · ⬤

**Fees:** £46–55; Second visit: £31–40
Northwood HA6
01923 827833

**Fiona Robertson GOsC, BOA**
⬤ · ⬤ · ⬤ · ⬤

**Fees:** £26–35; Second visit: £21–30
Northwood HA6
01923 828832

**C Mote GOsC**
O · ⬤ · ⬤ · ⬤ · ⬤

**Fees:** £36–45; Second visit: £21–30
Pinner HA5
020 8868 9315

**Jessica Ovett GOsC**
⬤ · ⬤ · ⬤ · ⬤

**Fees:** £36–45; Second visit: £21–30
Pinner HA5
020 8868 0239

**Kwok Yau GOsC**
⬤ · ⬤ · ⬤ · ⬤ · ⬤

**Fees:** £26–35; Second visit: £21–30
Pinner HA5
020 8202 2386

**Dani Godfrey GOsC, BOA**
⬤ · ⬤ · ⬤ · ⬤ · ⬤ · ⬤

**Fees:** £26–35; Second visit: £31–40
Ruislip HA4
020 8422 4163

**Anne Wright GOsC, BOA**
⬤ · ⬤ · ⬤ · ⬤

**Fees:** <£25; Second visit: £21–30
Ruislip HA4
01895 677179

**John Bird GOsC**
⬤ · ⬤ · ⬤ · ⬤

**Fees:** £36–45; Second visit: £31–40
Stanmore HA7
020 8907 3997

**Irving Boxer GOsC**
O · ⬤ · ⬤ · ⬤

**Fees:** £36–45; Second visit: £21–30
Stanmore HA7
020 8954 2254

**M Mirza GOsC, BOA,**
⬤ · O · ⬤ · ⬤ · ⬤ · ⬤

**Fees:** £36–45; Second visit: £31–40
Stanmore HA7
020 8427 3268

**Pragna Patel GOsC, BOA**
⬤ · ⬤ · ⬤ · ⬤

**Fees:** £26–35; Second visit: £21–30
Wembley HA0
020 8908 2979

## SOUTH EAST

**Vincent Barnes GOsC**
⬤ · O · ⬤ · ⬤

**Fees:** <£25; Second visit: £21–30
Beckenham BR3
020 8650 5001

**Jacqueline Ellison GOsC**
O · ⬤

**Fees:** £26–35; Second visit: £21–30
Beckenham BR3
020 8650 3831

# Osteopathy

**Lady Audrey Percival GOsC, BOA**
O ⬤ Ⓝ Ⓔ ❀
Fees: <£25; Second visit: <£20
Beckenham BR3
020 8650 4313

**Justin Sharp GOsC**
⊕ ❀
Fees: £26–35; Second visit: £21–30
Beckenham BR3
020 8658 3308

**James Smith GOsC**
⊕ Ⓝ ❀
Fees: <£25; Second visit: £21–30
Beckenham BR3
020 86505432

**John Roberts GOsC**
⊕ O Ⓝ ❀
Fees: £26–35; Second visit: £21–30
Belvedere DA17
01322 436436

**Remi Baudriboc GOsC, BOA**
⊕ ⊕ Ⓑ Ⓝ ❀
Fees: £26–35; Second visit: £21–30
Bexley DA5
01322 529326

**Dawn Draper GOsC**
⊕ O Ⓝ ❀
Fees: £26–35; Second visit: £21–30
Bexley DA5
01322 529326

**Jason Gunn GOsC, BOA**
⊕ Ⓑ Ⓝ ❀
Fees: £26–35; Second visit: £21–30
Bexley DA5
01322 527292

**Mayuri Kalidas GOsC, BOA**
⊕ ⊕ Ⓑ Ⓝ ⊘ ❀
Fees: £36–45; Second visit: £21–30
Bexley DA5
020 8882 2161

**Graeme Western GOsC, BOA**
⊕ Ⓝ ❀
Fees: £36–45; Second visit: £31–40
Bexley DA5
01322 529326

**Hilary Whitaker GOsC, BOA**
⊕ Ⓝ ❀
Fees: £26–35; Second visit: £21–30
Bexley DA5
01322 529326

**Rishi Angras GOsC**
⊕ ⊕ ❀
Fees: £26–35; Second visit: £21–30
Bromley BR1
020 8466 8844

**Anne Bones GOsC, BOA**
⊕ Ⓑ
Fees: £26–35; Second visit: £21–30
Bromley BR1
020 8313 1577

**Denise Callaghan GOsC, BOA**
⊕ O Ⓝ ❀
Fees: £26–35; Second visit: £21–30
Bromley BR1
020 8717 0510

**Charles Read GOsC, BOA**
⊕ Ⓑ Ⓝ ⊘ ❀
Fees: <£25; Second visit: £21–30
Bromley BR1
020 8467 4451

**Sylvie Falgairolle GOsC**
⊕ ❀
Fees: <£25; Second visit: £21–30
Bromley BR5
01689 827247

**Simon Tolson GOsC**
O ⬤ Ⓔ ❀
Fees: <£25; Second visit: £21–30
Bromley BR5
01689 827247

**Ruth Godec GOsC, BOA**
⊕ Ⓑ Ⓝ ❀
Fees: <£25; Second visit: £21–30
Chislehurst BR7
020 8295 0893

**Khalid Haq GOsC**
⊕ Ⓑ Ⓔ ❀
Fees: £26–35; Second visit: £21–30
Croydon CR2
020 8651 4071

**Hazel Silverstone GOsC, BOA**
➕ 🔵 Ⓔ
Fees: £26–35; Second visit: £31–40
Purley CR8
020 8660 6632

**John Silverstone GOsC, BOA**
➕ 🔵 Ⓔ 🔴
Fees: £26–35; Second visit: £31–40
Purley CR8
020 8660 6632

**Charles Smith GOsC, BOA**
➕ ⭕ ⊕ 🔵 ⊘ 🔴
Fees: £36–45; Second visit: £31–40
Purley CR8
020 8660 4086

**Jo-Anne Holmden GOsC**
⭕ 🔵 ⊘ 🔴
Fees: £26–35; Second visit: £21–30
Orpington BR6
01689 897354

**Nigel D Kettle GOsC, BOA**
➕ 🔵 🔴
Fees: <£25; Second visit: £21–30
Orpington BR6
01689 878508

**Julie Swann GOsC, BOA**
➕ ⊕ 🔵 ⊘ 🔴
Fees: £26–35; Second visit: £21–30
Orpington BR6
01634 878508

**Peter Sanders GOsC**
⭕ 🔵 🔴
Fees: £26–35; Second visit: £21–30
Orpington BR5
01689 876582

**Catherine Ashworth GOsC**
➕ 🔵 🔴
Fees: £26–35; Second visit: £21–30
Orpington BR6
01689 878508

**Moira Guth GOsC**
➕ ⊕ 🔵 ⊘ 🔴
Fees: £26–35; Second visit: £21–30
Sidcup DA14
020 8302 2624

**Ronald White GOsC, BOA**
➕ ⊕ 🔵 🔴
Fees: £26–35; Second visit: £21–30
Welling DA16
07811 842288

## SOUTH WEST

**L J Bailey GOsC, BOA**
➕ ⊕ 🔵 🔴
Fees: <£25; Second visit: £21–30
Carshalton SM5
020 8669 3818

**Nik Patel GOsC, BOA**
➕ 🔵 ⊘ 🔴
Fees: <£25; Second visit: £21–30
Feltham TW13
020 8890 3789

**Lesley Stockton GOsC, BOA**
⭕ 🔵 Ⓔ 🔴
Fees: £26–35; Second visit: £21–30
Feltham TW13
020 8890 3789

**Alan Patrick Burke GOsC, BOA**
➕ ⭕ ⊕ ⊕ 🔵 🔴
Fees: <£25; Second visit: £21–30
Feltham TW14
07932 040395

**Anthony Williams GOsC**
➕ ⭕ ⊕ ⊕ 🔵 🔴
Fees: £36–45; Second visit: £31–40
Hampton TW12
07958 745668

**Perry Lutz GOsC**
➕ 🔵 🔴
Fees: £36–45; Second visit: £21–30
Hampton TW12
020 8979 4519

**Gloria Elaine Best-John GOsC, BO**
⭕ 🔵 🔴
Fees: £26–35; Second visit: £21–30
Hayes UB3
020 8848 1425

**Suru Patel GOsC**
➕ ⭕ ⊕ 🔵
Fees: £26–35; Second visit: £21–30
Hayes UB3
020 8561 0819

# Osteopathy

**Satpal S Bansal GOsC**
⊕ ⊕ ⊘ ✿
Fees: £26–35; Second visit: £21–30
Hounslow TW3
020 8577 9731

**Gillian Craigie GOsC, BOA**
⊕ ⊕ ⊕ ⊕
Fees: £36–45; Second visit: £21–30
Hounslow TW3
020 8814 0894

**Anthony Walker GOsC**
Fees: £26–35; Second visit: £21–30
Isleworth TW7
Isleworth TW7
020 8560 7073

**Lisa A Gibbs GOsC, BOA**
⊕ ⊕ ✿
Fees: <£25; Second visit: £31–40
New Malden KT3
020 8942 1511

**Dominick Hussey GOsC**
⊕ ⊕ € ✿
Fees: £36–45; Second visit: £21–30
New Malden KT3
020 8942 3148

**Anne Faichney GOsC, BOA**
⊕ ⊕ ⊕ ⊕ ⊘ ✿
Fees: <£25; Second visit: £21–30
Richmond TW9
020 8332 6184

**Robert Kulesza GOsC, BOA**
⊕ O ⊘
Fees: £46–55; Second visit: £31–40
Richmond-upon-Thames TW9
020 8940 4861

**Brian Pattinson GOsC, BOA,**
⊕ ⊕ ✿
Fees: >£55; Second visit: >£50
Richmond-upon-Thames TW9
020 8332 6184

**Enayat-Ullah Erfan GOsC, BOA**
⊕ O ⊕ ⊘ ✿
Fees: £26–35; Second visit: £21–30
Southall UB1
020 8574 1459

**Basharat Ahmed Kaifi GOsC**
O ⊕ ⊘ ✿
Fees: <£25; Second visit: £21–30
Southall UB1
020 8813 8434

**Baldev Singh Dhillon GOsC, BOA**
O ⊕ ✿
Fees: <£25; Second visit: £21–30
Southall UB2
020 8574 0833

**John O'Connor GOsC, BOA**
⊕ O ⊘ ✿
Fees: £26–35; Second visit: £21–30
Staines TW18
01784 457364

**Helen Allport GOsC**
O
Fees: £36–45; Second visit: £31–40
Surbiton KT6
020 8398 2559

**Kathy O'Callaghan-Brown GOsC**
⊕ ⊕ ✿
Fees: <£25; Second visit: £21–30
Surbiton KT6
020 8397 5585

**Carolyn Peirce GOsC**
O ⊕ ⊕ ⊕ ✿
Fees: £26–35; Second visit: £31–40
Surbiton KT6
020 8399 2689

**Pinal Patel GOsC, BOA**
⊕ O
Fees: £26–35; Second visit: £21–30
Sutton SM6, London W1H
020 8669 3967

**David Penwarden GOsC**
O ⊕ ⊕ € ✿
Fees: <£25; Second visit: £21–30
Sutton SM2
020 8642 6639

**Martin Chorley GOsC, BOA**
⊕ ✿
Fees: £26–35; Second visit: £21–30
Teddington TW11
020 8977 2714

# Osteopathy

**Alexis Sims GOsC**
Fees: £26–35; Second visit: £21–30
Teddington TW11
020 8977 9859

**Jill Nickalls GOsC**
Fees: £36–45; Second visit: £31–40
Twickenham TW1
020 8892 8434

**Jenny Wolfenden GOsC**
Fees: £36–45; Second visit: £21–30
Twickenham TW1
020 8891 3400

**Katy Austin GOsC, BOA**
Fees: <£25; Second visit: £21–30
Twickenham TW1
020 8744 2450

**Rosalyn Foster GOsC**
Fees: <£25; Second visit: £21–30
Twickenham TW16
01932 789779

**Samantha Hurst GOsC**
Fees: £26–35; Second visit: £21–30
Twickenham TW2
020 8893 3084

**Nilesh Patel GOsC**
Fees: £26–35; Second visit: £21–30
Twickenham TW2
020 8755 3828

**Ferida Mistry GOsC**
Fees: £26–35; Second visit: £21–30
Twickenham TW7
020 8847 4542

**Joanna Wildy GOsC**
Fees: £26–35; Second visit: £31–40
Twickenham TW9
020 8940 1010

**Philip Allen GOsC, BOA**
Fees: £36–45; Second visit: £31–40
Twickenham TW9,Prestwood Great
Missenden HP16
020 8948 3144

**Janine Leach GOsC, BOA**
Fees: £26–35; Second visit: £21–30
Wallington SM6
020 8773 1106

**Carolyn Felton GOsC, BOA**
Fees: <£25; Second visit: £21–30
Worcester Park KT4
020 8715 1145

**Irene Phillips GOsC, BOA**
Fees: £46–55; Second visit: £31–40
Worcester Park KT4
020 8335 3787

**Zygmund Tatarkowski GOsC, BOA**
Fees: <£25; Second visit: £21–30
Croydon CR0
020 8680 2228

# Chiropractic

## NORTH EAST

**Wendy Hickleton GCC, BCA**
Fees: £26–35; Second visit: £21–30
Enfield EN4
020 8449 3300

**Paul Tibbitts GCC, MCA**
Fees: £36–45; Second visit: £21–30
Ilford IG10
020 8508 8257

# Chiropractic

## NORTH WEST

**Annette Dypping GCC, BCA**
➕ ⊕ ⓝ ⊘ ✿
Fees: £36–45; Second visit: £21–30
Barnet EN5
020 8441 0231

**Christopher A Pickard GCC, BCA**
➕ ⦿ ⓝ ✿
Fees: £36–45; Second visit: £21–30
Barnet EN4
020 8275 0656

**Rowen Simpson GCC, BCA**
➕ ✿
Fees: £36–45; Second visit: £21–30
East Barnet EN4,Barnet EN4
020 8275 0656

**Carl Irwin GCC, BCA**
➕ ⓝ ⊘ ✿ ⓔ
Fees: £26–35; Second visit: £21–30
Edgware HA8
020 8906 3323

**Sandra Richer GCC, BCA**
➕ ⓝ ⊘ ✿
Fees: £36–45; Second visit: £21–30
Edgware HA8
020 8343 1234

**Kishorelal Adatia GCC, BCA**
➕ ⊘ ✿
Fees: £26–35; Second visit: £21–30
Harrow HA5
020 8868 1631

**Richard Cook GCC, BCA**
⦿ ⓝ ⊘ ⓔ ✿
Fees: <£25; Second visit: £21–30
Harrow HA1
020 8864 6768

**Connell Carlin Dorrian GCC, BCA**
➕ ⓝ ⊘ ✿ ⓔ
Fees: £46–55; Second visit: £21–30
Harrow HA
020 8427 2133

**Lalit Sodha GCC, BCA**
➕ ⓝ ⊘ ⓔ
Fees: £36–45; Second visit: £21–30
Pinner HA5
020 8868 5020

**Gail Willmott GCC, BAAC**
➕ ⊕ ⓝ ✿
Fees: £36–45; Second visit: £31–40
Ruislip HA4,London WC2H
01895 634381

**Claudio Merkier GCC, BCA**
➕ ⓝ ⊘ ✿
Fees: £36–45; Second visit: £21–30
Watford WD6,Borehamwood WD6
020 8953 4515

## SOUTH EAST

**Kevin England GCC, MCA**
➕ ⦿ ⊕ ⓝ ⊘ ✿
Fees: £36–45; Second visit: £21–30
Croydon CR0
020 8654 4422

**Krisjanis Krumins GCC, BCA**
➕ ⓝ ✿
Fees: £36–45; Second visit: £21–30
Dartford DA7
020 8301 5859

**Liam McLaughlin GCC, BCA**
➕ ⓔ
Fees: £46–55; Second visit: £21–30
Purley CR8
020 8763 2629

## SOUTH WEST

**Joanne Archer GCC, MCA**
➕ ⦿ ⓝ ⊘ ✿
Fees: £36–45; Second visit: £21–30
Kingston-on-Thames KT2
020 8549 5669

**Helen Bartlett GCC, BCA**
➕ ⓝ ⓔ ✿
Fees: £46–55; Second visit: £21–30
Kingston-on-Thames KT21
01372 271970

**Dominic Metcalfe GCC, BCA**
➕ ⦿ ⓝ ⊘ ✿ ⓔ
Fees: £36–45; Second visit: £31–40
Kingston-on-Thames KT3,Bath BA1
020 8715 1133

# Chiropractic

**SophieCharlo Nielsen GCC, BCA**
**Fees:** £26–35; Second visit: £21–30
Kingston-on-Thames KT2
020 8549 6696

**Simon Norton GCC, BCA**
**Fees:** £46–55; Second visit: £21–30
Kingston-on-Thames KT17
01372 741151

**Linda Schiller GCC, BCA**
**Fees:** £36–45; Second visit: £21–30
Kingston-on-Thames KT17
01372 741151

**Julian Welch GCC, BCA**
**Fees:** £36–45; Second visit: £21–30
Kingston-on-Thames KT12
01932 227360

**G T Van Der Walt GCC, BCA**
**Fees:** £26–35; Second visit: £21–30
Morden SM4
020 8646 3139

**Paul Danford GCC, BCA**
**Fees:** £46–55; Second visit: £21–30
Richmond TW9
020 8948 2744

**Jason Foggo GCC, BCA**
**Fees:** £26–35; Second visit: £21–30
Sutton SM2
020 8661 1614

**Katriona Heaslip GCC, BCA**
**Fees:** £46–55; Second visit: £21–30
Sutton SM2
020 8661 1613

**Sern Kjellberg GCC, BCA**
**Fees:** £26–35; Second visit: £21–30
Sutton SM2
020 8661 1613

**Thomas Greenway GCC, BCA**
**Fees:** >£55; Second visit: £31–40
Teddington TW11
020 8943 2424

**Nicholas Loftus GCC, BCA**
**Fees:** >£55; Second visit: £31–40
Teddington TW11
020 8943 2424

**Anthony M Metcalfe GCC, BCA**
**Fees:** £26–35; Second visit: £31–40
Teddington TW11
020 8943 2424

**Emma Morris GCC, BCA**
**Fees:** £26–35; Second visit: £31–40
Teddington TW11
020 8943 2424

**Patrick Molloy GCC, BAAC, MCA**
**Fees:** £26–35; Second visit: £21–30
Worcester Park KT4
020 8335 3433

# Western Herbal Medicine

**NORTH EAST**

**C Anderson MNIMH**
Enfield EN3
020 8804 1318

**M Courtenay-Luck MNIMH**
**Fees:** £26–35; Second visit: £21–30
Enfield EN1
020 8482 1112

# Western Herbal Medicine

**H Bradley MNIMH**
⊕ ✿
**Fees:** £26–35; Second visit: <£20
Ilford IG1
020 8518 1977

**G Leddy MNIMH**
O ⊕ ⓜ ⊘ ✿
**Fees:** £26–35; Second visit: <£20
Ilford IG1
020 8518 1442

## NORTH WEST

**B A Pendry MNIMH**
O ⊕ ⓔ ✿
**Fees:** £26–35; Second visit: <£20
Barnet EN5,Enfield EN3
020 8906 4841

**M Hyland MNIMH,**
O ⓔ ✿
**Fees:** £36–45; Second visit: £21–30
Bushey WD23
020 8950 1251

**I Middleton MNIMH**
⊕ ⊕ ✿
**Fees:** £26–35; Second visit: £21–30
Edgware HA8
020 8952 9566

**F M Campbell-Atkinson MNIMH**
⊕ ⊕ ⊕ ⓝ ⊘ ✿
**Fees:** £36–45; Second visit: £21–30
Harrow HA1
020 8861 1221

**Anand Marshall MNIMH**
⊕ O ⊕ ⊕ ⓔ ✿
**Fees:** £36–45; Second visit: £21–30
Harrow HA2,London NW8
020 8861 4280

**S Nugent MNIMH**
⊕ ⊕ ✿
**Fees:** £26–35; Second visit: £21–30
Hadley Wood EN4
020 8441 8352

**B K Sond MNIMH**
O ⓝ ✿
**Fees:** £26–35; Second visit: £21–30
Southall UB1
020 8575 2393

## SOUTH EAST

**S Tawse MNIMH**
O
**Fees:** £26–35; Second visit: <£20
Croydon CR2,Surbiton KT6
020 8686 1950

**K Hevezi MNIMH**
O ✿
**Fees:** £26–35; Second visit: <£20
West Wickham BR4
020 8777 6769

## SOUTH WEST

**J Mitchell MNIMH**
⊕ ⊕ ⓔ ✿
**Fees:** £26–35; Second visit: <£20
Chessington KT9
020 8287 6577

**J-A Dunbar MNIMH**
⊕ ⊕ ⓝ ✿
**Fees:** £36–45; Second visit: £21–30
Kingston-on-Thames KT10
01372 464659

**David Melrose MNIMH**
⊕ ⊕ ⓝ ✿
**Fees:** £46–55; Second visit: £41–50
New Malden KT3, London W1N
020 8942 3148

**N Nissen MNIMH**
⊕ ⊕ ⓝ ✿
**Fees:** £26–35; Second visit: £21–30
Richmond TW9
0208 948 9248

**A Christie MNIMH**
O ⓝ ⓔ ✿
**Fees:** £26–35; Second visit: £21–30
Teddington TW11
020 8977 8468

**D Austin MNIMH**
⊕ O ⊕ ⊕ ⓝ ✿
**Fees:** £26–35; Second visit: <£20
Twickenham TW2
020 8977 2947

# Chinese Herbal Medicine

## NORTH EAST

**Daniela Matal RCHM**
✚ ⊕ ⓜ ❀
Fees: £26–35; Second visit: £21–30
Dagenham RM8
020 8599 2628

## SOUTH EAST
✚ ⊕ ❀
Fees: £36–45; Second visit: £21–30
Beckenham BR3,London SE16
020 8402 7265

**Matthew Whale RCHM**
✚ O ⊕ ⊕ ⓜ ❀
Fees: £26–35; Second visit: £21–30
Croydon CR2
020 8645 0589

**Lifei Zhang RCHM,**
✚ ⊕ ⓜ ❀
Fees: <£25; Second visit: <£20
Purley CR8
020 8763 1119

## SOUTH WEST

**Chi Kin Po RCHM**
O ❀
Fees: <£25; Second visit: <£20
Carshalton SM5
020 8646 7697

**S Wei-Fen Zhu RCHM**
✚ ⓜ ⊘ ❀
Fees: <£25; Second visit: <£20
Hounslow TW3,Pinner HA5
020 8570 9998

**Susan Sutton RCHM**
O ⓜ ❀
Fees: £36–45; Second visit: £21–30
Kingston-on-Thames KT13
01932 221268

**Guang Xu RCHM**
✚ ⓜ ❀
Fees: £26–35; Second visit: <£20
Kingston-on-Thames KT8

**Wai Kwan Che RCHM**
✚ ⓜ ⓔ ❀
Fees: £26–35
Surbiton KT6
020 8390 1758

# Ayurvedic Medicine

## NORTH WEST

**Lata Joshi AMAUK**
O
Fees: <£25
Wembley HA0
020 8902 3897

**B Patel AMAUK**
O ❀
Fees: £26–35; Second visit: <£20
Wembley HA0
020 8902 4381

## SOUTH EAST

**N Sathiyamoorthy AMAUK**
✚ ⓜ ❀
Fees: £36–45; Second visit: £31–40
Croydon CR2
020 8681 1756

# Ayurvedic Medicine

**Maggi Talmadge GOsC, BOA**
🔆 ⭕ 🔵 ❄
**Fees:** £26–35; Second visit: £21–30
Purley CR8
020 8763 8279

**A F Alvi AMAUK**
🔆 ⭕ 🔵 🔵 ❄
**Fees:** <£25
Welling DA16
020 8303 4175

# North

Cumbria
Durham
East Riding of Yorkshire
Northumberland
North Yorkshire
Teesside (inc Darlington)
Tyne & Wear
West Yorkshire

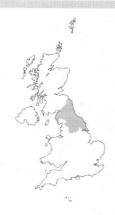

## Acupuncture

### CUMBRIA

**Simon Rogerson BMAS,**
Fees: £26–35; Second visit: £21–30
Barrow-in-Furness LA14
01229 822024

**Frederick D H Carson BAcC**
Fees: £26–35; Second visit: £21–30
Carlisle CA1
01228 515078

**Eric Duncan BAcC**
Fees: £26–35; Second visit: £21–30
Cockermouth CA13,Keswick CA12
01900 827377

**Kerrie Evans BAcC, AACP**
Fees: <£25; Second visit: £21–30
Cockermouth CA13
01900 828810

**Dianne Allan AACP**
Fees: £36–45; Second visit: £41–50
Egremont CA22
01946 825402

**Graham Dyer BAcC**
Fees: <£25; Second visit: £21–30
Grange-over-Sands LA11
01539 558132

**Janet Conway BAcC**
Fees: £36–45; Second visit: £21–30
Kendal LA9
01539 741447

**Judith Leigh BAcC**
Fees: £26–35; Second visit: £21–30
Kendal LA9
01539 725220

**June M Parker BAcC**
Fees: £26–35; Second visit: £21–30
Sedbergh LA10,Kirkby Stephen
CA17,Lancaster LA1
01539 620972

**Lilla Cooper BAcC**
Fees: <£25; Second visit: <£20
Ulverston LA12,Kendal
01229 716197

# Acupuncture

### John Boyd BAcC
🌀 ⭕ 🌐 🍀 🔵
**Fees:** £26–35; Second visit: £21–30
Whitehaven CA28, Carlisle CA2
01946 692597

### Jenny Craig BAcC
🌀 🍀 🔵
**Fees:** £36–45; Second visit: £21–30
Windermere LA23
01539 447888

### Janet E Smedley AACP
🌀 🔵
**Fees:** £26–35; Second visit: £21–30
Windermere LA23
07831 219849

## DURHAM

### Anthonia Andreadis BAcC
🌀 🌀 🌐 🔵 🍀 🔵
**Fees:** £26–35; Second visit: £21–30
Durham DH1
0191 383 2090

### Karen Raine AACP
🌀 🌐 🔵 🍀 🔵
**Fees:** £26–35; Second visit: £21–30
Durham DH7, Blaydon-on-Tyne
NE21, Washington NE38
0191 377 9256

### Gillian Rhind BAcC
🌀 🌐 🔵
**Fees:** £26–35; Second visit: £21–30
Durham DH1
0191 383 0677

### Pamela Todd BAcC
🌀 🔵 ⊘ 🔵
**Fees:** £26–35; Second visit: £21–30
Stanley DH9
0191 511 0214

## EAST RIDING OF YORKSHIRE

### Michael Stephenson BAcC
⭕ 🔵 🍀 🔵
**Fees:** £26–35; Second visit: £21–30
Bridlington YO15
01262 677032

### Deborah Sutcliffe BAcC
🌀 🍀 🔵
**Fees:** <£25; Second visit: <£20
Hornsea HU18
01964 536416

### Michael Ward BAcC
🌀 🌐 🔵
**Fees:** £26–35; Second visit: £21–30
Hull HU5
01964 550822

## NORTHUMBERLAND

### Reginald Carr BMAS
🌀 ⊘ 🍀 🔵
**Fees:** £26–35; Second visit: £21–30
Blyth NE24
01670 363334

### Wendy Marie Burrows BAcC
🌀 🌐 ⊘ 🍀 🔵
**Fees:** £26–35; Second visit: £21–30
Hexham NE46
01434 609494

## NORTH YORKSHIRE

### Laurine Murison BAcC
⭕ 🍀 🔵
**Fees:** £26–35; Second visit: £21–30
Harrogate HG3
01423 340480

### Nicola Wood BAcC
🌀 ⭕ 🍀 🔵
**Fees:** £26–35; Second visit: £21–30
Harrogate HG2, Wetherby LS22
01423 810272

### Kath Tuck BAcC
🌀 ⭕ 🌐 🔵
**Fees:** £36–45; Second visit: £21–30
Knaresborough HG5
01423 865738

### Mandy Metcalfe BAcC
🌀 🌐 🍀 🔵
**Fees:** £26–35; Second visit: £21–30
Northallerton DL6, York YO61
01609 783600

**Mark Young BAcC**
✚ ⊕ ✿ ✪
Fees: £36–45; Second visit: £21–30
Ripon HG4
01765 601447

**Roger William Coles BMAS,**
O ✿ ✪
Fees: £26–35; Second visit: £21–30
Scarborough YO12
01723 367021

**Christopher Gibson BAcC**
✚ ⊕ ✿ ✪
Fees: £26–35; Second visit: £21–30
Scarborough YO12
01723 366455

**D F Jones BMAS,**
✚ ⊕ ⊘ ✿ ✪
Fees: £26–35; Second visit: £21–30
Scarborough YO11
01723 365363

**Brendan O Sullivan BAcC**
O ⊕ ✿ ✪
Fees: <£25; Second visit: <£20
Scarborough YO11
01723 366747

**Jane Parkinson AACP**
✚ ⊕ ⊕ ✪ ✪
Fees: £36–45; Second visit: £41–50
Selby YO8
01757 704152

**Christine Swales BAcC**
✪ ✿ ✪
Fees: £26–35; Second visit: <£20
Whitby YO21
01947 820720

**Vincent Lyles AACP**
✚ ⊕ ✪ ⊘ ✿ ✪
Fees: £26–35; Second visit: £21–30
York YO24
01904 784055

**Michael Burgess BAcC**
✚ O ⊕ ✪ ✿ ✪
Fees: £36–45; Second visit: £21–30
York YO31
01904 421032

**Michael Cordel BAcC**
✚ ⊕ ✿ ✪
Fees: £26–35; Second visit: £21–30
York YO62
01751 430335

**Sarah Dixon BAcC**
✚ ✚ ⊘ ✿ ✪
Fees: £26–35; Second visit: £21–30
York YO31, York YO32
01904 627807

**Alison Gould BAcC**
O ✿ ✪
Fees: £36–45; Second visit: £21–30
York YO31
01904 421032

**Harriet Lansdown BAcC**
O ✿ ✪
Fees: £26–35; Second visit: £21–30
York YO23
01904 651884

**Hugh MacPherson BAcC**
✚ ⊕ ✿ ✪
Fees: £36–45; Second visit: £21–30
York YO24
01904 709688

**Robert N Mason BAcC**
✚ O ✿ ✪
Fees: £36–45; Second visit: £21–30
York YO23
01904 651367

**Annie Milles BAcC**
✚ ⊕ ✪
Fees: £26–35; Second visit: £21–30
York YO24
01904 709688

**June Tranmer BAcC**
✚ ⊕ ✪ ✿ ✪
Fees: £36–45; Second visit: £21–30
York YO10
01904 679868

## TEESSIDE

**Simon Robey BAcC**
✚ ⊕ ✿ ✪
Fees: £26–35; Second visit: £21–30
Darlington DL3
01325 467287

# Acupuncture

**Jane Sutton AACP**
⊕ ⊕ ⊕ ⊕ ⊕ ⊕
**Fees:** £26–35; Second visit: £21–30
Guisborough TS14
01287 635478

**Andrew Cross BAcC**
⊕ ○ ⊕ ⊕
**Fees:** £36–45; Second visit: £21–30
Middlesbrough TS4
01642 253515

**Keith Thomas BAcC**
⊕ ⊕ ⊕ ⊕ ⊕
**Fees:** £26–35; Second visit: £21–30
Middlesbrough TS4
01642 246385

**Stewart Anthony Chilton BMAS,**
○ ⊕ ⊘ ⊕
**Fees:** £26–35; Second visit: £21–30
Middlesbrough TS7
01642 313508

## TYNE & WEAR

**Angel Powell AACP**
⊕ ⊘ ⊕ ⊕
**Fees:** £26–35; Second visit: £31–40
Newcastle Upon Tyne NE3
0191 284 0087

**W W Feng BAcC**
⊕ ⊘ ⊕ ⊕
**Fees:** <£25; Second visit: <£20
Newcastle Upon Tyne NE1
0191 221 0090

**Feras Jerjis BAcC**
⊕ ⊕ ⊕ ⊕ ⊕
**Fees:** £26–35; Second visit: £21–30
Newcastle Upon Tyne NE1
0191 233 0500

**Anne Palmer BAcC**
○ ⊕
**Fees:** £36–45; Second visit: £21–30
Newcastle Upon Tyne NE2
0191 281 8201

**Leonie Walker BAcC**
⊕ ⊕ ⓔ ⊕ ⊕
North Shields NE1
0191 290 0300

**Margaret Moore BAcC**
⊕ ⊕ ⊕ ⊕
**Fees:** £26–35; Second visit: £21–30
Ryton NE40
0191 413 4003

**Steve May BAcC**
○ ⓔ ⊕ ⊕
**Fees:** £26–35; Second visit: £21–30
Sunderland
0191 567 8003

## WEST YORKSHIRE

**Mark Popplewell BAcC**
○ ⊕ ⓔ ⊕ ⊕
**Fees:** £26–35; Second visit: <£20
Batley WF17
01924 443527

**Hilary Coles BAcC**
⊕ ○ ⊕ ⓔ ⊕ ⊕
**Fees:** £26–35; Second visit: £21–30
Bradford BD15, Skipton BD23
01274 409338

**Shashi Champaneria BAcC**
⊕ ⊕ ⊕ ⊕ ⊕
**Fees:** £36–45; Second visit: £21–30
Bradford BD8
01274 783811

**M Samuel BAcC**
⊕ ⊕ ⊕ ⊕ ⊕
**Fees:** >£55; Second visit: £31–40
Bradford BD8
01274 547020

**Stan Switala BAcC**
⊕ ⊕ ⊕
**Fees:** £26–35; Second visit: £21–30
Bradford BD8
01274 484514

**Liping Han BAcC**
⊕ ⊕ ⊕ ⊕
**Fees:** £26–35; Second visit: £21–30
Bradford BD8, Newcastle Upon Tyne
NE3, York YO24
01274 484514

**David S O'Kell  AACP**
Fees: £36–45; Second visit: >£50
Dewsbury WF12
01924 450183

**Anna Bitelli BAcC**
Fees: £36–45; Second visit: £21–30
Dewsbury WF12,Leeds LS27
01924 430770

**Angela Johnson AACP**
Fees: £36–45; Second visit: £31–40
Halifax HX3
01422 250362

**John Barry Landale BAcC**
Fees: £36–45; Second visit: £21–30
Hebden Bridge HX7
01422 843123

**Stacey Ash BAcC**
Fees: £26–35; Second visit: £21–30
Holmfirth HD9,Huddersfield HD5
01484 684245

**Rebecca Hunter BAcC**
Fees: £36–45; Second visit: £21–30
Huddersfield HD1
01484 480841

**Ruth Johnson AACP**
Fees: £36–45; Second visit: £21–30
Huddersfield HD2
01484 533131

**Elizabeth Chapman BAcC**
Fees: £36–45; Second visit: £21–30
Ilkley LS29
01943 602177

**Yves E Dereix AACP**
Fees: £26–35; Second visit: £21–30
Ilkley LS29
01943 431999

**Stephen Hunter BAcC**
Fees: £26–35; Second visit: £21–30
Ilkley LS29
01943 602177

**Liuqing Wang BAcC**
Fees: £26–35; Second visit: £21–30
Leeds LS15,Wakefield WF1,Leeds LS13
0113 260 1177

**Don Clarke BAcC**
Fees: £36–45; Second visit: £21–30
Leeds LS18
0113 295 9752

**Cathryn Spengeler BAcC**
Fees: £26–35; Second visit: £21–30
Leeds LS19
0113 261 3562

**Margaret Davis BAcC**
Fees: £26–35; Second visit: £21–30
Leeds LS25,Castleford WF10
0113 286 4778

**John P Heptonstall BAcC**
Fees: £26–35; Second visit: <£20
Leeds LS27
0113 238 0208

**Lester Ward AACP**
Fees: £36–45; Second visit: £31–40
Leeds LS5
0113 295 1160

**Louise Attwood BAcC**
Fees: £36–45; Second visit: £21–30
Leeds LS7
0113 228 4996

**Sally Howarth BAcC**
Fees: £26–35; Second visit: £21–30
Otley LS21
01943 462811

# Acupuncture

**Caroline Haigh BAcC**
♣ ☺
**Fees:** £26–35; Second visit: £21–30
Pudsey LS28
0113 256 3262

**Stella King BAcC**
⊕ ♣ ☺
**Fees:** £36–45; Second visit: £21–30
Todmorden OL14
01706 813527

**Alison West BAcC**
⊕ © ♣ ☺
**Fees:** £36–45; Second visit: £21–30
Todmorden OL14
01706 813527

**Jacqueline Clelland BAcC**
⊕ ⊕ ♣ ☺
**Fees:** £36–45; Second visit: £21–30
Wakefield
01924 373353

**Ian C Wood BAcC**
⊕ ☺
**Fees:** £36–45; Second visit: £21–30
Wetherby LS23
01937 573381

**Julia Barnett BAcC, BMAS,**
⊕ ⊕ ⊕ ☺
**Fees:** £36–45; Second visit: £21–30
Leeds LS8
0113 237 1173

**Sarah Nolan BAcC**
⊕ ⊕ ♣ ☺
**Fees:** £36–45; Second visit: £21–30
Leeds LS7,Leeds LS16
0113 269 4448

**Giles Watts BAcC**
⊕ ⊕ ♣ ☺
**Fees:** £26–35; Second visit: £21–30
Leeds LS7
0113 274 3439

# Homeopathy

## CUMBRIA

**David Evans RSHom**
⊕ ⊕ ∅ ©
**Fees:** £36–45; Second visit: £20–30
Ambleside LA22
01539 431766

**Alice Bondi RSHom**
⊕ O ♣
**Fees:** £36–45; Second visit: £20–30
Carlisle CA2
01434 381504

**Raymond Sevar MFHom**
O ⊕ ∅ ♣
**Fees:** >£55; Second visit: £31–40
Carlisle CA3
01228 531691

**Deirdre Moon RSHom**
⊕ ⊕ ⊕ ©
**Fees:** £46–55; Second visit: £20–30
Cockermouth CA13,Dalton-in-Furness
LA15
01900 821122

**Sheila Wood RSHom**
⊕ ⊕ ⊕ ⊕ ©
**Fees:** £36–45; Second visit: £20–30
Cockermouth CA13
01900 821122

**Angela Jackson RSHom**
⊕ ⊕ ⊕ ©
**Fees:** £36–45; Second visit: £20–30
Kendal LA9
01539 824099

**Pamela Moon RSHom**
⊕ ⊕ ⊕ ♣
**Fees:** £25–35; Second visit: £20–30
Ulverston LA12
01229 861646

## DURHAM

**Angela Morse RSHom**
⊕ ⊕ © ♣
**Fees:** £46–55; Second visit: £31–40
Chester-le-Street DH3
0191 388 4929

**Caroline Melody RSHom**
⊕ ⊕ ⊛ © ❀
**Fees:** £46–55; Second visit: £20–30
Durham DH1,Durham DH1
0191 383 9189

## EAST RIDING OF YORKSHIRE

**Pauline Darling RSHom**
O ⊕ ⊛ © ❀
**Fees:** £25–35; Second visit: £20–30
Beverley HU17
01482 882811

**Sally Stephenson RSHom**
⊕ O ⊕ ⊛ © ❀
**Fees:** £36–45; Second visit: <£20
Bridlington YO15
01262 677032

**James Rogers RSHom**
⊕ O ⊛ ❀
**Fees:** £25–35; Second visit: <£20
Willerby HU10
01482 650567

## NORTHUMBERLAND

**Dolores Armstrong RSHom**
⊕ ⊕ ⊛ ©
**Fees:** £25–35; Second visit: £20–30
Alnwick NE66,North Shields NE30
01665 576024

**Julie Horrocks RSHom**
⊕ O ⊕ ⊛ © ❀
**Fees:** £36–45; Second visit: £20–30
Corbridge NE45
01434 381064

**Audrey-Gail Parkin RSHom**
⊕ O ⊕ ⊛ ⊘ ❀
**Fees:** £36–45; Second visit: £20–30
Hexham NE46
01434 601577

**Jennifer Fowler RSHom**
O ⊛
**Fees:** £36–45; Second visit: £31–40
Morpeth NE61
01670 787391

**Valerie Vaughan RSHom**
O ⊛ ⊘ ©
**Fees:** £36–45; Second visit: £20–30
Morpeth NE61
01670 772686

## NORTH YORKSHIRE

**Brenda Adey RSHom**
O ⊛ ❀
**Fees:** £46–55; Second visit: £20–30
Richmond DL10
01239 654969

**Mark Young RSHom**
⊕ ⊕ ⊛ ❀
**Fees:** £36–45; Second visit: £20–30
Ripon HG4
01765 601447

**Jocelyn Young RSHom**
⊕ ⊕ ⊛ ❀
**Fees:** £36–45; Second visit: £20–30
Ripon HG4
01765 601447

**Sally Cook RSHom**
O ⊛
**Fees:** £46–55; Second visit: £20–30
Tadcaster LS24
01937 833669

**Wendy Bousfield RSHom**
O ⊛ © ❀
**Fees:** £46–55; Second visit: £31–40
Thirsk YO7
01845 525859

**Tricia Griffin RSHom**
⊕ ⊕ ⊕ ⊛ ©
**Fees:** £36–45; Second visit: £20–30
Whitby YO21,Whitby YO22,York YO62
01947 821747

**Tricia Murthwaite RSHom**
⊕ ⊕ ⊛ © ❀
**Fees:** £36–45; Second visit: £20–30
York YO61,York YO62
01347 868152

**Shirley Riley RSHom**
⊕ O ⊕ ⊛ © ❀
**Fees:** £36–45; Second visit: <£20
York YO43,Cottingham HU16
01430 860690

# Homeopathy

**Madeline Evans RSHom**
⊕ ⓝ
**Fees:** >£55; Second visit: £20–30
York YO10
01904 784274

**Eva Fox-Gal RSHom**
O ⓝ ❀
**Fees:** >£55; Second visit: £31–40
York YO10
01904 411696

**Maggie Gravells RSHom**
⊕ ⓔ ❀
**Fees:** £46–55; Second visit: £20–30
York YO1
01904 431244

**Angela King RSHom**
ⓝ ❀
**Fees:** £36–45; Second visit: £20–30
York YO1
01904 679612

**Paula Leszczuk RSHom**
⊕ O ⊕ ❀
**Fees:** £25–35; Second visit: £20–30
York YO19,York YO10,York YO61
01759 372563

**David Sault RSHom**
O ⓝ ⓔ ❀
**Fees:** £36–45; Second visit: £20–30
York YO24
01904 635366

## TEESSIDE

**Olwen Grieves RSHom**
O ⓝ
**Fees:** £46–55; Second visit: £20–30
Darlington DL3
01325 464705

**Richard Laver RSHom**
O ⓝ ⓔ
**Fees:** £46–55; Second visit: £20–30
Darlington DL1
01325 467544

**Carol Hudson RSHom**
⊕ ⊕ ⓔ ❀
**Fees:** £46–55; Second visit: £20–30
Middlesbrough TS1
01642 244337

**Elizabeth Stewart RSHom**
O ⊕ ⓝ ⊘ ❀
**Fees:** £36–45; Second visit: £20–30
Sunderland SR6
0191 529 2135

## TYNE & WEAR

**Christine Conyers RSHom**
⊕ ⊕ ⓝ ⊘ ⓔ
**Fees:** £46–55; Second visit: £31–40
Gateshead NE8
01661 834855

**Glynis Ingram RSHom**
⊕ ⓝ ⓔ ❀
**Fees:** £46–55; Second visit: £31–40
Gateshead NE8
0191 490 0274

**Rhoda Lewis RSHom**
O ⓝ ⓔ ❀
**Fees:** £36–45; Second visit: £20–30
Jarrow NE32
0191 421 2416

**Jade Swain RSHom**
⊕ ⊕ ⓝ ⓔ ❀
**Fees:** £36–45; Second visit: £20–30
Newcastle Upon Tyne NE1
0191 281 4888

**Anna Thorley RSHom**
ⓝ ❀
**Fees:** £36–45; Second visit: £31–40
Newcastle Upon Tyne NE1
0191 261 7643

**Irene Forshaw RSHom**
⊕ ⊕ ⊕ ⓝ ⓔ ❀
**Fees:** >£55; Second visit: £41–50
Newcastle Upon Tyne NE2
0191 281 2636

**Margaret Reid MFHom**
O ⓝ ❀
**Fees:** >£55; Second visit: £41–50
Newcastle Upon Tyne NE2
0191 284 0484

# Homeopathy

**Madeleine van Zwanenberg RSHom**
Fees: >£55; Second visit: £41–50
Newcastle Upon Tyne NE2,Newcastle
Upon Tyne NE1
0191 281 2636

**Ruth Sadler RSHom**
Fees: £36–45; Second visit: £20–30
Newcastle Upon Tyne NE20,
Morpeth NE65
01661 881654

**Beth MacEoin RSHom**
Fees: £36–45; Second visit: £20–30
Newcastle Upon Tyne NE3
0191 236 6935

**Elisabeth Edmundson RSHom**
Fees: £36–45; Second visit: £20–30
Newcastle-upon-tyne NE3
0191 286 5053

**Hazel White-Cooper RSHom**
Fees: £36–45; Second visit: £20–30
Newcastle-upon-tyne NE3
0191- 2865053

**Dorothy Cragg RSHom**
Fees: £25–35; Second visit: £20–30
North Shields NE29
0191 257 6740

**Joy Nancarrow RSHom**
Fees: £25–35; Second visit: £20–30
North Shields NE29
0191 290 0300

**Annie Gray FFHom, RSHom**
Fees: £36–45; Second visit: £31–40
North Shields NE30
0191 296 0026

**Judith Marshall RSHom**
Fees: £36–45; Second visit: £20–30
South Shields NE33
0191 455 4885

**Elizabeth Barrow RSHom**
Fees: £25–35; Second visit: £20–30
Tyne & Wear NE37
0191 417 8075

**Caroline White RSHom**
Fees: £36–45; Second visit: £20–30
Washington NE38
0191 416 4911

## WEST YORKSHIRE

**Catherine Presto RSHom**
Fees: <£25; Second visit: <£20
Bradford BD8
07720 448771

**Gabriela Rieberer MFHom**
Fees: >£55; Second visit: £41–50
Bradford BD9
01274 774055

**Diana Seymour RSHom**
Fees: £36–45; Second visit: £20–30
Hebden Bridge HX7
01422 846554

**Janette Batty RSHom**
Fees: £46–55; Second visit: £20–30
Holmfirth HD7
01484 845959

**Virginia Crompton RSHom**
Fees: £46–55; Second visit: £20–30
Huddersfield HD7
01484 645616

**Alistair Dempster RSHom**
Fees: £46–55; Second visit: £31–40
Huddersfield HD4
01484 327049

**Carolyn Garland RSHom**
Fees: >£55; Second visit: £20–30
Huddersfield HD3
01484 654751

# Homeopathy

**Clare Walters RSHom**
➊ O ⊕ ⊕ NHS ⊘ ✿
Fees: £46–55; Second visit: £20–30
Huddersfield HD5 ,Huddersfield HD8
01484 452788

**Anne Grey RSHom**
O NHS
Fees: >£55; Second visit: £31–40
Ilkley LS29
01943 609818

**Annetta Kershaw RSHom**
➊ ⊕ NHS € ✿
Fees: £25–35; Second visit: £20–30
Ilkley LS29
01943 862841

**Carol Wise RSHom**
➊ O ⊕ NHS €
Fees: £46–55; Second visit: £20–30
Ilkley LS29
01943 863213

**Krystyna Hilton RSHom**
➊ ⊕ ⊕ NHS €
Fees: £36–45; Second visit: £20–30
Keighley BD21
01535 690055

**Catherine Barker RSHom**
➊ ⊕ ⊕ NHS €
Fees: £46–55; Second visit: £31–40
Leeds LS8
0113 237 1173

**Andrea Bartig RSHom**
➊ O ⊕ NHS € ✿
Fees: £46–55; Second visit: £31–40
Leeds LS15,Leeds LS8
0113 293 0345

**Helen Bowcock RSHom**
➊ O ⊕ NHS € ✿
Fees: £36–45; Second visit: £20–30
Leeds LS8,Halifax HX1
0113 262 1693

**Jane Brown RSHom**
O NHS ✿
Fees: >£55; Second visit: £31–40
Leeds LS6
0113 278 7346

**Nette Humphreys RSHom**
NHS € ✿
Fees: £36–45; Second visit: £20–30
Leeds LS6
0113 305 0272

**Elizabeth Dunford RSHom**
O NHS € ✿
Fees: £46–55; Second visit: £20–30
Leeds LS6
07946 410837

**Joanna More RSHom**
O NHS € ✿
Fees: £36–45; Second visit: £20–30
Leeds LS17
0113 269 7850

**Georgina Ramseyer RSHom**
➊ O ⊕ NHS € ✿
Fees: £46–55; Second visit: £20–30
Leeds LS7
0113 2744894

**Marion Stephens RSHom**
O NHS
Fees: £46–55; Second visit: £31–40
Leeds LS27,Leeds LS27
0113 252 5218

**Khan Hamidullah MFHom**
➊ O ⊕ NHS ⊘ € ✿
Fees: >£55; Second visit: £41–50
Liversedge WF17
01924 479251

**Gill Scott RSHom**
➊ O ⊕ NHS €
Fees: £46–55; Second visit: £20–30
Otley LS21
01943 461784

**Richard Kenchington RSHom**
➊ O NHS € ✿
Fees: £25–35; Second visit: £31–40
Settle BD24
01729 822786

**Barbara McLoughlin RSHom**
➊ O NHS €
Fees: £36–45; Second visit: £20–30
Settle BD24
01729 822197

**Christine DeHeera RSHom**
☯ ⊕ ⓝ ⓔ
Fees: >£55; Second visit: £20–30
Shipley BD18
01274 532661

**David Fairfax RSHom**
⊕ ⊕ ⓝ ⓔ ✳
Fees: >£55; Second visit: £31–40
Shipley BD18
01274 638167

**Sue Asquith RSHom**
☯ ⊕ ⓝ ⓔ ✳
Fees: £25–35; Second visit: £20–30
Skipton BD23
01756 796690

**Jan Edgar RSHom**
☯ ◯ ⓝ ✳
Fees: £46–55; Second visit: £20–30
Wakefield WF2
01924 381562

**Lindsay Harper RSHom**
ⓝ ⓔ ✳
Fees: £46–55; Second visit: £20–30
Wakefield WF4
01924 860366

**Judith Scott RSHom**
☯ ◯ ⊕ ⓝ ✳
Fees: £36–45; Second visit: £20–30
Wetherby LS23
01937 842471

**Angela Zajac RSHom**
☯ ◯ ⊕ ⓝ ⓔ ✳
Fees: £46–55; Second visit: £20–30
Wetherby LS23
01937 541418

## CUMBRIA

**Timothy Marris GOsC**
☯ ⊕ ⓝ
Fees: <£25; Second visit: £21–30
Ambleside LA22
01539 433220

**Mary-Clare Scragg GOsC**
☯ ⓝ
Fees: <£25; Second visit: £21–30
Barrow-in-Furness LA14
01229 823516

**Val Makinson GOsC, BOA**
☯ ⓝ ⊘
Fees: <£25; Second visit: £21–30
Barrow-in-Furness LA14
01229 812002

**Stephen Bolger GOsC, BOA**
☯ ⓝ ✳
Fees: £26–35; Second visit: £21–30
Carlisle CA1
01228 524701

**Frederick Carson GOsC**
☯ ⊕
Fees: £26–35; Second visit: £21–30
Carlisle CA1
01228 515078

**Richard N Lloyd GOsC, BOA**
☯ ⊕ ⓝ
Fees: <£25; Second visit: £21–30
Carlisle CA1
01228 524701

# Osteopathy

**Elizabeth Wake GOsC**
✛ ⓝ
**Fees:** £26–35; Second visit: £21–30
Carlisle CA1
01228 524701

**Eric Duncan GOsC**
✛ Ⓞ ⓝ ✿
**Fees:** £26–35; Second visit: £21–30
Cockermouth CA13
01900 827377

**Geoffrey Smith GOsC**
✛ ⓝ ✿
**Fees:** £26–35; Second visit: £21–30
Grange-over-Sands LA11
01539 535314

**Jolyon Wardle GOsC, BOA**
✛ ⓝ ✿
**Fees:** <£25; Second visit: £21–30
Grange-over-Sands LA11
015395 58647

**Clifford Conway GOsC, BOA**
ⓝ ⊘ ⓔ
**Fees:** £36–45; Second visit: £21–30
Kendal LA9
01539 730102

**Daphne Jackson GOsC, BOA**
✛ Ⓞ ⓝ
**Fees:** <£25; Second visit: <£20
Kendal LA9
01539 740452

**Josephine Luard GOsC, BOA**
✛ ⓑ ⓝ ⊘ ✿
**Fees:** <£25; Second visit: £31–40
Kingswood CA1
07956 509922

**Adam Hill GOsC, BOA**
✛ ⊕ ⓑ ⓝ ✿
**Fees:** £26–35; Second visit: £21–30
Penrith CA11
01768 890800

**Margaret Towson GOsC, BOA**
✛ ⓝ
**Fees:** £26–35; Second visit: £21–30
Penrith CA11
01768 890800

**Ralph Sutton GOsC, BOA**
✛ ⊕ ⊘ ✿
Windermere LA23
01539 444383

## DURHAM

**Peter W Hairsine GOsC, BOA**
✛ ⓑ ⓝ ⓔ ✿
**Fees:** <£25; Second visit: £21–30
Barnard Castle DL12
01833 630640

**Iluminado Claveras-Gil GOsC, BOA**
✛ ⓝ ✿
**Fees:** £26–35; Second visit: £21–30
Durham DH3
0191 410 2320

**Kevin Kirkup GOsC, BOA**
✛ ⓝ ✿
**Fees:** £36–45; Second visit: £21–30
Durham DH3
0191 492 1448

**Fiona Birnie GOsC**
✛ Ⓞ ⓝ ✿
**Fees:** £26–35; Second visit: £21–30
Durham DH7
0191 378 2141

**Sian Greeves GOsC, BOA**
✛ ⓑ ⓝ ⓔ
**Fees:** £26–35; Second visit: £21–30
Durham DH1
0191 383 0677

**Melanie Rowland GOsC, BOA**
✛ ⊕ ⓝ ⊘ ⓔ ✿
**Fees:** £26–35; Second visit: £21–30
Newton Aycliffe DL5
01325 319183

## EAST RIDING OF YORKSHIRE

**Neil Evans GOsC**
✛ ⓑ ⓝ ⊘ ✿
**Fees:** <£25; Second visit: £21–30
Beverley HU17
01482 869678

### Irene Baker GOsC, BOA
Fees: £26–35; Second visit: £21–30
Driffield YO25
01377 256835

### David Harvey GOsC, BOA
Fees: <£25; Second visit: £21–30
Kingston upon Hull HU10
01482 651575

### Gerard Vallely GOsC
Fees: £26–35; Second visit: £21–30
Kingston upon Hull HU1
01482 580560

## NORTHUMBERLAND

### Christopher Gelson GOsC, BOA
Fees: £26–35; Second visit: £21–30
Corbridge NE45
01434 632427

## NORTH YORKSHIRE

### Jocelyn Ashley GOsC
Fees: £26–35; Second visit: £21–30
Harrogate HG1
01423 521164

### Thomas Miller Cree GOsC, BOA
Fees: <£25; Second visit: £21–30
Harrogate HG1
01423 561566

### Kathryn Elliott GOsC, BOA
Fees: £26–35; Second visit: £21–30
Knaresborough HG5
01423 868388

### Suzanne Hibberd GOsC, BOA
Fees: £26–35; Second visit: £21–30
Northallerton DL6
01609 783600

### Joanna Waterworth GOsC, BOA
Fees: <£25; Second visit: £21–30
Northallerton DL6
01609 783600

### Claire MacDonald GOsC, BOA
Fees: £36–45; Second visit: £21–30
Ripon HG14
01765 601447

### Mark H Young GOsC, BOA
Fees: £36–45; Second visit: £21–30
Ripon HG4
01765 601447

### Thomas Cullen GOsC
Fees: <£25; Second visit: £21–30
Scarborough YO11
01723 371248

### Jo Moretta GOsC
Fees: <£25; Second visit: £21–30
Scarborough YO12
01723 366455

### Martin J Rose GOsC
Fees: £26–35; Second visit: £21–30
Whitby YO22
01947 821235

### Trevor MacArthur GOsC
Fees: <£25; Second visit: £31–40
York YO1
01904 659588

### Pamela O'Sullivan GOsC
Fees: <£25; Second visit: <£20
York YO11
01723 366747

### Roger Kingston GOsC, BOA
Fees: £36–45; Second visit: £21–30
York YO24
01904 790567

# Osteopathy

**Nicholas Sheehan GOsC**
➕ ⓝ
**Fees:** <£25; Second visit: £21–30
York YO31
01904 431335

**Simon Barnard GOsC, BOA**
➕ ⭕ ⓖ ⓝ ⊘ ✿
**Fees:** <£25; Second visit: £21–30
York YO61
01347 822946

## TEESSIDE

**Philip Hambly GOsC**
➕ ⓝ ✿
**Fees:** <£25; Second visit: <£20
Darlington DL1
01325 381326

**Timothy Corbishley GOsC**
➕ ⓝ ✿
**Fees:** £36–45; Second visit: £21–30
Darlington DL3
01325 466022

**Stephen Castleton GOsC**
➕ ⊕ ⓝ ⊘
**Fees:** <£25; Second visit: £21–30
Middlesbrough TS1
01642 217557

**Andrew Cross GOsC**
➕ ⭕ ⓖ ⓝ ⊘ ✿
**Fees:** £26–35; Second visit: £21–30
Middlesbrough TS4
01642 253515

**W Keith Birks GOsC, BOA**
⭕ ⓝ
**Fees:** £26–35; Second visit: £21–30
Middlesbrough TS5
01642 850018

**Peter Ayton GOsC, BOA**
➕ ⓝ ⊘ ✿
**Fees:** <£25; Second visit: £21–30
Stockton-on-Tees TS20
01642 559690

## TYNE & WEAR

**Michael Bannister GOsC**
➕
**Fees:** £26–35; Second visit: £21–30
Newcastle Upon Tyne NE2
0191 281 2204

**Fiona Ellis GOsC**
➕ ⓝ
**Fees:** £36–45; Second visit: £21–30
Newcastle Upon Tyne NE11
0191 264 9828

**Ann Farthing GOsC, BOA**
➕ ⓝ ✿
**Fees:** £36–45; Second visit: £21–30
Newcastle Upon Tyne NE30
0191 296 2159

**Robin Watkins GOsC, BOA**
➕ ⭕
**Fees:** £26–35; Second visit: £21–30
Newcastle Upon Tyne NE3
0191 284 3678

**Fiona Birnle GOsC**
➕ ⭕ ⓝ
**Fees:** £26–35; Second visit: £21–30
Sunderland SR2
0191 510 0555

**Peter Buxton GOsC**
➕ ✿
**Fees:** <£25; Second visit: <£20
Sunderland SR6
0191 548 6294

**K Francis GOsC**
➕ ⓝ ✿
**Fees:** <£25; Second visit: <£20
Sunderland SR6
0191 536 7224

**Jane Dent GOsC, BOA**
➕ ⓝ ⊘ ✿
**Fees:** £26–35; Second visit: £21–30
Whitley Bay NE26
0191 252 1555

**Simone Rose GOsC**
➕ ⓝ ✿
**Fees:** £26–35; Second visit: £21–30
Whitley Bay NE26
0191 252 1555

## WEST YORKSHIRE

**Suzanne Austin GOsC, BOA**
➕ ⓝ ⊘ ✤
Fees: <£25; Second visit: <£20
Bingley BD16
01274 562525

**Mary McMahon GOsC**
➕ ⓞ ⓝ ✤
Fees: £26–35; Second visit: £21–30
Bradford BD6
01274 600659

**Oliver Bell GOsC, BOA**
➕ ⓝ
Fees: <£25; Second visit: <£20
Castleford WF10
01977 515108

**Ginette Bennett GOsC, BOA**
➕ ⓑ ⓝ ✤
Fees: <£25; Second visit: <£20
Castleford WF10
01977 513642

**Andrew Cunnington GOsC, BOA**
➕ ⓑ ⓝ
Fees: <£25; Second visit: £21–30
Halifax HX1
01422 320225

**Lee M Blackburn GOsC, BOA**
➕ ⓝ ✤
Fees: <£25; Second visit: £21–30
Huddersfield HD1
01484 469143

**David Ellwood GOsC, BOA**
➕ ⊕ ⓑ ⓝ ⓒ ✤
Fees: <£25; Second visit: £21–30
Huddersfield HD1
07867 523240

**Nina V Gallagher GOsC, BOA**
ⓞ ⓝ ⊘ ✤
Fees: <£25; Second visit: £21–30
Huddersfield HD2
01484 454845

**Timothy McClune GOsC**
➕ ⊕ ⓝ ⊘ ⓒ
Fees: £26–35; Second visit: £21–30
Huddersfield HD1
01484 424329

**Peter Nash GOsC, BOA**
➕ ⓝ ✤
Fees: <£25; Second visit: £21–30
Huddersfield HD1
01484 423918

**Agnieszka Sykes GOsC, BOA**
➕ ⓝ ⓒ
Fees: £26–35; Second visit: £21–30
Huddersfield HD1
01484 424329

**David Sykes GOsC, BOA**
➕ ⓝ ⓒ
Fees: £26–35; Second visit: £21–30
Huddersfield HD1
01484 424329

**Roberta Grech-Cini GOsC**
➕ ⓝ ✤
Fees: £26–35; Second visit: £21–30
Ilkley LS29
01943 817117

**Amos Grech-Cini GOsC**
➕ ⊘ ✤
Fees: £26–35; Second visit: £21–30
Ilkley LS29
01943 817117

**John Brewster GOsC, BOA**
➕ ⊕ ⓑ ⓝ ⊘ ✤
Fees: <£25; Second visit: £21–30
Keighley BD21
01535 690055

**Katherine Brewster GOsC, BOA**
➕ ⊕ ⓑ ⓝ
Fees: £26–35; Second visit: £21–30
Keighley BD21
01535 690055

**Stuart Cooper GOsC, BOA**
➕ ⊕ ⓑ ⓝ ⊘
Fees: <£25; Second visit: £21–30
Keighley BD21
01535 690055

**Jim Winterborn GOsC**
➕ ⊕ ⓑ ⓝ
Fees: <£25; Second visit: £21–30
Keighley BD21
01535 690055

# Osteopathy

**Paul Cairns GOsC, BOA**
➊ ➍ ⓝ ✻
Fees: £36–45; Second visit: £31–40
Leeds LS1
0845 121 9003

**David Davies GOsC**
➊ ➕ ⓝ ⊘ ✻
Fees: £26–35; Second visit: £21–30
Leeds LS18
0113 2589687

**Louise Elliott GOsC**
➊ ➍ ⓝ
Fees: £26–35; Second visit: £21–30
Leeds LS20,Roundhay LS8
01943 872278

**Peter Fenton GOsC, BOA**
◯ ⓝ ✻
Fees: <£25; Second visit: £21–30
Leeds LS17
0113 268 5992

**Jane Goodall GOsC, BOA**
➊ ➕ ➍ ⓝ ⊘ ✻
Fees: £26–35; Second visit: £21–30
Leeds LS8
0113 237 1173

**Wendy Holtham GOsC**
➊ ➍ ⓜ ✻
Fees: £26–35; Second visit: £21–30
Leeds LS20
01943 872278

**Sarah Izzard GOsC, BOA**
➊ ➍ ⓝ ⊘ ✻
Fees: <£25; Second visit: £21–30
Leeds LS1
0113 243 6066

**Andrew Pallas GOsC, BOA**
◯ ➕ ⓝ ✻
Fees: <£25; Second visit: £21–30
Leeds LS20
01943 878363

**Nathan Reynolds GOsC**
➊ ➍ ⓝ ✻
Fees: <£25; Second visit: £21–30
Leeds LS16
0113 2745126

**Nicola Sell GOsC, BOA**
➊ ➍ ⓝ ✻
Fees: <£25; Second visit: £21–30
Leeds LS16
0113 274 5126

**A Sevi GOsC, BOA**
➊ ➕ ➍ ⓝ ⊘ ✻
Fees: <£25; Second visit: £21–30
Leeds LS8
0113 237 1173

**Martyn B Speight GOsC, BOA,**
➊ ➍ ⓝ ⊘ ✻
Fees: £46–55; Second visit: £31–40
Leeds LS18
0870 078 0589

**Alan Apling GOsC**
➊ ➍ ⓝ ⊘ ✻
Fees: £26–35; Second visit: £21–30
Leeds LS6
0113 275 3692

**Kerrie Barker GOsC, BOA**
➊ ⓝ Ⓔ
Fees: <£25; Second visit: £21–30
Leeds LS6
0113 2786606

**James Beck GOsC**
➊ ➕ ⓝ ✻
Fees: <£25; Second visit: £21–30
Leeds LS6
0113 278 6606

**Christopher Huyton GOsC, BOA**
➊ ⓝ Ⓔ ✻
Fees: <£25; Second visit: £21–30
Leeds LS6
0113 278 6606

**S Persaud GOsC**
➊ ➍ ⓝ ⊘ ✻
Fees: <£25; Second visit: £21–30
Skipton BD23
01756 792610

**Alexia Cook GOsC**
➊ ◯ ⓝ ⊘
Fees: <£25; Second visit: £41–50
Wakefield WF1
01924 369077

**Lisa Harris GOsC, BOA**
✛ NHS ✿
Fees: £26–35; Second visit: £21–30
Wakefield WF1
01924 369077

**Mark Wilcox GOsC, BOA**
✛ O ⊕ NHS ✿
Fees: £26–35; Second visit: <£20
Wakefield WF1
01924 369077

**Mary Bridger GOsC, BOA**
✛ NHS
Fees: £26–35; Second visit: £21–30
Wetherby LS22
01937 584775

# Chiropractic

## CUMBRIA

**Ruth Brittain-Dodd GCC, MCA**
✛ O NHS ✿
Fees: £26–35; Second visit: £21–30
Carlisle CA6
01228 675819

**Claire Duplock GCC, BCA**
✛ O ⊕ NHS ⊘ € ✿
Fees: £26–35; Second visit: £21–30
Kendal LA9
01539 733000

## DURHAM

**David Stott GCC, MCA**
✛ O ⊕ ✿
Fees: £36–45; Second visit: £21–30
Darlington DL1
01325 486485

**Steffan H Abel GCC, BCA**
✛ ⊕ NHS ✿
Fees: £36–45; Second visit: £21–30
Durham DH3
0191 389 1866

**Marie Allan GCC, BCA**
✛ NHS ✿
Fees: £36–45; Second visit: £21–30
Durham DH3
0191 389 1866

## EAST RIDING OF YORKSHIRE

**Paul Allison GCC, BCA**
✛ NHS ✿
Fees: £26–35; Second visit: £21–30
Beverley HU17
01482 870934

## NORTHUMBERLAND

**The Hon Richard Arthur GCC, MCA**
O NHS
Fees: <£25; Second visit: £21–30
Hallington NE19
01434 672219

**Richard Millo GCC**
✛ NHS ✿
Fees: £36–45; Second visit: £21–30
Heaton NE6
0191 209 4511

**Sonya Floreani GCC**
✛ NHS € ✿ ⊜
Fees: £36–45; Second visit: <£20
Hexham NE46
01434 602666

**Vincent Sharkey GCC, BCA**
✛ O NHS € ✿
Fees: £36–45; Second visit: <£20
Morpeth NE61, Ashington NE63
01670 511066

# Chiropractic

**Matthew Bailey GCC, BCA**
✦ 🔵 ⊘
**Fees:** £36–45
Newcastle Upon Tyne NE2
0191 281 3711

**Stephen Henderson GCC**
✦ ✚ ✦ 🔵 ⊘ ✿
**Fees:** £26–35; Second visit: £21–30
Newcastle Upon Tyne NE1
0191 245 3790

**Adam Kasar GCC, BAAC**
○ ✿
**Fees:** £26–35; Second visit: £21–30
Newcastle Upon Tyne NE4
0191 273 2040

**Alan Scott GCC, BCA**
✦ 🔵 Ⓔ ✿
**Fees:** £36–45; Second visit: £21–30
Newcastle Upon Tyne NE3
0191 217 0387

## NORTH YORKSHIRE

**Paul Cheung GCC, BCA**
✦ 🔵 ⊘ ✿
**Fees:** £46–55; Second visit: £21–30
Harrogate HG2
01423 701777

**Debbie Saxton GCC, BCA**
✦ 🔵 Ⓔ ✿
**Fees:** £46–55; Second visit: £21–30
Harrogate HG2
01423 701777

**Christopher John Smith GCC, BCA**
✦ 🔵
**Fees:** £36–45; Second visit: <£20
Skipton BD23
01756 797838

**Mrs Sue Brown GCC, MCA**
✦ ✚ ✦ 🔵 ⊘ ✿
**Fees:** £36–45; Second visit: £21–30
York YO62
01751 430335

**Helen Knowles GCC, MCA**
○ 🔵 ✿
**Fees:** £36–45; Second visit: £21–30
York YO61
01347 810346

**Jessica Johnson GCC, BCA**
✦ 🔵 ⊘ 🔴
**Fees:** £36–45; Second visit: £21–30
York YO7
01845 522242

**Richard Skippings GCC, BCA**
✦ 🔵 ⊘ 🔴
**Fees:** £36–45; Second visit: £21–30
York YO7
01845 522242

**M Weatherstone MNIMH**
✦ ○ 🔵 ✿
**Fees:** £26–35; Second visit: <£20
York YO23
01904 613644

## TEESSIDE

**Amanda Corbishley GCC, BCA**
✦ ✦ 🔵
**Fees:** £36–45; Second visit: £21–30
Darlington DL3
01325 466022

**Maria Fletcher GCC, BAAC**
✦ 🔵 ✿
**Fees:** <£25; Second visit: £21–30
Hartlepool TS26
01429 860460

**Rosemary Ellenor GCC, BAAC**
✦ 🔵 ✿
**Fees:** <£25; Second visit: £21–30
Middlesbrough TS3
01642 501111

**Anne Laursen GCC, BCA**
✦ 🔵 ⊘
**Fees:** £36–45; Second visit: £21–30
Stockton-on-Tees TS17
01642 633888

## TYNE & WEAR

**Luke R Ramsay GCC, BCA**
✦ 🔵 ✿
**Fees:** £36–45; Second visit: £21–30
Monkseaton NE25
0191 252 2170

**Debbie Thomson GCC, BCA**
✚ ⓝ ✿
**Fees:** £36–45; Second visit: £21–30
South Shields NE33
0191 455 8735

## WEST YORKSHIRE

**Jacqueline Beer GCC, BCA**
✚ ⓝ ⊘
**Fees:** £36–45; Second visit: £21–30
Bradford BD9
01274 545510

**Martin Vesely GCC, BCA**
✚ ⓝ ⊘ ✿
**Fees:** £36–45; Second visit: £21–30
Bradford BD9
01274 545510

**Roland Berman GCC**
✚ ⓝ ✿ ⓔ
**Fees:** £36–45; Second visit: £21–30
Halifax HX1
01422 252625

**Fiona Driver GCC, MCA**
✚ ⓞ ⊕ ⓝ ✿
**Fees:** £36–45; Second visit: £21–30
Huddersfield HD8
01484 865459

**A Vesela GCC, BCA**
✚ ⓝ ⊘
**Fees:** £36–45; Second visit: £21–30
Huddersfield HD3
01484 461440

**Martin Andersen GCC, BCA**
ⓝ ⊘ ✿
**Fees:** £36–45; Second visit: £21–30
Leeds LS27,Bradford BD4
0113 295 1666

**Mark Butterworth GCC, BCA**
✚ ⓝ ⓔ ✿
**Fees:** £36–45; Second visit: £21–30
Leeds LS16
0113 228 9888

**Christine Waterer GCC, MCA**
✚ ⓞ ⊕ ⊘ ✿
**Fees:** £36–45; Second visit: £21–30
Marsden HD7
01484 841176

**Mark Holbek GCC, BCA**
✚ ⓝ ✿ ⓔ
**Fees:** £26–35; Second visit: <£20
Roundhay LS8
0113 266 1419

**Barry McQuire GCC, BCA**
✚ ⓝ ⓔ
**Fees:** £46–55; Second visit: £21–30
Roundhay LS8
0113 266 1419

**Nicola Morrison-Poole GCC, BCA**
✚ ⓝ ⓔ ✿ ⓔ
**Fees:** £26–35; Second visit: <£20
Roundhay LS8
0113 266 1419

**D Corlet GCC, BCA**
✚ ⓝ ⓔ
**Fees:** £26–35; Second visit: £21–30
Wakefield WF1,Wakefield WF1
01924 200805

**Ann Byrgren GCC, BCA**
✚ ⓝ ⊘ ✿
**Fees:** <£25; Second visit: <£20
Wakefield WF8
01977 690333

# Western Herbal Medicine

## CUMBRIA

**L M Hodgkinson MNIMH**
ⓝ ✿
**Fees:** £26–35; Second visit: <£20
Cockermouth CA13
01900 826392

**J Ainsworth MNIMH**
ⓞ
**Fees:** £26–35; Second visit: <£20
Wigton CA7
01697 320116

# Western Herbal Medicine

## EAST RIDING OF YORKSHIRE

**Margaret E Garner IRCH**
⊕ ⓝ ❀
**Fees:** £26–35; Second visit: <£20
Driffield YO25
01377 241800

**Elizabeth King MNIMH**
⊕ ⓖ ⓝ ❀
**Fees:** <£25; Second visit: <£20
Hull HU17
01482 869678

## NORTHUMBERLAND

**Ross Menzies IRCH**
⊕ ⓖ ⓝ ❀
**Fees:** £26–35; Second visit: £21–30
Hexham NE46
01434 606619

**A Romer MNIMH**
○ ⓔ ❀
**Fees:** £36–45; Second visit: <£20
Seaton Sluice NE26
0191 237 1063

## NORTH YORKSHIRE

**C A Haughton MNIMH**
⊕ ○ ⓝ
**Fees:** £26–35; Second visit: <£20
Malton YO17
01944 728441

## WEST YORKSHIRE

**S Cahill MNIMH**
⊕ ⓔ
**Fees:** £26–35; Second visit: <£20
Halifax HX1
01422 357009

**S Goodwin MNIMH**
⊕ ⓖ ❀
**Fees:** £26–35; Second visit: <£20
Hebden Bridge HX7
01422 843517

**P A Jones MNIMH**
⊕ ○ ⊕ ⓖ ⓝ ⓔ ❀
**Fees:** £26–35; Second visit: <£20
Huddersfield HD9,Huddersfield HD5
01484 682196

**T Wightman MNIMH**
⊕ ○ ⓖ ❀
**Fees:** £26–35; Second visit: <£20
Leeds LS18,Wakefield WF1
0113 258 9332

# Chinese Herbal Medicine

## NORTH YORKSHIRE

**Michael Burgess RCHM**
⊕ ⓖ ❀
**Fees:** £36–45; Second visit: £21–30
York YO31
01904 421032

**Alison Gould RCHM**
○ ❀
**Fees:** £36–45; Second visit: £21–30
York YO31
01904 421032

## TEESSIDE

**Keith Thomas RCHM**
⊕ ⓖ ⓝ ❀
**Fees:** £36–45; Second visit: £21–30
Middlesbrough TS4
01642 246385

**Clifton Wicks RCHM**
⊕ ⓖ ⓝ ⊘ ❀
**Fees:** £26–35; Second visit: <£20
Middlesbrough TS4
01642 818241

## TYNE & WEAR

**Neil Thompson RCHM**
O ❀
Fees: £26–35; Second visit: £21–30
Newcastle Upon Tyne NE6
0191 265 0202

## WEST YORKSHIRE

**Liping Han RCHM**
⊕ ⊕ ⓔ
Fees: £26–35
Bradford BD8,Newcastle Upon Tyne
NE3,York YO24
01274 484514

**Mary Samuel RCHM**
⊕ ⊕ ⊕ ⓝ ❀
Fees: >£55; Second visit: £31–40
Bradford BD8
01274 547020

**Stan Switala RCHM**
⊕ ⊕
Fees: £26–35; Second visit: £21–30
Bradford BD8
01274 484514

**Louise Attwood RCHM**
⊕ ⓝ ⊘
Fees: £36–45; Second visit: £21–30
Leeds LS7
0113 228 4996

**Jacqueline Clelland RCHM**
⊕ ⊕ ⊘ ❀
Fees: £36–45; Second visit: <£20
Wakefield WF10
01924 373353

# North West

Cheshire
Greater Manchester
Lancashire
Merseyside

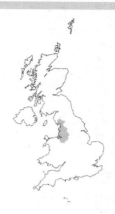

## Acupuncture

### CHESHIRE

**Charles Buck BAcC**
Fees: >£55; Second visit: £21–30
Chester CH2
01244 390411

**Marianne Buck BAcC**
Fees: £36–45; Second visit: £21–30
Chester CH2
01244 390411

**Trish Hunter BAcC, AACP**
Fees: £36–45; Second visit: £21–30
Chester CH2
01244 390411

**Carl Reynolds BAcC**
Fees: £26–35; Second visit: £21–30
Chester CH3
01244 344131

**Peter Thompson BAcC**
Fees: Second visit: £21–30
Crewe CW1
01270 505558

**S E Shaw AACP**
Fees: £26–35; Second visit: £31–40
Deeside CH5
01244 535548

**David M Jones BAcC**
Fees: £46–55; Second visit: £21–30
Knutsford WA16
01565 633967

**Joanne Middleton BAcC**
Fees: £26–35; Second visit: £21–30
Knutsford WA16
01565 750081

**Jacqueline Hu BAcC**
Fees: £26–35; Second visit: £21–30
Nantwich CW5
01270 629222

**Stephen Macallan BAcC**
Fees: £46–55; Second visit: £21–30
Nantwich CW5
01270 629933

# Acupuncture

**Jinty Keating BAcC, BMAS**
🜨 🅞 🜨 🜨
**Fees:** £26–35; Second visit: £21–30
Tarporley CW6,Sandbach CW11
01829 752472

**N G O'Callaghan BMAS,**
🜨 🜨 🜨 🜨 🜨
**Fees:** <£25; Second visit: £21–30
Tarporley CW6
01829 733456

**Paula Simm BAcC**
🜨 🜨 🜨 🜨
**Fees:** £26–35; Second visit: £21–30
Widnes WA8
0151 420 3398

## GREATER MANCHESTER

**Zhuang Kang BAcC**
🜨 🜨 🜨 🜨 🜨
**Fees:** <£25; Second visit: <£20
Ashton-under-Lyne OL6
0161 343 2480

**Andrew Strinyce BAcC,**
🜨 🜨
**Fees:** £26–35; Second visit: <£20
Ashton-under-Lyne OL6
0161 339 4292

**Jieqi Hui BAcC**
🜨 🜨 🜨
**Fees:** <£25; Second visit: <£20
Altrincham WA15
0161 973 2107

**Diana E Grogan BAcC**
🜨 🜨 🜨 🜨
**Fees:** £26–35; Second visit: £21–30
Blackburn BB2
01254 263728

**Ann Marie James BAcC**
🜨 🜨 🜨
**Fees:** £26–35; Second visit: £21–30
Blackburn BB2
01254 52143

**F Ding BAcC**
🜨 🅞 🜨 🜨 🜨 🜨
**Fees:** £26–35; Second visit: £21–30
Blackpool FY4,Kendal LA9
01253 344115

**Hanna HM Huo BAcC**
🜨 🅞 🜨 🜨 🜨 🜨
**Fees:** £26–35; Second visit: £21–30
Blackpool FY4,Kendal LA9
01253 344115

**Helen Rocca AACP**
🜨 🜨 🜨 🜨 🜨
**Fees:** £26–35; Second visit: £21–30
Blackpool FY1
01253 699444

**Karen Willcock BAcC, AACP**
🜨 🜨 🜨 🜨 🜨
**Fees:** £26–35; Second visit: £21–30
Bolton BL1
01204 386170

**Junkun Bai BAcC**
🜨 🜨 🜨
**Fees:** £36–45; Second visit: £21–30
Bolton BL2
0161 905 3666

**Alasdair Carter BMAS**
🜨 🜨 🜨 🜨 🜨
**Fees:** £26–35; Second visit: £21–30
Clitheroe BB7
01200 421888

**James Hampson BAcC**
🅞 🜨
**Fees:** <£25; Second visit: <£20
Fleetwood FY7
01253 872331

**Cherith Adams BAcC**
🅞 🜨 🜨
**Fees:** £26–35; Second visit: £21–30
Lancaster LA2,Kendal LA8
01524 811066

**Susan M Keady BAcC**
🜨 🜨 🜨 🜨
**Fees:** £26–35; Second visit: £21–30
Leyland PR25
01772 456657

**Catherine Swales BAcC**
🜨 🜨 🜨 🜨
**Fees:** £26–35; Second visit: £21–30
Leyland PR25
01772 456657

**Susan Martin AACP**
⊕ ✿ 🔘
Fees: £36–45; Second visit: £31–40
Ormskirk L40
01695 729019

**Steve Harris BAcC**
⊕ ⊕ ⊕ ✿ 🔘
Fees: £26–35; Second visit: £21–30
Preston PR3
01729 840670

**Anthony Mark Smith BAcC**
O ⊘ ✿ 🔘
Fees: £36–45; Second visit: £21–30
Preston PR5
01254 854809

**Sheila M Crisp AACP**
O ⊕ 🔘 ⊘ ✿ 🔘
Fees: £36–45; Second visit: £31–40
Rossendale BB4
01706 215836

**Xuan He BAcC**
⊕ 🔘 ✿ 🔘
Fees: £36–45; Second visit: £21–30
Bolton BL2,Preston PR2,
Stoke-on-Trent ST1
01204 399116

**Vivien Onslow BAcC**
⊕ O ✿ 🔘
Fees: £36–45; Second visit: £21–30
Bolton BL3,Chorley PR7,Bury BL9
01204 658532

**Hilary Evans AACP**
O ✿ 🔘
Fees: £36–45; Second visit: £31–40
Bury BL9
0161 761 6400

**Xiaohong Kang BAcC**
⊕ ⊕ 🔘 ⊘ ✿ 🔘
Fees: £26–35; Second visit: £21–30
Cheadle SK8,Alderley Edge SK9
0161 428 4222

**Lingsoong Wong BAcC**
⊕ O ⊕ ⊘ ✿ 🔘
Fees: £26–35; Second visit: £21–30
Cheadle SK8
0161 491 4667

**Karen Devlin BAcC**
⊕ ⊕ ✿ 🔘
Fees: £26–35; Second visit: £21–30
High Peak SK22
01663 742282

**Allison Sumner AACP**
⊕ ⊕ 🔘
Fees: £26–35; Second visit: £21–30
Leigh WN7
01942 260714

**Ann Bromley BAcC**
O ⓔ ✿ 🔘
Fees: £26–35; Second visit: £21–30
Manchester M20
0161 445 7998

**Joshua Enkin BAcC**
⊕ O ⊕ ⊘ ✿ 🔘
Fees: £46–55; Second visit: £31–40
Manchester M20,Stockport SK7
0161 434 0195

**Tejapushpa Entwistle BAcC**
⊕ ⊕ ✿ 🔘
Fees: £36–45; Second visit: £21–30
Manchester M4
0161 833 2528

**Janne Foster BAcC**
⊕ ⊕ 🔘
Fees: £36–45; Second visit: £21–30
Manchester M21
0161 881 2128

**Tracey Kennedy BAcC**
O ⊕ 🔘 ✿ 🔘
Fees: £26–35; Second visit: £21–30
Manchester M9
0161 702 1278

**Chris Nortley BAcC**
⊕ 🔘 ⊘ 🔘
Manchester M8
0161 720 2466

**John Spencer AACP**
⊕ 🔘 🔘
Fees: £26–35; Second visit: £21–30
Manchester M4
0161 8346050

# Acupuncture

**Jian Lan Suen BAcC**
⊕ 🔵 ✿ 🔵
**Fees:** £26–35; Second visit: £21–30
Manchester M1
0161 2361319

**Jane Sweet BAcC**
⊕ ⊕ ⊕ ✿ 🔵
**Fees:** £36–45; Second visit: £21–30
Manchester M2,Ashton-under-Lyne
OL6
0161 834 7899

**Shulan Tang BAcC**
⊕ 🔵 ✿ 🔵
**Fees:** £26–35
Manchester M21
0161 8810088

**Linda Greenwood BAcC**
O ✿ 🔵
**Fees:** £36–45; Second visit: £21–30
Rochdale OL12
01706 377073

**Jennifer Train AACP**
O ⊘ 🔵
**Fees:** £26–35; Second visit: £31–40
Rochdale OL12
01706 359947

**Christine White AACP**
⊕ O ⊘ 🔵
**Fees:** £36–45; Second visit: £31–40
Rochdale OL11
01706 522277

**Zeng Fu Peng BAcC**
⊕ 🔵 ⊘ ✿ 🔵
**Fees:** £26–35; Second visit: £21–30
Stockport SK1
0161 480 7060

**Robert Powell BAcC**
O ✿ 🔵
**Fees:** £26–35; Second visit: £21–30
Stockport SK7
0161 439 8605

**Marion Fisher BAcC**
O ✿ 🔵
**Fees:** £26–35; Second visit: <£20
Warrington WA2
01925 812263

**Madeleine Soderstrom BAcC**
⊕ ⊕ ⊘ ✿ 🔵
**Fees:** <£25; Second visit: <£20
Wigan WN1
01942 321235

**Lynne M Dean BAcC**
O ✿ 🔵
**Fees:** £26–35; Second visit: £21–30
Wigan WN4
01942 271425

## MERSEYSIDE

**Ian James Griffiths BAcC**
⊕ ✿ 🔵
**Fees:** £26–35; Second visit: £21–30
Birkenhead CH42
0151 645 9073

**Peter A Pang BAcC**
⊕ 🔵 ✿ 🔵
**Fees:** £36–45; Second visit: £21–30
Bootle L20
0151 922 2873

**Kate Anderson BAcC**
⊕ O ⊕ ⊕ ✿ 🔵
**Fees:** £26–35; Second visit: £21–30
Liverpool L15
0151 734 4918

**Wendy Bland BAcC**
⊕ ⊕ 🔵 ✿ 🔵
**Fees:** £26–35; Second visit: £21–30
Liverpool L15
0151 734 5909

**Ylping Fang BAcC**
⊕ ⊕ 🔵 ✿ 🔵
**Fees:** £26–35; Second visit: £21–30
Liverpool L1
0151 708 8088

**Keith Milner BAcC**
⊕ O ⊕ 🔵 ✿ 🔵
**Fees:** £26–35; Second visit: £21–30
Liverpool L1,Newtown SY16
0151 707 1311

# Acupuncture

**Hal Brittain BAcC**
○ ⊙
**Fees:** £26–35; Second visit: £21–30
Southport PR9
01704 501271

**Sarah Green AACP**
⊕ ⬤ ✴ ⬤
**Fees:** £36–45; Second visit: £21–30
Wirral CH61
0151 929 5260

# Homeopathy

## CHESHIRE

**Angela Needham RSHom**
⊕ ○ ⊕ ⬤ © ✴
**Fees:** £36–45; Second visit: £20–30
Chester CH2,Neston CH64
01244 311952

**Carol Reynolds RSHom**
⊕ ○ ⊕ ⬤ © ✴
**Fees:** £36–45; Second visit: £20–30
Chester CH3
01244 344131

**Kathleen Kerry RSHom**
⊕ ○ ⊕ ⬤ ©
**Fees:** £46–55; Second visit: £20–30
Helsby WA6
01928 722356

**Helen Whalley RSHom**
⊕ ⬤ © ✴
**Fees:** £36–45; Second visit: £20–30
Knutsford WA16
01270 528116

**Elizabeth Kinsey RSHom**
⊕ ⬤ ©
**Fees:** >£55; Second visit: £31–40
Macclesfield SK11
01625 431480

**Cos Petrondas RSHom**
⊕ ⊕ ⬤ ©
**Fees:** >£55; Second visit: £20–30
Macclesfield SK10
01625 500778

**Susan Petrondas RSHom**
⊕ ⊕ ⬤ ©
**Fees:** >£55; Second visit: £20–30
Macclesfield SK10
01625 500778

## GREATER MANCHESTER

**Carmel Searson RSHom**
⊕ ○ ⊕ © ✴
**Fees:** £46–55; Second visit: £20–30
Bolton BL1
01204 386170

**Karen A Bridgwater RSHom**
⊕ ⊕ ⊕ ⬤ ✴
**Fees:** £46–55; Second visit: £20–30
Bolton BL5
01942 810318

**Carole Gimson RSHom**
○ ⬤ ✴
**Fees:** £46–55; Second visit: £20–30
Bolton BL5
01942 797193

**Jonathan Jones MFHom**
⊕ ⬤ ✴
**Fees:** £36–45; Second visit: £20–30
Bolton BL7
01204 853869

**Andrew Demetriou MFHom**
⊕ ⊕ ⬤ ⊘ © ✴
**Fees:** >£55; Second visit: £41–50
Bury BL9,Rochdale OL11
0161 761 6677

**Prunella Elizabeth Caville MFHom**
⊕ ⊕ ⊕ ⬤ ⊘ ©
**Fees:** >£55; Second visit: £41–50
Cheadle SK8
0161 428 4222

**Annette Bond RSHom**
○ ⬤ ©
**Fees:** £36–45; Second visit: £20–30
Manchester M16
0161 860 6716

# Homeopathy

**Nancy Green RSHom**
➕ 🅞 🏥 Ⓔ
**Fees:** £46–55; Second visit: £20–30
Manchester M21
0161 881 0733

**Liz Hennel RSHom**
➕ ➕ ⊘ ❈
**Fees:** £36–45; Second visit: £20–30
Manchester M27,Littleborough
OL15,Oldham OL4
0161 794 0665

**Annie Manogue RSHom**
➕ 🅞 🏥 Ⓔ ❈
**Fees:** £36–45; Second visit: £20–30
Manchester M14,Sale M33
0161 225 7352

**Steffie Price RSHom**
➕ ➕
**Fees:** £46–55; Second visit: £20–30
Manchester M14
0161 257 2445

**Kathy Ryan MFHom**
➕ ➕ 🏥 ⊘
**Fees:** £46–55; Second visit: £31–40
Manchester M1
0845 121 9005

**Anne Rydeheard RSHom**
➕ 🅞 ➕ 🏥 Ⓔ ❈
**Fees:** £36–45; Second visit: £20–30
Manchester M20
0161 445 9122

**Ann Donaldson RSHom**
➕ ➕ 🏥 ❈
**Fees:** £46–55; Second visit: £20–30
Manchester M29
0161 211 9685

**Sarah Roberts RSHom**
➕ ➕ Ⓔ ❈
**Fees:** £46–55; Second visit: £20–30
Manchester M14
0161 226 2237

**Ernest Roberts RSHom**
🅞 🏥
**Fees:** >£55; Second visit: £31–40
Manchester M14
0161 257 2445

**Catherine Donovan RSHom**
➕ 🅞 🏥 Ⓔ ❈
**Fees:** £36–45; Second visit: £20–30
Sale M33
0161 973 3116

**Ian MacLure MFHom**
➕ ➕ ⊘ ❈
**Fees:** >£55; Second visit: £20–30
Stockport SK6
0161 494 1452

**Gail Moore RSHom**
➕ 🏥 ❈
**Fees:** £36–45; Second visit: £20–30
Stockport SK6
0161 430 5980

**Gillian Scott Zukovskis RSHom**
➕ ➕ 🏥 Ⓔ ❈
**Fees:** £46–55; Second visit: £20–30
Stockport SK4
0161 431 6991

**Joy Lucas RSHom**
🅞 🏥 Ⓔ ❈
**Fees:** £36–45; Second visit: £20–30
Saddleworth OL3
01457 873349

**Jean Sharples RSHom**
➕ ➕ 🏥 ❈
**Fees:** >£55; Second visit: £20–30
Oldham OL12
01942 819832

## LANCASHIRE

**Valerie Colley RSHom**
🅞 🏥 Ⓔ ❈
**Fees:** £25–35; Second visit: <£20
Accrington BB5
01254 395902

**Jean Duckworth RSHom**
➕ 🅞 ➕ 🏥 ⊘ Ⓔ ❈
**Fees:** £46–55; Second visit: £20–30
Blackburn BB1
01254 249970

**Terence E J Ryan RSHom**
➕ ➕ 🏥 ❈
**Fees:** £36–45; Second visit: £20–30
Blackburn BB2,Preston PR2
01254 55526

**Amanda Bingley RSHom**
O Ⓔ ❀
Fees: £46–55; Second visit: £20–30
Carnforth LA5
01524 781375

**Agnes Moodie RSHom**
⊕ O ⊕ ⓦ Ⓔ ❀
Fees: £36–45; Second visit: £20–30
Carnforth LA6
01524 241753

**Robert A Duddell RSHom**
O ⓦ Ⓔ ❀
Fees: £36–45; Second visit: £20–30
Lancaster LA5
01524 701166

**Margaret Ecclestone RSHom**
O ⊕ ⓦ Ⓔ ❀
Fees: £46–55; Second visit: £20–30
Lancaster LA1
01524 68378

**Kate Chatfield RSHom**
⊕ ⊕ ⓦ ❀
Fees: £46–55; Second visit: £20–30
Preston PR2
01772 761166

**Janet Harding RSHom**
⊕ ⊕ ⊕ ⓦ Ⓔ ❀
Fees: £46–55; Second visit: £20–30
Preston PR2
01772 761166

**Margaret Livesey RSHom**
⊕ O ⊕ ⊕ ⓦ Ⓔ ❀
Fees: £46–55; Second visit: £20–30
Preston PR5
01772 629569

**Hazel Partington RSHom**
⊕ O ⓦ Ⓔ ❀
Fees: £36–45; Second visit: £20–30
Preston PR5
01772 626194

**Karen Goodman MFHom**
⊕ ⓦ ∅
Fees: £36–45; Second visit: <£20
Salford M6
0161 736 7422

**Archana Gandhi RSHom**
⊕ O ⊕ ⊕ ⓦ Ⓔ ❀
Fees: £46–55; Second visit: £31–40
Wigan WN5,Southport PR8
01695 625900

## MERSEYSIDE

**Hilary Hampel RSHom**
⊕ O ⊕ Ⓔ ❀
Fees: £46–55; Second visit: £31–40
Birkdale PR8,Liverpool L18,Liverpool
L22
0151 931 4116

**Anna Pawley RSHom**
O ⓦ ❀
Fees: £25–35; Second visit: £20–30
Lydiate L31
0151 526 2001

**Som Singh Chana MFHom**
⊕ ⊕ ⓦ Ⓔ ❀
Fees: >£55; Second visit: £20–30
Prescot L34,Prescot L35
0151 430 9223

**Anne Campbell Biezanek MFHom**
O
Fees: £46–55; Second visit: £20–30
Wallasey CH45
0151 630 4000

# Osteopathy

## CHESHIRE

**Thomas Walter GOsC**
⊕ ⊕ Ⓝ Ⓔ ✿
Fees: £26–35; Second visit: £21–30
Alderley Edge SK9
01625 586229

**Sally Devereux GOsC, BOA**
⊕
Fees: £36–45; Second visit: £31–40
Chester CH1
01244 371820

**Elizabeth Ellis GOsC, BOA**
O Ⓝ ⊘ ✿
Fees: <£25; Second visit: £21–30
Chester CH4
01244 678322

**Yvonne McCarthy GOsC, BOA**
⊕ O ⊕ ⊕ Ⓝ ⊘ Ⓔ ✿
Fees: £36–45; Second visit: £21–30
Chester CH65
0151 356 1394

**Deirdre Stubbs GOsC, BOA**
⊕ ⊕ Ⓝ
Fees: £36–45; Second visit: £31–40
Chester CH1
01244 371820

**Maziar Vaezzadeh GOsC**
⊕ O ⊕ ⊕ Ⓝ Ⓔ ✿
Fees: £26–35; Second visit: £21–30
Chester CH2
01244 321885

**Georgina Vere GOsC, BOA**
⊕ Ⓝ ⊘ ✿
Fees: £36–45; Second visit: £31–40
Chester CH1
01244 371820

**Margaret Horner GOsC, BOA**
⊕ Ⓝ ⊘ Ⓔ ✿
Fees: <£25; Second visit: £21–30
Congleton CW12
01260 280444

**Suzette Pulman GOsC, BOA**
⊕ ⊕ Ⓝ ⊘ ✿
Fees: £36–45; Second visit: £21–30
Lymm WA13
01925 752264

**Susan M Coupe GOsC, BOA**
⊕ ⊕ ✿
Fees: <£25; Second visit: £21–30
Nantwich CW5
01270 629933

**Martin Davies GOsC, BOA**
⊕ ⊕ ⊕ Ⓝ ⊘ ✿
Fees: <£25; Second visit: £21–30
Nantwich CW5
01270 610288

**Jason Le Roy GOsC**
⊕ ⊕ Ⓝ ✿
Fees: <£25; Second visit: £21–30
Nantwich CW5
01270 629933

**John Constantine GOsC, BOA**
O Ⓝ Ⓔ ✿
Fees: £26–35; Second visit: £21–30
Northwich CW8
01606 74746

**Charlotte OToole GOsC, BOA**
⊕ O ⊕ Ⓝ Ⓔ ✿
Fees: £26–35; Second visit: £21–30
Sale M33
0101 969 6555

**Elizabeth Curphey GOsC, BOA**
⊕ ⊕ Ⓝ ⊘
Fees: £26–35; Second visit: £21–30
Sandbach CW11
01270 763926

**Louise Potter GOsC**
⊕ ⊕ Ⓝ ⊘ ✿
Fees: £26–35; Second visit: £21–30
Sandbach CW11
01270 763926

**Elizabeth Spiby GOsC, BOA**
⊕ O ⊕ Ⓝ Ⓔ ✿
Fees: <£25; Second visit: <£20
Sandbach CW11
01270 753146

**Brian McCormick GOsC, BOA**
⊕ Ⓝ ⊘ ✿
Fees: <£25; Second visit: £21–30
Warrington WA3
01925 766666

Osteopathy

## Martin Murgatroyd GOsC, BOA
➕ 🔵 ⊘ ❄
**Fees:** £36–45; Second visit: £21–30
Warrington WA1
01925 635670

## Nicholas 'Jadon' Smith GOsC, BOA
➕ 🔵 🔵 ❄
**Fees:** <£25; Second visit: £21–30
Widnes WA8
0151 420 3398

## Julia Gaze GOsC
⭕ 🔵 ⊘ ❄
**Fees:** £26–35; Second visit: £21–30
Wilmslow SK9
01625 533813

## Margaret Gul GOsC, BOA
➕ 🔵 ❄
**Fees:** £26–35; Second visit: £21–30
Wilmslow SK9
01625 526875

## Andrew N F Kerr GOsC
➕ ⊘ ❄
**Fees:** £36–45; Second visit: £31–40
Wilmslow SK9
01625 530977

## Adam Mark Tilstone GOsC, BOA
➕ 🔵 🔵 ⊘ ❄
**Fees:** <£25; Second visit: £21–30
Nantwich CW5
01270 629933

## GREATER MANCHESTER

## John Ibbetson GOsC
➕ ⭕ ⊕ 🔵 🔵 ⊘ ⒠ ❄
**Fees:** £26–35; Second visit: £21–30
Bolton BL1
01204 360010

## Philippe Raffit GOsC
➕ 🔵 ❄
**Fees:** <£25; Second visit: £21–30
Bolton BL6
01204 668686

## Debra Stackwood GOsC
➕ ⊕ 🔵 ❄
**Fees:** <£25; Second visit: £21–30
Bolton BL1
01204 841060

## Zoe Sutcliffe GOsC
➕ 🔵
**Fees:** £26–35; Second visit: £21–30
Bolton BL1
01204 522133

## Joanna Cheaney GOsC, BOA
➕ 🔵 ❄
**Fees:** £36–45; Second visit: £31–40
Bramhall SK7
0161 440 0298

## Maureen Pickup GOsC, BOA
➕ 🔵 ⒠
**Fees:** £36–45; Second visit: £31–40
Bramhall SK7
0161 440 0298

## Michael Taylor GOsC
➕ ⊕ 🔵
**Fees:** £26–35; Second visit: £21–30
Bury BL9
0161 797 7770

## Philip Owen GOsC, BOA
➕ ⊕ 🔵 ❄
**Fees:** >£55; Second visit: £41–50
Cheadle SK8
0161 428 4222

## Nicholas Vine GOsC
➕ ⊕ 🔵 ⒠ ❄
**Fees:** £26–35; Second visit: £21–30
Didsbury M20
0161 445 1018

## Denis Brown GOsC, BOA
➕ 🔵 ⊘ ❄
**Fees:** <£25; Second visit: £21–30
Manchester M3
0161 834 4076

## Dharmendra Gogia GOsC, BOA
➕ ⭕ 🔵 ⊘
**Fees:** £46–55
Manchester M3
0161 834 3090

## Richard Griffiths GOsC
➕ ⊕ 🔵
**Fees:** £26–35; Second visit: £21–30
Manchester M21
0161 881 2128

# Osteopathy

**Christopher Heslop GOsC, BOA**
⊕ ⊕ ⊕ ⊛ ⊘ ❈
Fees: <£25; Second visit: £21–30
Manchester M41
0161 747 2443

**Jonathan Poston GOsC, BOA**
⊕ ⊛
Fees: <£25; Second visit: £21–30
Manchester M25
0161 798 6352

**Simon Turgoose GOsC**
⊕ O ⊕ ⊛ ⊘ ❈
Fees: £26–35; Second visit: £21–30
Manchester M21
0161 434 0947

**Kay Barker GOsC**
⊕ O ⊛ ❈
Fees: £36–45; Second visit: £21–30
Manchester M25,Liverpool
L1,Southport PR8
0161 773 0123

**Tara Ascott GOsC, BOA**
⊕ O ⊕ ⊘ ❈
Fees: <£25; Second visit: £21–30
Manchester M27
0161 728 2857

**Janet Fowler GOsC, BOA**
⊕ ⊕ ⊛ ⊘
Fees: <£25; Second visit: £21–30
Manchester M13
0161 276 4102

**Andrew Murray GOsC**
⊕ ⊕ ⊘ ⓔ ❈
Manchester OL6
0161 330 4089

**Alan Joy GOsC**
⊕ ⊕ ⊛ ⓔ ❈
Fees: £26–35; Second visit: £21–30
Oldham OL2
0161 652 6781

**Iain McGregor GOsC, BOA**
⊕ ⊛ ❈
Fees: £26–35; Second visit: £21–30
Rochdale OL16
01706 642390

**Alexandra Langdon GOsC, BOA**
⊕ ⊕ ⊛ ❈
Fees: £26–35; Second visit: £21–30
Sale M33
0161 969 6555

**Carolyn Greenhalgh GOsC, BOA**
⊕ ⊕ ⊛ ❈
Fees: <£25; Second visit: £21–30
Stockport SK6
0161 427 8577

**Clifford Lomas GOsC, BOA**
⊕ ⊛ ⓔ ❈
Fees: £26–35; Second visit: £21–30
Stockport SK2,Glossop SK13
0161 456 2087

**Neil Chestock GOsC**
⊕ ⊛ ❈
Fees: <£25; Second visit: £31–40
Stockport SK4
0161 432 2986

**Adrian Murray GOsC**
⊕ O ⊛ ⓔ ❈
Fees: £36–45; Second visit: £31–40
Stockport SK7
0161 440 0298

**Brian Walker GOsC, BOA**
⊕ ⊛
Fees: £26–35; Second visit: £21–30
Stockport SK6
0161 427 8577

**Jason A Gaskill GOsC, BOA**
⊕ O ⊕ ⊛ ⊘ ❈
Fees: £26–35; Second visit: £21–30
Stockport SK4
0161 432 8215

## LANCASHIRE

**John Bradley GOsC, BOA**
⊕ ⊛ ⊘ ❈
Fees: <£25; Second visit: £21–30
Accrington BB5
01254 381545

**Martin Dixon GOsC, BOA**
⊕ ⊕ ⊛ ⊘ ❈
Fees: <£25; Second visit: £21–30
Accrington BB5
01254 399915

**John Walsh GOsC, BOA**
✚ ⓝ ⊘
Fees: <£25; Second visit: £21–30
Accrington BB5
01254 381545

**Allan Mooney GOsC**
✚ ⓝ ✿
Fees: <£25; Second visit: £21–30
Ashton-under-Lyne OL6
0161 330 9926

**David H Gutteridge GOsC, BOA**
✚ ⓑ ⊘
Fees: <£25; Second visit: £41–50
Blackburn BB2
01254 52143

**Keith Nicol GOsC**
✚ ⓝ
Fees: £26–35; Second visit: £21–30
Blackpool FY1
01253 625578

**George Owen GOsC, BOA**
✚ ⓝ ✿
Fees: <£25; Second visit: £21–30
Blackpool FY4
01253 342712

**Sarah Wheildon GOsC**
✚ ⓑ ⓝ ✿
Fees: £26–35; Second visit: £21–30
Blackpool FY5
01253 822948

**Ryan O'Shea GOsC, BOA**
✚ ⓑ ⓝ ✿
Fees: <£25; Second visit: £21–30
Chorley PR7
01257 260520

**Helen Allison GOsC**
✚ ⓑ ⓝ ⊘ © ✿
Fees: £26–35; Second visit: £21–30
Clitheroe BB7
01200 424901

**Richard Freeman GOsC, BOA,**
⊘
Fees: £26–35; Second visit: £21–30
Clitheroe BB7
01200 421900

**Martien Jonkers GOsC**
✚
Fees: £26–35; Second visit: £21–30
Clitheroe BB7
01200 424901

**Robin W Percival GOsC, BOA**
✚ ⓑ ⓝ ⊘ © ✿
Fees: £26–35; Second visit: £21–30
Clitheroe BB7
01200 424901

**Hilary Percival GOsC, BOA**
✚ ⓝ ⊘ © ✿
Fees: <£25; Second visit: £31–40
Clitheroe BB7
01200 424901

**Charles Tisdall GOsC**
✚ ⓑ ⓝ ✿
Fees: £36–45; Second visit: £21–30
Lancaster LA1
01524 69864

**Mary Vale GOsC**
O ⓝ ✿
Fees: <£25; Second visit: £21–30
Lancaster LA2
01524 822501

**Joanne Danby GOsC, BOA**
✚ ⓑ ⓝ ✿
Fees: £26–35; Second visit: £21–30
Preston PR2
01772 733007

**Michael Gregson GOsC, BOA**
✚ ⓑ
Fees: £26–35; Second visit: £21–30
Preston PR2
01772 712048

**Dorothy J Griffiths GOsC, BOA**
✚ ⓑ ⓝ
Fees: <£25; Second visit: £21–30
Preston PR2
01772 761166

**Russell Oakes GOsC, BOA**
✚ ✚ ⓑ ⓝ ⊘ ✿
Fees: £26–35; Second visit: £21–30
Standish WN5
01257 405406

# Osteopathy

## MERSEYSIDE

**Philip Howard GOsC, BOA**
Fees: <£25; Second visit: £21–30
Formby L37
01704 543532

**Caroline Robinson GOsC**
Fees: £26–35; Second visit: £21–30
Formby L37
01704 877001

**Michael Hammond GOsC**
Fees: <£25; Second visit: <£20
Liverpool L18
0151 733 7632

**Valerie Makinson GOsC, BOA**
Fees: £26–35; Second visit: £21–30
Liverpool L23
0151 924 7238

**Christina Parsons GOsC, BOA**
Fees: £36–45; Second visit: £21–30
Liverpool L1
0151 709 6639

**Nicholas Jason Smith GOsC, BOA**
Fees: <£25; Second visit: £21–30
Liverpool L9
0151 284 5016

**Philip Thomas GOsC, BOA**
Fees: <£25; Second visit: £21–30
Liverpool L9
0151 284 5016

**Jolyon Wardle GOsC, BOA**
Fees: £26–35; Second visit: £21–30
Liverpool L23
0151 924 7238

**Christopher Dixon GOsC**
Fees: £26–35; Second visit: £21–30
Liverpool L37
01704 877001

**Andrew C Woodhouse GOsC**
Fees: <£25; Second visit: £21–30
Neston CH64
0151 336 6222

**Patrick Phillips GOsC**
Fees: £26–35; Second visit: £21–30
Prescot L34
0151 431 1549

**Jonathan Bell GOsC, BOA**
Fees: <£25; Second visit: £21–30
Rainhill L35,Southport PR8
0151 431 1700

**H A Brittain GOsC, BOA**
Fees: <£25; Second visit: £41–50
Southport PR9
01704 501271

**Judith Jenkins GOsC, BOA**
Fees: £26–35; Second visit: £21–30
Southport PR8
01704 550694

**Martin Morris GOsC, BOA**
Fees: £26–35; Second visit: £21–30
St Helens WA10
01744 28103

**Peter Lloyd GOsC, BOA**
Fees: £46–55; Second visit: £21–30
Wallasey CH45
0151 638 9132

**Sylvain Gateaud GOsC, BOA**
Fees: £26–35; Second visit: £21–30
West Kirby CH48
0151 625 0030

**Margaret Lavender GOsC, BOA**
Fees: £26–35; Second visit: £21–30
Wirral CH61
0151 648 6870

**Melanie Wright GOsC**
⊕ ⊕ ⦿ ⦿ ✿
**Fees:** £26–35; Second visit: £21–30
Wirral CH60
0151 342 5538

## Chiropractic

### CHESHIRE

**Eevamaria Heinonen GCC, BCA**
⊕ ⦿ ✿
**Fees:** £46–55; Second visit: £21–30
Alderley Edge SK9
01565 651133

**L Cooper GCC, BCA**
⊕ ⦿ ⦿
**Fees:** £36–45; Second visit: £21–30
Chester CH2
01244 343236

**Howard Gardener GCC, BCA**
⊕ ⦿ ✿
**Fees:** £36–45; Second visit: £21–30
Chester CH2
01244 343236

**Peter Gordon GCC, BCA**
⊕ ⦿ ⦿ ✿ ⦿
**Fees:** £36–45; Second visit: £21–30
Chester CH2
01244 343236

**Tana Williams GCC, MCA**
O ⦿ ✿
**Fees:** £36–45; Second visit: £21–30
Mottram St Andrew SK10
01625 828140

**Clare Sheehan GCC, MCA**
⊕ O ⊕ ⦿ ⦿
**Fees:** £26–35; Second visit: £21–30
Nantwich CW5
01270 520404

**Claire Mather-Dodd GCC, BCA**
⊕ ⦿ ⦿ ✿
**Fees:** <£25; Second visit: £21–30
Rudheath CW9
01606 47776

**Monica Handa GCC, BCA**
⊕ ⦿ ✿ ⦿
**Fees:** £46–55; Second visit: £21–30
Warrington WA2
01925 417817

**Caroline Shanks GCC, BCA**
⊕ ⦿ ⦿ ⦿
**Fees:** £36–45; Second visit: £21–30
Warrington WA10
01744 22441

**Scott Middleton GCC, BCA**
⊕ ⊕ ⊕ ⦿ ⦿ ⦿
**Fees:** >£55; Second visit: £21–30
Wilmslow SK9
01625 531164

### GREATER MANCHESTER

**Carrie Phillips GCC, MCA**
O ⦿ ✿
**Fees:** £26–35; Second visit: £21–30
Altrincham WA14
0161 928 9016

**Stephen Roberts GCC, BCA**
⊕ ⊕ ⦿ ⦿ Ⓔ ✿
**Fees:** £36–45; Second visit: £21–30
Manchester M20
0161 4462009

**David Middleton GCC, BCA**
⊕ O ⦿ ✿
**Fees:** £26–35; Second visit: £41–50
Stockport SK12
01625 850300

**James Doherty GCC, BAAC**
⊕ ✿
**Fees:** £36–45; Second visit: £21–30
Stockport SK8,Manchester M3
0800 956 1890

# Chiropractic

**Gowan Robinson GCC, BCA**
➊ ⊜
**Fees:** >£55; Second visit: £21–30
Stockport SK9
01625 531164

**Lorna Mills GCC**
➊ ⊛
**Fees:** £36–45; Second visit: £21–30
Oldham OL4
0161 678 1824

**Adam Wilkey GCC, BCA**
➊ ⊛ ⊘ Ⓔ ❈
**Fees:** £36–45; Second visit: £21–30
Oldham OL4
0161 628 7319

## LANCASHIRE

**Gordon Winter GCC, BCA**
➊ ⊛ ❈
**Fees:** £36–45; Second visit: £21–30
Chorley PR6
01257 226821

**Peter Doleman GCC, BCA**
➊ ➊ ⊛ ❈
**Fees:** £26–35; Second visit: <£20
Lancaster LA1
01524 33146

**John Parsons GCC, BAAC**
➊ ⊕ ⊛ ❈
**Fees:** £36–45; Second visit: £21–30
Leyland PR5
01655 55412

**Louis T Westerbeek GCC, BCA**
➊ ⊛ ⊘ ❈
**Fees:** £46–55; Second visit: £21–30
Blackpool FY8
07870 135743

**Gareth Jones GCC, BCA**
⊕ ⊛
**Fees:** £26–35; Second visit: £21–30
Queensway FY6
01253 882513

**Catherine Corcoran GCC, MCA**
➊ ⊛ ⊘ ❈
**Fees:** £36–45; Second visit: £21–30
Skelmersdale WN8
01695 732538

**Jeffrey Shurr GCC, BCA**
➊ ⊕ ⊛ ⊘ Ⓔ ❈
**Fees:** £46–55; Second visit: £21–30
Preston PR5
01772 696611

## MERSEYSIDE

**Ida Moos GCC, BCA**
➊ ⊛ ⊘ ❈
**Fees:** £26–35; Second visit: £21–30
Birkenhead CH41
0151 647 7989

**Neil Bray GCC, BCA**
➊ ⊛ Ⓔ ❈
**Fees:** £26–35; Second visit: £21–30
Southport PR8, Chorley PR6
01704 569695

**J Scott Fullwood GCC, BCA**
➊ ⊛ ❈
**Fees:** £26–35; Second visit: £21–30
Southport PR8
01704 569695

**David Shacklady GCC, BCA**
➊ ⊕ ⊕ ⊛ ⊘ ❈ ⊜
**Fees:** £36–45; Second visit: £21–30
Warrington WA10
01744 22441

**Deirdre Concannon GCC**
➊ ➊ ❈
**Fees:** £36–45; Second visit: £41–50
Wirral CH61
0151 648 7236

## Western Herbal Medicine

### CHESHIRE

**C W Thomas MNIMH**
✪ ⓓ ⓔ
**Fees:** £26–35; Second visit: £21–30
Chester CH2
01244 390411

**A Cooper MNIMH**
✪ ⊕ ⓓ ⊘
**Fees:** £26–35; Second visit: <£20
Crewe CW2
01270 669215

**J A Spicer MNIMH**
✪ ◯ ⓜ
**Fees:** £26–35; Second visit: <£20
Warrington WA2
01925 652656

### GREATER MANCHESTER

**F Kershner MNIMH**
✪ ⓓ ⓜ
**Fees:** £26–35; Second visit: <£20
Manchester M1
0161 228 0220

**J Gray MNIMH**
✪ ◯ ⓜ ✿
**Fees:** £36–45; Second visit: £21–30
Stockport SK3
0161 476 4179

### LANCASHIRE

**H M Duxbury MNIMH**
✪ ⓓ ⓜ ⓔ ✿
**Fees:** £26–35; Second visit: <£20
Blackburn BB2
01254 52143

**A L Denney MNIMH**
✪ ⓜ ✿
**Fees:** £26–35; Second visit: <£20
Chorley PR6
01257 482264

**J Manwaring MNIMH**
◯
**Fees:** £26–35; Second visit: £21–30
Chorley PR7
01257 451327

**C S Potter MNIMH**
◯ ✿
**Fees:** £26–35; Second visit: <£20
Clitheroe BB7
01282 776189

**Sarah Atkinson MNIMH**
✪ ◯ ⓓ ⓜ
**Fees:** £26–35; Second visit: <£20
Lancaster LA20, Ulverston LA12
01229 716023

**A Green MNIMH**
◯ ⓓ
**Fees:** £36–45; Second visit: £21–30
Lancaster LA1
01524 67631

**M Whitelegg MNIMH**
✪ ⓓ ✿
**Fees:** £36–45; Second visit: £21–30
Lancaster LA1
01524 39450

**J E Wilby MNIMH**
✪ ⓓ ⓜ
**Fees:** £26–35; Second visit: <£20
Preston PR2
01772 725200

### MERSEYSIDE

**Kate Butler MNIMH**
✪ ◯ ⓜ ⊘ ✿
Liverpool L8
0151 734 0866

**H A Davies MNIMH**
✪ ⓓ ⓜ ✿
**Fees:** <£25; Second visit: <£20
St Helens WA10
01744 29119

**M Knowles MNIMH**
◯
**Fees:** £26–35; Second visit: <£20
St Helens WA11
01744 23322

# Chinese Herbal Medicine

## CHESHIRE

**Charles Buck RCHM**
⊕  ⊕
Fees: >£55; Second visit: <£20
Chester CH2
01244 390411

**Jacqueline Hu RCHM**
⊕  ✿
Fees: £26–35; Second visit: £21–30
Nantwich CW5
01270 629222

## GREATER MANCHESTER

**Junkun Bai RCHM**
⊕  ⦾  ✿
Fees: <£25; Second visit: £21–30
Sale M33,Warrington WA1,Chester
CH3
0161 905 3666

**Anne Signol RCHM**
⊕  ⊘  ✿
Stockport SK6
0161 430 3697

## LANCASHIRE

**Julie Almond RCHM**
⊕  ✿
Fees: <£25; Second visit: <£20
Blackpool FY8
01253 724920

**Fang Ding RCHM**
⊕  O  ⊕  ⦾  ✿
Fees: £26–35; Second visit: £21–30
Blackpool FY4,Kendal LA9
01253 344115

**Xiaoming Zhou RCHM**
⊕  ⦾  ✿
Fees: £36–45; Second visit: £21–30
Blackpool FY4
01253 341644

## MERSEYSIDE

**Peter Pang RCHM**
⊕
Fees: £36–45; Second visit: <£20
Bootle L20
0151 922 2873

**Xiao Yan Zhang RCHM**
O  ✿
Fees: <£25; Second visit: <£20
Liverpool L14
0151 292 4028

# Ayurvedic Medicine

## CHESHIRE

**Himagauri Deshmukh AMAUK**
O  ✿
Fees: <£25; Second visit: <£20
Warrington WA5
01925 453672

## GREATER MANCHESTER

**Kailashben Patel AMAUK**
⊕  O  ✿
Rochdale OL16,Rochdale OL16
01706 718337

# South East

Berkshire
Buckinghamshire
Channel Islands
Dorset
Hampshire
Hertfordshire
Isle of Wight

Kent
Milton Keynes
Northamptonshire
Oxfordshire
Surrey
Sussex

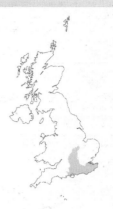

## Acupuncture

### BERKSHIRE

**Nicola Breedon BAcC**
Fees: £26–35; Second visit: £31–40
Ascot SL5
01344 620174

**Jane Flynn BAcC**
Fees: £36–45; Second visit: £31–40
Ascot SL5
01344 620174

**Katie Scampton BAcC**
Fees: £26–35; Second visit: £21–30
Ascot SL5
01344 620174

**Victoria Irwin BAcC**
Fees: £26–35; Second visit: £21–30
Bracknell RG26
07779 003636

**Maureen Dennis BAcC, AACP**
Fees: £26–35; Second visit: £21–30
Maidenhead SL6
01628 603935

**Malcolm Gibson BAcC**
Fees: £36–45; Second visit: £21–30
Maidenhead SL6,Bracknell RG42
01344 423860

**Margaret Rawlinson BAcC**
Fees: £36–45; Second visit: £21–30
Maidenhead SL6
01628 770796

**Julia Sommerville BAcC**
Fees: £36–45; Second visit: £21–30
Newbury RG14
01635 48452

**Lesley Boardman BAcC**
Fees: £36–45; Second visit: £31–40
Reading RG7
0118 9883155

**Sean Cleere BAcC**
Fees: £36–45; Second visit: £21–30
Reading RG1
0118 986 0879

# Acupuncture

**Diana Eckersley BAcC**
⊕ ⊕ 🔵 🔵
Fees: £36–45; Second visit: £21–30
Reading RG1,Newbury RG14
0118 950 8889

**Judith Elliott BAcC**
⊕ O ⊕ ⊕ ⊘ 🔵 🔵
Fees: £36–45; Second visit: £31–40
Reading RG7
01488 608361

**Karen Hall BAcC**
⊕ ⊕ Ⓒ 🔵 🔵
Fees: £36–45; Second visit: £21–30
Reading RG1
0118 950 8880

**Sigyta Hart BAcC**
⊕ O ⊕ ⊕ ⊘ 🔵 🔵
Fees: £36–45; Second visit: £31–40
Reading RG8
01491 873972

**Angela Hicks BAcC**
⊕ 🔵
Fees: £36–45; Second visit: £21–30
Reading RG1
0118 950 8880

**Amanda Kemp AACP**
⊕ ⊕ 🔵 🔵
Fees: £26–35; Second visit: £21–30
Reading RG6,Reading RG10
0118 966 4585

**Magdalena Koc BAcC**
⊕ ⊕ 🔵
Fees: £36–45; Second visit: £21–30
Reading RG1
0118 9508889

**Marcus Senior BAcC**
⊕ 🔵 🔵
Fees: £36–45; Second visit: £21–30
Reading RG1
0118 975 7475

**Jackie Shaw BAcC**
⊕ 🔵 🔵
Fees: £36–45; Second visit: £21–30
Reading RG1
01635 579412

**Lynne Wilkes BAcC**
O 🔵
Fees: £36–45; Second visit: £31–40
Reading RG6
0118 966 7433

**Tristan Bishop BAcC**
O 🔵 🔵
Fees: £26–35; Second visit: £21–30
Slough SL2
01753 648567

**Dena Robertson BAcC**
O 🔵 🔵
Fees: £36–45; Second visit: £21–30
Windsor SL4
01753 853493

**Jane Wessely BAcC**
O 🔵 🔵
Fees: >£55; Second visit: £21–30
Winkfield Row RG32
01344 886301

**Lorraine Canning BAcC**
⊕ O ⊕ 🔵 🔵
Fees: £26–35; Second visit: £21–30
Wokingham RG40
0118 978 6145

### BUCKINGHAMSHIRE

**Nicholas Eden Grove AACP, BAcC**
O ⊘ 🔵 🔵
Fees: £26–35; Second visit: £21–30
Aylesbury HP22
01296 622363

**Andre Yee Gan Lai Man Chun BAcC**
🔵
Fees: £36–45; Second visit: £21–30
Aylesbury HP21
01296 487686

**Penny Upchurch-Davies BAcC**
⊕ ⊕ 🔵 🔵 🔵
Fees: £26–35; Second visit: £21–30
Aylesbury HP21
01296 612361

**Joy Dutta BMAS**
O 🔵 🔵
Fees: £36–45; Second visit: £31–40
Beaconsfield HP9
01494 676972

**Susan Cady AACP**

Fees: £36–45; Second visit: £31–40
Chesham HP5
07958 799128

**Damon Fewster BAcC**

Fees: £36–45; Second visit: £21–30
Great Missenden HP16
01494 862713

**Fraser N Jackson AACP**

Fees: £36–45; Second visit: £21–30
High Wycombe HP13
01494 438554

**Liz Keens AACP**

Fees: £26–35; Second visit: £21–30
High Wycombe HP11
01494 464094

**Susanne Keil BAcC**

Fees: £36–45; Second visit: £31–40
High Wycombe HP13
01494 445282

**Sandra King BAcC**

Fees: £26–35; Second visit: £21–30
High Wycombe HP10
01494 680847

**Michele Marsland BAcC**

Fees: £26–35; Second visit: £21–30
High Wycombe HP13
01494 530004

**Gillian Morgan AACP**

Fees: £26–35; Second visit: £21–30
Marlow SL7
01628 481866

**Richard Nutting BAcC**

Fees: £36–45; Second visit: £21–30
Marlow SL7
01628 487719

**Alexandra Reynolds BAcC, AACP**

Fees: £36–45; Second visit: £31–40
Marlow SL7
01628 476443

**E J Whelpton BAcC**

Fees: £26–35; Second visit: £21–30
Marlow SL7
01628 474061

## CHANNEL ISLANDS

**Johanna Vessey BAcC**

Fees: £26–35; Second visit: £21–30
Guernsey GY1
01481 724184

**Polly Ashton BAcC**

Fees: £46–55; Second visit: £31–40
St Helier JE2
01534 618285

**Jenny Matthews BAcC**

Fees: £46–55; Second visit: £31–40
St Helier JE2
01534 727145

## DORSET

**Frances Mason BAcC**

Fees: £36–45; Second visit: £21–30
Broadstone BH18
01202 692493

**Rachel Dufft BAcC**

Fees: <£25; Second visit: £21–30
Bournemouth BH4
01202 540088

**Michael Edmondson BAcC**

Fees: <£25; Second visit: £21–30
Bournemouth BH5
01202 512394

# Acupuncture

**Gary Hussey BAcC**
➊ ➓ 🔵
**Fees:** £26–35
Bournemouth BH1
01202 295128

**Phillipa Johnson AACP**
◯ 🔵 ✸ 🔵
**Fees:** £36–45; Second visit: £31–40
Bournemouth BH4
01202 761137

**Kate Rowe-Jones AACP**
🔵
**Fees:** £26–35; Second visit: £21–30
Bournemouth BH8
01202 391144

**Susan Tows AACP**
➊ ➕ 🔵
**Fees:** £26–35; Second visit: £21–30
Bournemouth BH1
01202 702813

**Hilary Sharp BAcC**
◯ ✸ 🔵
**Fees:** £26–35; Second visit: £21–30
Bridport DT6
01297 560639

**Alison Booth AACP**
➊ ➕ ⊘ 🔵
**Fees:** £36–45; Second visit: £21–30
Christchurch BH23
01202 477335

**Mark Dale BAcC**
◯ ✸ 🔵
**Fees:** £26–35; Second visit: £21–30
Christchurch BH23
01202 481490

**Liz Hawk BAcC**
➊ ◯ ➓ ✸ 🔵
**Fees:** £26–35; Second visit: £21–30
Christchurch BH23
01202 245310

**Tony Campbell BAcC**
➊ ✸ 🔵
**Fees:** £26–35; Second visit: £21–30
Dorchester DT1,Gillingham
SP8,Blandford Forum DT11
01305 250110

**Robert Lock BAcC**
➊ ➓ ✸ 🔵
**Fees:** £26–35; Second visit: £21–30
Dorchester DT1
01305 267069

**Geoffrey Wadlow BAcC**
➊ ◯ ➕ ➓ 🔵
**Fees:** £36–45; Second visit: £21–30
Dorchester DT1
01305 262626

**Dwara Young BAcC**
➊ ◯ ➓ ✸ 🔵
**Fees:** £46–55; Second visit: £31–40
Dorchester DT1,Shaftesbury SP7
01305 262626

**Janie Prince BAcC**
◯ 🔵
**Fees:** £46–55; Second visit: £21–30
Lyme Regis DT7
01297 445952

**Dianna Jazwinski AACP**
➊ ➕ ✸ 🔵
**Fees:** £26–35; Second visit: £21–30
Poole BH15
01202 244200

**Debra Todd BMAS, AACP**
➊ ➕ ➓ 🔵 🔵
**Fees:** £26–35; Second visit: £21–30
Poole BH14
01202 749514

**Georgina Rhodes BAcC**
➊ ➓ 🔵 ✸ 🔵
**Fees:** £46–55; Second visit: £31–40
Sherborne DT9
01935 817442

**M G Cripps BMAS**
➕ 🔵 ⊘ ✸ 🔵
**Fees:** £26–35; Second visit: £21–30
Sturminster Newton DT10
01258 474500

**Teresa Fennell AACP**
➕ 🔵 ⊘ 🔵
**Fees:** £26–35; Second visit: £21–30
Swanage BH19
01929 422282

**Paul Savage AACP**
⊕ ⊕ ⓜ ✿ 🔟
Fees: £25–35; Second visit: £20–30
Verwood BH31
07976 419813

**Ulla Johari BAcC**
⊕ O ✿ 🔟
Fees: <£25; Second visit: <£20
Wareham BH20
01929 400581

**Sue Branch BAcC**
ⓜ ✿ 🔟
Fees: £36–45; Second visit: £21–30
Weymouth DT3
01305 834583

**Sue Horne BAcC**
⊕ O ⊕ ⓜ ✿ 🔟
Fees: £36–45; Second visit: £21–30
Wimborne BH21,Ringwood BH24
01725 517883

## HAMPSHIRE

**Kevin Watts BAcC**
O ⓔ ✿ 🔟
Fees: £36–45; Second visit: £21–30
Alton GU34
01420 588316

**Christine R Ball AACP**
O ⊕ ⓜ ✿ 🔟
Fees: £36–45; Second visit: £31–40
Andover SP11
07790 392981

**Nicholas R Bowden BAcC**
⊕ O ⊕ ⊕ ✿ 🔟
Fees: £36–45; Second visit: £21–30
Andover SP10
01264 335333

**Lynn Bird BAcC**
O ✿ 🔟
Fees: £26–35; Second visit: £21–30
Basingstoke RG23
01256 780202

**Caroline Mountford BAcC**
⊕ ⊕ ✿ 🔟
Fees: £46–55; Second visit: £21–30
Basingstoke RG21
01256 479500

**Linda A Tagg AACP**
O ⊕ ⊘ ✿ 🔟
Fees: £36–45; Second visit: £31–40
Basingstoke RG24
01256 351080

**Johanna Adriana van Hoorn BAcC**
O ⊕ 🔟
Fees: £26–35; Second visit: £31–40
Chichester PO19
01243 778159

**Gillian Carpenter BAcC**
⊕ O ⊕ ⊘ ✿
Fees: £36–45; Second visit: £21–30
Emsworth PO10
01243 374855

**Sunette Greeff AACP**
⊕ ⊕ ✿ 🔟
Fees: £36–45; Second visit: £21–30
Havant PO9
023 9245 6000

**Jan Henriksson AACP**
⊕ ⊕ ⓜ ✿ 🔟
Fees: £36–45; Second visit: £31–40
Havant PO9
023 9295 6066

**K Nilsen AACP**
⊕ 🔟
Fees: £36–45; Second visit: £31–40
Havant PO9
023 9247 0345

**Jacqui McCann BAcC**
O ⊕ ⊕ ✿ 🔟
Fees: £36–45; Second visit: £21–30
Hollycombe GU30
01428 725474

**Justin Hextall BAcC**
⊕ ✿ 🔟
Fees: £46–55; Second visit: £21–30
Lymington SO41,Bournemouth BH4
07767 221910

**Louise Corello BAcC**
O ✿ 🔟
Fees: £36–45; Second visit: £21–30
Petersfield GU32
01730 268301

# Acupuncture

### Tamara Kircher BAcC
⊕ ⊕ ⊘
**Fees:** £26–35; Second visit: £21–30
Petersfield GU32
01730 231655

### Na Lian BAcC
⊕ ⓝ ⊘ ✿ ⊕
Petersfield GU32
01730 710020

### Sari Avis BAcC
⊕ ⊕ ⓝ ✿ ⊕
**Fees:** £36–45; Second visit: £21–30
Ringwood BH24
01425 472776

### Margaret Burgess AACP
⊕ ⊕
**Fees:** £26–35; Second visit: £21–30
Ringwood BH24
01425 472202

### Paul Baker AACP
⊕ ✿ ⊕
**Fees:** £26–35; Second visit: £21–30
Southampton SO16
023 8074 7182

### Michael Clark BMAS
⊕ ⓝ ⊘ ✿ ⊕
**Fees:** <£25; Second visit: £21–30
Southampton SO15,London NW1
023 8033 4752

### Grahame Coleman BAcC
O ⊘ ✿ ⊕
**Fees:** £26–35; Second visit: £31–40
Southampton SO16
023 8076 0149

### Peter Hewitt BAcC
⊕ ⊕ ✿ ⊕
**Fees:** £46–55; Second visit: £21–30
Southampton SO17,Sherborne
DT9,Ringwood BH24
07973 558782

### Elizabeth Tong AACP
O ⊕
**Fees:** £36–45; Second visit: £21–30
Southampton SO15
023 8077 2511

### Tracey Curry BAcC
O
**Fees:** £46–55; Second visit: £31–40
Southampton SO32
01329 835512

### Ruth Tayler AACP
⊕ ⓝ ⊘ ⊕
**Fees:** £26–35; Second visit: £21–30
Southampton SO31
01489 584297

### Nigel Willett BAcC
O ✿ ⊕
**Fees:** <£25; Second visit: <£20
Southsea PO5
023 9261 2293

### Paul Wilson BAcC
⊕ ⊕ ✿ ⊕
**Fees:** £26–35; Second visit: £21–30
Southsea PO5
023 9287 4748

### Neil Allardyce BAcC
⊕ ⊕ ✿ ⊕
**Fees:** £26–35; Second visit: £21–30
Winchester SO21
023 8023 3764

### Claire Johnson BAcC
⊕ ⊕ ✿ ⊕
**Fees:** £36–45; Second visit: £21–30
Winchester SO23
01962 864641

## HERTFORDSHIRE

### Melvyn Epstein BAcC
⊕ O ⊕ ✿ ⊕
**Fees:** £36–45; Second visit: £21–30
Berkhamsted HP4,Leighton Buzzard
LU7
01442 863430

### Maureen Lovesey BAcC, AACP
✿ ⊕
**Fees:** £36–45; Second visit: £31–40
Berkhamsted HP4
01442 864243

**Wendy Emberson BAcC, AACP**
O ⊕ 🌑 🔴
Fees: £36–45; Second visit: £31–40
Bishop's Stortford CM22
01279 654020

**Diana Griffin BAcC**
O 🌑
Fees: £46–55; Second visit: £21–30
Bishop's Stortford CM23
01279 658629

**Clare Wang BAcC**
🌑 O 🌑 🌑 🌑 🌑
Fees: £26–35
Bishop's Stortford CM23
01279 505315

**Paul Johnson BAcC**
🌑 O 🌑 🌑 🌑
Fees: £36–45; Second visit: £31–40
Borehamwood WD6,London WC2H
020 8953 6964

**Lall Aubeeluck BAcC**
🌑 🌑
Fees: £26–35; Second visit: £21–30
Harpenden AL5
01582 621880

**Nicola Kerins AACP**
⊕ 🌑 🌑 🌑
Fees: £36–45; Second visit: £21–30
Harpenden AL5
01582 714441

**Nicola Smith AACP**
🌑 ⊘ 🌑
Fees: £26–35; Second visit: £21–30
Hatfield AL10,Norwich NR2
01707 284461

**Suzanne Reid BAcC**
🌑 🌑 🌑 🌑
Fees: £36–45; Second visit: £31–40
Hertford SG14
01992 505306

**Emma Banks BAcC**
🌑 ⊕ 🌑 ⊘ 🌑 🌑
Fees: £26–35; Second visit: £21–30
Hitchin SG5
01462 459595

**Jethro Rowland BAcC**
🌑 O 🌑 🌑 🌑
Fees: £26–35; Second visit: £21–30
Hitchin SG4
01462 440762

**Tim Stillwell BAcC**
🌑 O ⊕ 🌑 🌑 🌑 🌑
Fees: £26–35; Second visit: £21–30
Hitchin SG5
01462 434424

**Julie Tant BAcC**
🌑 🌑 🌑 🌑 🌑
Fees: £46–55; Second visit: £21–30
Hitchin SG5
01462 459020

**Martin Storrie AACP**
🌑 O ⊕ 🌑 ⊘ 🌑 🌑
Fees: £36–45; Second visit: £21–30
Kings Langley WD4
01923 261974

**Joanne & Paul Carnell BAcC, AACP**
🌑 🌑 🌑
Fees: £36–45; Second visit: £21–30
Much Hadham SG10
01279 843558

**Elaine Everitt BAcC**
🌑 ⊘ 🌑 🌑
Fees: £26–35; Second visit: £21–30
Potters Bar EN6
01707 661411

**Vivien Fish BAcC**
🌑 O 🌑 🌑 🌑
Fees: >£55; Second visit: £31–40
Royston SG8
01763 247440

**J Brouwer BAcC**
🌑 O 🌑 🌑
Fees: £46–55; Second visit: £21–30
St Albans AL4
01727 836478

**Helen Thomas BAcC**
🌑 O 🌑 🌑 🌑
Fees: £36–45; Second visit: £31–40
St Albans AL1
01727 860737

# Acupuncture

**Magid Yusefi AACP**
✛ Ⓜ Ⓞ 🔟
Fees: <£25
St Albans AL1
01727 850925

**Jidong Wu BAcC**
✛ ✿ 🔟
Fees: £36–45; Second visit: £21–30
Waltham Cross EN8
01992 711772

**Liang Ji BAcC**
✛ Ⓜ Ⓞ ✿ 🔟
Fees: <£25; Second visit: <£20
Watford WD17
01923 244635

**Anna McCann AACP**
✛ ✛ Ⓜ ✿ 🔟
Fees: £26–35; Second visit: £21–30
Watford WD19
01923 218082

**Rachel Thomas AACP**
✛ Ⓞ ✛ Ⓜ Ⓞ ✿ 🔟
Fees: £26–35; Second visit: £21–30
Welwyn AL6
01438 716838

**Kathy H Winsor AACP**
✛ ✛ 🔟
Fees: £26–35; Second visit: £21–30
Welwyn AL6
01438 716838

**David F Mayor BAcC, AACP**
Ⓞ ✿ 🔟
Fees: £36–45; Second visit: £21–30
Welwyn Garden City AL8
01707 320782

**Jill Spence BAcC**
Ⓞ Ⓞ Ⓔ ✿ 🔟
Fees: £36–45; Second visit: £21–30
Welwyn Garden City AL7
01707 390833

**Noreen Todd BAcC**
Ⓞ ✿ 🔟
Fees: £26–35; Second visit: £21–30
Welwyn Garden City AL7
01707 320449

## ISLE OF WIGHT

**Peter Munt-Davies BAcC**
✛ ✛ ✛ Ⓞ 🔟
Fees: £36–45; Second visit: £21–30
Ryde PO33
01983 563539

## KENT

**Carol Kerr BAcC**
✛ ✛ 🔟
Fees: £26–35; Second visit: £21–30
Ashford TN27
01622 890803

**Cecile Kiener BAcC**
✛ ✛ ✛ Ⓜ ✿
Fees: £26–35; Second visit: £21–30
Ashford TN25
01303 813712

**Cliff Hill BMAS, AACP**
✛ Ⓜ ✿ 🔟
Fees: £36–45; Second visit: £31–40
Broadstairs CT10
01843 298408

**C J Brian BMAS**
✛ ✛ Ⓜ Ⓞ 🔟
Fees: <£25; Second visit: £21–30
Canterbury CT4
01227 455466

**Robert Esser BAcC**
✛ ✛ Ⓜ ✿ 🔟
Fees: £36–45; Second visit: £21–30
Canterbury CT1,Hythe CT21
01227 454404

**Philippa Nice BAcC**
✛ Ⓞ ✛ ✿ 🔟
Fees: £46–55; Second visit: £21–30
Canterbury CT1
01304 842343

**Pippa Sequeira BAcC**
✛ Ⓞ ✛ ✿ 🔟
Fees: £36–45; Second visit: £21–30
Canterbury CT1
01227 738816

**Dianne Stewart BAcC**
⊕ ⊕ ✿
Fees: £36–45; Second visit: £21–30
Canterbury CT1,Hythe CT21,Ashford
TN24
01227 454404

**Sue Thompson AACP**
⊕ ⊕ ✿ ⊛
Fees: £36–45; Second visit: £21–30
Canterbury CT4
01227 709240

**Paul Blacker BAcC**
⊕ ⊕ ⊕ ⊜ ✿ ⊛
Fees: £26–35; Second visit: £21–30
Dartford DA1,Gravesend
DA12,Gravesend DA13
01322 284898

**Lucy Bagley BAcC**
○ ⊛
Fees: £26–35; Second visit: £21–30
Deal CT14
01304 373920

**Linda Wilson BAcC**
⊕ ⊕ ⊜ ✿ ⊛
Fees: £26–35; Second visit: £21–30
Deal CT14
01304 381478

**K C Wong BAcC**
○ ✿ ⊛
Fees: £26–35; Second visit: £21–30
Gillingham ME7
01634 574432

**Renate Blacker BAcC**
⊕ ⊕ ✿ ⊛
Fees: £26–35; Second visit: £21–30
Gravesend DA13
01474 812135

**P R Hammond BAcC**
⊕ ○ ⊕ ⊛
Fees: <£25; Second visit: <£20
Maidstone ME15
01622 741598

**Susan Macfarlane BAcC, AACP**
⊕ ⊛
Fees: £26–35; Second visit: £21–30
Maidstone ME14
01622 762628

**Colin Waldock AACP**
⊕ ⊜ ⊛
Fees: £26–35; Second visit: £21–30
Rochester ME1
01634 817217

**Claire Hollobon BAcC**
⊕ ⊕ ⊘ ✿ ⊛
Fees: £26–35; Second visit: £21–30
Sevenoaks TN13
01732 464109

**Robert Hughes BAcC**
⊕ ⊕ ✿ ⊛
Fees: £26–35; Second visit: £21–30
Sevenoaks TN13
01732 450049

**Susan Jane Murray AACP**
⊕ ⊕ ⊘ ✿ ⊛
Fees: £26–35; Second visit: £21–30
Sittingbourne ME10
01795 439911

**Sandie Cameron AACP**
⊕ ○ ⊕ ⊜ ✿ ⊛
Fees: £36–45; Second visit: £41–50
Tonbridge TN9
01732 354578

**Karen Elsworth AACP**
⊕ ⊕ ⊕ ⊘ ✿ ⊛
Fees: £26–35; Second visit: £31–40
Tonbridge TN12
01892 724377

**Gordon Peck BAcC**
⊕ ⊛
Fees: £36–45; Second visit: £31–40
Tunbridge Wells TN4
01892 546237

**Susan J Rowland AACP**
⊕ ⊕ ⊜ ⊘ ✿ ⊛
Fees: £26–35; Second visit: £21–30
Tunbridge Wells TN3,East Grinstead
RH19,Tunbridge Wells TN2
01892 740047

**Susan Tosoni BAcC**
⊕ ⊕ ✿ ⊛
Fees: £36–45; Second visit: £21–30
Tunbridge Wells TN1,Tonbridge
TN10,West Malling ME19
01892 510950

# Acupuncture

**Joanne Inman AACP**
🔵 🔵 🔵 🔵
**Fees:** £36–45; Second visit: £21–30
Whitstable CT5
01795 539410

**Pippa Zintilis BAcC**
🔵 🔵
**Fees:** £26–35; Second visit: £21–30
Whitstable CT5
01227 792452

## MILTON KEYNES

**Susan Alexander BAcC**
🔵 🔵 🔵 🔵 🔵
**Fees:** £26–35; Second visit: £21–30
Milton Keynes MK6
01908 690705

**Shantha Godagama BAcC**
🔵 🔵 🔵 🔵 🔵 🔵
**Fees:** £26–35; Second visit: £21–30
Milton Keynes MK7
01908 604666

**Jane Lambert BAcC**
🔵 🔵 🔵 🔵 🔵
**Fees:** £36–45; Second visit: £21–30
Milton Keynes MK5
01908 526524

**Maxwell I Naiken BAcC**
🔵 🔵 🔵 🔵 🔵
**Fees:** £26–35; Second visit: £21–30
Bletchley MK3
01234 212788

**Gabriele Stutz BAcC**
🔵 🔵 🔵 🔵
**Fees:** £36–45; Second visit: £21–30
Milton Keynes MK12
01908 225051

**Helen Taylor-Weekes BAcC**
🔵 🔵 🔵 🔵 🔵 🔵
**Fees:** £26–35; Second visit: £21–30
Milton Keynes MK17
01908 584350

**Carla Smith AACP**
🔵 🔵 🔵 🔵
**Fees:** £26–35; Second visit: £21–30
Newport Pagnell MK16
01908 611767

**John Chadwick BAcC**
🔵 🔵 🔵
**Fees:** £36–45; Second visit: £21–30
Olney MK46
01234 241459

**Ruth Clarke BAcC**
🔵 🔵
**Fees:** £36–45; Second visit: £21–30
Olney MK46
01234 241200

## NORTHAMPTONSHIRE

**Jean Simmonds AACP**
🔵 🔵 🔵 🔵 🔵 🔵
**Fees:** £26–35; Second visit: £21–30
Brackley NN13
01295 760498

**Rosanna Price BAcC**
🔵 🔵 🔵
**Fees:** £46–55; Second visit: £31–40
Daventry NN11
01327 311507

**Sheena M Ross BMAS**
🔵 🔵 🔵 🔵 🔵
**Fees:** £36–45; Second visit: £21–30
Kettering NN14
01832 735392

**Jane Spencer BAcC**
🔵 🔵 🔵 🔵
**Fees:** £36–45; Second visit: £21–30
Kettering NN15
01536 512927

**Maxine Chimes BAcC**
🔵 🔵 🔵 🔵 🔵
**Fees:** £26–35; Second visit: £21–30
Northampton NN3
01604 451200

**Steve Kent AACP**
🔵 🔵 🔵 🔵 🔵 🔵
**Fees:** £26–35; Second visit: £31–40
Northampton NN2,Northampton NN1
01604 722272

**Stephen Lee BAcC**
🔵 🔵 🔵
**Fees:** £26–35; Second visit: £21–30
Northampton NN1
01604 717585

# Acupuncture

**Guy Levi BAcC**
➕ ⊕ ✿ ☻
Fees: £26–35; Second visit: £31–40
Northampton NN1
01604 632129

**Hina Patel BAcC**
➕ ⊕ ⊕ ✿ ☻
Fees: £36–45; Second visit: £21–30
Northampton NN1,Kettering
NN15,East Haddon
01604 622999

**S Reynolds BAcC**
○ ⊕ ✿ ☻
Fees: £26–35; Second visit: £21–30
Northampton NN2
01604 713135

**Soh-Eng Lim BAcC**
○ ☻ ✿ ☻
Fees: £46–55; Second visit: £21–30
Wellingborough NN8
01933 279586

## OXFORDSHIRE

**Michael David Baker BAcC**
➕ ⊕ ☻ ⊘ © ✿ ☻
Fees: £36–45; Second visit: £21–30
Abingdon OX14
01235 531021

**Fiona Farmer AACP**
➕ ✿ ☻
Fees: £26–35; Second visit: £21–30
Bampton OX18
01993 851753

**Clare Brannigan BAcC**
➕ ⊕ ✿ ☻
Fees: £46–55; Second visit: £21–30
Banbury OX16
01295 257746

**Sarah Brown Higgins BAcC**
➕ ⊕ ⊕ ✿ ☻
Fees: £46–55; Second visit: £31–40
Banbury OX15
07957 335398

**Carol Horner BAcC**
➕ ○ ⊕ ☻ ⊘ ✿ ☻
Fees: £26–35; Second visit: £21–30
Banbury OX16,High Wycombe
HP11,High Wycombe HP12
01295 266807

**Katherine Hutchings BAcC**
○ ✿ ☻
Fees: £36–45; Second visit: £21–30
Banbury OX15
01295 268836

**Gill Randall AACP**
○ ➕ ☻ ☻
Fees: £36–45; Second visit: £31–40
Banbury OX17
01295 812552

**Sharon Wallace-Shanks BAcC**
➕ ✿ ☻
Fees: £36–45; Second visit: £21–30
Banbury OX16,Boston PE21
01295 277494

**Tania Duby BAcC**
➕ ○ ✿ ☻
Fees: £26–35; Second visit: £21–30
Bicester OX26
01869 325088

**Claire Lindley AACP**
☻
Fees: £36–45; Second visit: £31–40
Bicester OX26
01869 326747

**Lorna Hipkins BAcC**
○ ☻ ✿ ☻
Fees: £36–45; Second visit: £21–30
Chipping Norton OX7
01993 868003

**Michael McIntyre BAcC**
➕ ✿ ☻
Fees: £36–45; Second visit: £21–30
Chipping Norton OX7
01993 830419

**Clare Blakeway-Phillips BAcC**
➕ ✿ ☻
Fees: £36–45; Second visit: £21–30
Oxford OX33
01865 872448

# Acupuncture

**Josephine Clegg BAcC**
O 🏥 ✿ 🌐
**Fees:** £46–55; Second visit: £21–30
Oxford OX2
01865 865318

**Mary Coombs BAcC**
⊕ ⊕ ⊛ ✿ 🌐
**Fees:** £36–45; Second visit: £31–40
Oxford OX2
01865 318338

**Pam Geggus BAcC**
O ✿ 🌐
**Fees:** £36–45; Second visit: £21–30
Oxford OX2
01865 554005

**Jeremy Hill BAcC**
⊕ ⊛ ✿ 🌐
**Fees:** <£25; Second visit: £21–30
Oxford OX2
01865 747844

**Gabriele Hock BAcC**
⊕ ⊛ ✿ 🌐
**Fees:** £46–55; Second visit: £31–40
Oxford OX4
01865 247851

**Amber Hodges BAcC**
O ✿ 🌐
**Fees:** £36–45; Second visit: £21–30
Oxford OX3
01865 779489

**Thomas Jennings BAcC**
⊕ ⊕ ⊛ ✿ 🌐
**Fees:** £46–55; Second visit: £21–30
Oxford OX4
01865 715615

**Christopher Kear BAcC**
⊕ ⊛ 🏥 ✿ 🌐
**Fees:** £36–45; Second visit: £21–30
Oxford OX2
01865 200365

**Jacqueline Mangold BAcC**
⊕ ⊛ ✿ 🌐
**Fees:** £46–55; Second visit: £21–30
Oxford OX2
01865 200365

**Peter Mole BAcC**
⊕ ⊛ 🌐
**Fees:** £46–55; Second visit: £21–30
Oxford OX2
01865 715615

**Maeve O'Donnell BAcC**
⊕ ⊛ ✿ 🌐
**Fees:** £36–45; Second visit: £21–30
Oxford OX4
01865 749842

**Linda Paris BAcC**
⊕ O ⊛ ✿ 🌐
**Fees:** £26–35; Second visit: £21–30
Oxford OX3
01865 763410

**Sue Pennington BAcC**
O 🌐
**Fees:** £46–55; Second visit: £21–30
Oxford OX4
01865 776759

**Jane Roberts BAcC**
⊕ ⊛ ✿ 🌐
**Fees:** £46–55; Second visit: £21–30
Oxford OX4,Oxford OX2
01865 715615

**David Ruddick BAcC**
⊕ ⊛
**Fees:** £36–45; Second visit: £31–40
Oxford OX2
01865 558561

**Vivien Shaw BAcC**
⊕ O ⊛ ⊘ © 🌐
**Fees:** £26–35; Second visit: £21–30
Oxford OX2
01865 250200

**Clare Stephenson BAcC,**
⊕ ⊛ © ✿ 🌐
**Fees:** £46–55; Second visit: £21–30
Oxford OX4
01865 715615

**James Unsworth BAcC**
⊕ ⊛ ✿ 🌐
**Fees:** £46–55; Second visit: £21–30
Oxford OX4
01865 715615

# Acupuncture

**Jani White BAcC**
➊ ⊕ ⊕ ❀ ☺
Fees: £46–55; Second visit: £21–30
Oxford OX2
07713 808789

**Allegra Wint BAcC**
O ☺
Fees: £46–55; Second visit: £31–40
Oxford OX2
01865 512299

**Andrew Roscoe BAcC**
➊ ⊕ ☺
Fees: £26–35; Second visit: £21–30
Thame OX9,Oxford OX4
01844 215555

**Mary Kaspar BAcC**
O ☺
Fees: £46–55; Second visit: £21–30
Wallingford OX10
01491 832552

**Vanessa Lampert BAcC**
❀ ☺
Fees: £36–45; Second visit: £21–30
Wallingford OX10
01491 201372

**Fiona Piddock BAcC**
➊ ⊕ ❀ ☺
Fees: £36–45; Second visit: £21–30
Wallingford OX10
01491 824724

**Stephanie Ross AACP**
➊ O ⊕ ⊕ ◍ ❀ ☺
Fees: £36–45; Second visit: £31–40
Wantage OX12
01235 760079

**John Herbert BAcC**
O ◍ ☺
Fees: £26–35; Second visit: £21–30
Witney OX29
01865 881623

**Samantha Jessel BAcC**
O ⊕ ❀ ☺
Fees: £26–35; Second visit: £31–40
Woodstock OX20
01993 812353

## SURREY

**Heather Bingham AACP**
⊕ ❀ ☺
Fees: £36–45; Second visit: £21–30
Ashtead KT21
01372 722402

**Saumeel Patel BAcC**
➊ O ⊕ ❀ ☺
Fees: £36–45; Second visit: £31–40
Banstead SM7,East Grinstead RH19
01737 360996

**Michael Hutchings BAcC**
➊ ⊕ ⊕ ❀ ☺
Fees: £36–45; Second visit: £21–30
Blackwater GU17
01276 64401

**Lynette Marchant BAcC**
➊ O ⊕ ⊕ ◍ ❀ ☺
Fees: £36–45; Second visit: £21–30
Camberley GU15,London SE1
01276 503354

**Michael Robey BAcC**
➊ ⊕ ❀ ☺
Fees: £36–45; Second visit: £21–30
Camberley GU17
01276 504979

**Janetta Bensouilah BAcC**
⊘ ❀ ☺
Fees: £26–35; Second visit: £21–30
Cobham KT11
01932 867491

**Karina Jeetoo AACP**
➊ ⊕ ◍ ⊘ ❀ ☺
Fees: £36–45; Second visit: £21–30
Cranleigh GU6
01483 267747

**David Reynolds BAcC**
➊ ⊕ ⊘ ❀ ☺
Fees: £36–45; Second visit: £31–40
Cranleigh GU6
01483 275500

**Sara Friday AACP**
➊ ☺
Fees: £26–35; Second visit: £21–30
Dorking RH4
01306 880488

# Acupuncture

**Andrew Sordyl BAcC**
☺ ⊕ ⊕ ⦿ ✿ ☻
Fees: £36–45; Second visit: £31–40
Dorking RH4
01306 742150

**Martine Faure-Alderson BAcC**
O ⊘ ✿ ☻
Fees: £36–45; Second visit: £21–30
East Molesey KT8
020 8398 6943

**Sue Gaastra AACP**
☺ ⊕ ☻
Fees: £26–35; Second visit: £31–40
Egham TW20
01784 433973

**Kevin M Young BAcC**
☺ ✿ ☻
Fees: £26–35; Second visit: £21–30
Egham TW20
01784 470480

**Royston Low BAcC, AACP**
O ☻
Fees: £26–35; Second visit: £21–30
Esher KT10
01372 464171

**Penelope Dadd AACP**
☺ ⦿ ☻
Fees: £26–35; Second visit: £21–30
Farnham GU10,Hook RG29
01252 726479

**Michael C K Ng BAcC**
☺ O ⊕ ☻
Fees: £36–45; Second visit: £21–30
Farnham GU10,Emsworth PO10
01252 794353

**Binh Thien Phung BAcC**
O ⓔ ☻
Fees: <£25; Second visit: <£20
Farnham GU9
01252 726868

**E Gaynor Wilson AACP**
⊘ ☻
Fees: £36–45; Second visit: £21–30
Godalming GU8
01483 424505

**Jadwiga Palmer BAcC**
☺ O ⊕ ⓔ ✿ ☻
Fees: £36–45; Second visit: £21–30
Godalming GU7
01485 418103

**Colin Lewis BMAS,**
☺ ⊘ ✿ ☻
Fees: £26–35; Second visit: £21–30
Guildford GU3
01483 569637

**Susan Thorne BAcC**
☺ ✿ ☻
Fees: >£55; Second visit: £31–40
Guildford GU5
01483 893373

**Erwen Zhou BAcC**
☺ ⊕ ⦿ ☻
Fees: £26–35; Second visit: £21–30
Guildford GU2
01483 823094

**Pauline Giesberts BAcC**
☺ O ⊘ ☻
Fees: £46–55; Second visit: £41–50
Haslemere GU27
01428 643015

**J D van Buren BAcC**
O
Fees: £46–55; Second visit: >£50
Haslemere GU27
01428 643015

**Elaine Williams BAcC**
⊕ ✿ ☻
Fees: £36–45; Second visit: £21–30
Hindhead GU26
01428 602066

**Susan Anastasiadis AACP, BAcC**
☺ O ⊕ ⦿ ✿ ☻
Fees: £36–45; Second visit: £31–40
Leatherhead KT24
01483 281685

**Sandie Moore AACP**
O ✿ ☻
Fees: £36–45; Second visit: £31–40
Leatherhead KT22
01372 374612

# Acupuncture

**Richard Cross BAcC**
✚ ❄ ☻
**Fees:** £26–35; Second visit: £21–30
Oxted RH8
01883 714036

**Claire Mindham BAcC**
✚ O ❄ ☻ ☻
**Fees:** £26–35; Second visit: £21–30
Oxted RH8
01883 717277

**Gwendolen Stamp BAcC**
O © ❄ ☻
**Fees:** <£25; Second visit: <£20
Oxted RH8
01883 713617

**Christine Eade BAcC, BMAS, AACP**
⊕ ◐ ⊘ ❄ ☻
**Fees:** £26–35; Second visit: £21–30
Redhill RH1
01737 231688

**Jane Straker AACP**
✚ ⊘ ☻
**Fees:** £26–35; Second visit: £21–30
Redhill RH1
01737 763632

**Galit Hughes BAcC**
✚ O ⊕ ☻
**Fees:** £26–35; Second visit: £21–30
Sevenoaks RH19
01732 450049

**Rosie Temple BAcC**
O ❄
**Fees:** £26–35; Second visit: £21–30
Staines TW19
01344 628298

**Suky Bains BAcC**
✚ O ⊕ © ❄ ☻
**Fees:** £36–45; Second visit: £31–40
West Byfleet KT14,London N6,London E3
01932 354535

**Susan Sutton BAcC**
O ❄ ☻
**Fees:** £36–45; Second visit: £21–30
Weybridge KT13
01932 221268

**Annie Hall BAcC**
O ◐ ⊘ ☻
**Fees:** £26–35; Second visit: £21–30
Woking GU22
01483 829048

**Sallie Hone BAcC**
✚ © ☻
**Fees:** £36–45; Second visit: <£20
Woking GU23
01483 224166

**Stuart Revell BAcC**
✚ O ⊕ ❄ ☻
**Fees:** £26–35; Second visit: £21–30
Woking GU22
01483 715730

**S N Shohet BAcC**
✚ ☻
**Fees:** >£55; Second visit: £41–50
Woking GU22
01483 726644

## SUSSEX

**David Bennett BAcC**
✚ ⊕ ❄ ☻
**Fees:** £36–45; Second visit: £21–30
Brighton BN2
01273 307001

**Christopher John Fish BAcC**
✚ ⊕ ❄ ☻
**Fees:** £26–35; Second visit: £21–30
Brighton BN2
01273 626644

**Elaine Gibbons BAcC**
O ⊕ ❄ ☻
**Fees:** £36–45; Second visit: £21–30
Brighton BN2
01273 562676

**Deborah Woolf BAcC**
O ⊕ ⊕ ☻
**Fees:** £26–35; Second visit: £21–30
Brighton BN2, Brighton BN1
01273 239466

**Sara Baxter AACP**
✚ ⊕ ❄ ☻
**Fees:** £36–45; Second visit: £31–40
Brighton BN3
01273 621248

# Acupuncture

**Helen Galindo AACP**
⊕ 🌑 🔴
**Fees:** £36–45; Second visit: £21–30
Brighton BN1
01273 207001

**Roger Murray BAcC**
● ○ ⊕ ✿ 🔴
**Fees:** £26–35; Second visit: £21–30
Brighton BN7
01323 873866

**Merriel Woodward BAcC**
⊕ ⊕ ✿ 🔴
**Fees:** £26–35; Second visit: £21–30
Crowborough TN6
01892 862308

**Richard Alan Hurn BAcC**
● ⊕ 🌑 🔴
**Fees:** £26–35; Second visit: £21–30
Eastbourne BN21
01323 727785

**Andrew Parfitt BAcC**
● ⊕ ✿ 🔴
**Fees:** £26–35; Second visit: £21–30
Eastbourne BN20,Eastbourne
BN20,Eastbourne BN21
01323 649439

**Ann Rambaut AACP**
● ⊕ ⊘ ✿ 🔴
**Fees:** £26–35; Second visit: £31–40
Eastbourne BN21
01323 411900

**Jing Ying Wang BAcC**
● ⊕ 🌑 ✿ 🔴
**Fees:** £36–45; Second visit: £21–30
Eastbourne BN21
01323 641576

**Deirdre Parrinder BAcC**
● ○ ⊕ ⊕ ✿ 🔴
**Fees:** £26–35; Second visit: £21–30
Etchingham TN19, London SE14
01580 861269

**David Cocks BAcC**
● ⊕ ⊕ ✿ 🔴
**Fees:** £36–45; Second visit: £31–40
Forest Row RH18, London W11,
Twickenham TW1
01342 824305

**Amanda Edwards BAcC**
● ○ ⊕ ✿ 🔴
**Fees:** £26–35; Second visit: £21–30
Forest Row RH18
01342 826581

**Irene Zalewska BAcC**
○ ✿ 🔴
**Fees:** £36–45; Second visit: £21–30
Forest Row RH18
01342 822087

**Deborah Cosbey BAcC**
● ⊕ 🔴
**Fees:** £26–35; Second visit: £21–30
Hastings TN35
01273 476211

**Yuko Nakamura BAcC**
○ 🌑 ⊘ ✿ 🔴
**Fees:** £26–35; Second visit: £21–30
Hastings TN34,London SE21
07960 915775

**Justin Xiaoyong Wu BAcC**
● ⊕ 🌑 ✿ 🔴
**Fees:** £26–35; Second visit: £21–30
Heathfield TN21
01435 812323

**Ian Appleyard BAcC**
● ⊕ 🔴
**Fees:** £26–35; Second visit: £21–30
Hove BN3
01273 776499

**Peter Helps BAcC,**
● ⊕ 🔴
**Fees:** £26–35; Second visit: £21–30
Hove BN3
01273 776499

**Nicholas Tilling BAcC**
● ⊕ ⊕ ✿ 🔴
**Fees:** £26–35; Second visit: £21–30
Hove BN3
01273 776499

**Stuart Wright BAcC**
○ 🌑 ✿ 🔴
**Fees:** £26–35; Second visit: £21–30
Hove BN3
01273 777768

**Kevin Baker BAcC,**
⊕ ⊕ ⊕ ✿ ⊜
Fees: £26–35; Second visit: £31–40
Lewes BN7, Brighton BN2
01273 474428

**Andrew Flower BAcC**
O ⊕ ⊕ ✿ ⊜
Fees: £26–35; Second visit: £21–30
Lewes BN7
01273 488547

**Keith Wright BAcC**
⊕ O ⊕ ⊛ ⊜
Fees: £36–45; Second visit: £31–40
Uckfield TN22
01825 712895

**Paul Hambly BAcC**
⊕ ⊕ ✿ ⊜
Fees: £36–45; Second visit: £21–30
Wadhurst TN5
01892 783027
**SUSSEX**

**Elaine Cook BAcC**
⊕ ⊕ ⊜
Fees: £36–45; Second visit: £21–30
Brighton BN1
01273 561844

**Deborah Ridley BAcC**
⊕ O ⊕ ⊛ ✿ ⊜
Fees: £26–35; Second visit: £21–30
Brighton BN42,Horsham
RH12,Horsham RH13
01273 596560

**Thomas Sydenham BAcC**
⊕ ⊕ ✿ ⊜
Fees: £36–45; Second visit: £21–30
Brighton BN1
01273 202221

**Anne-Marie Urbanowicz BAcC**
⊕ ⊕ ✿ ⊜
Fees: £36–45; Second visit: £21–30
Brighton BN1
01273 202221

**Dianna Crook AACP**
⊕ ⊕
Fees: £26–35; Second visit: £31–40
Bognor Regis PO21
01243 262126

**David John Soper BAcC**
⊕ ⊕ ⊕ ✿ ⊜
Fees: >£55; Second visit: >£50
Burgess Hill RH15
01444 232251

**Jayne Storer BAcC**
⊕ O ⊕ ⊕ ✿
Burgess Hill RH15
01273 843780

**Christine Dorricott AACP**
⊕ ✿ ⊜
Fees: £26–35; Second visit: £21–30
Chichester PO20
01243 603442

**Gabriella Kispal BAcC**
⊕ ⊕ ⊛ ✿ ⊜
Fees: £46–55; Second visit: £21–30
Chichester PO19
01243 786946

**Sue-Ellen Nicholls AACP**
O ⊕ ⊛ ⊜
Fees: £36–45; Second visit: £31–40
Chichester PO19
01243 788122

**Gary Brooks AACP**
⊕ ✿ ⊜
Fees: £26–35; Second visit: £21–30
Crawley RH10
01293 884488

**Tim Burrows BAcC**
⊕ ⊕ ⊕ ✿ ⊜
Fees: £26–35; Second visit: £21–30
Crawley RH10
01293 550079

**Greta Goodeve BAcC**
⊕ ⊕ ⊛ ✿ ⊜
Fees: £26–35; Second visit: £21–30
Crawley RH10
01293 562601

**Francesca Diebschlag BAcC**
O ⊜
Fees: £46–55; Second visit: £31–40
East Grinstead RH19
01342 313973

# Acupuncture

**Sarah Major BAcC**
⊕ ⊕ 🌸 🌿
**Fees:** £36–45; Second visit: £21–30
East Grinstead RH19
01342 324375

**Ninette Sapir BAcC**
⊕ O ⊕ ⓒ 🌸 🌿
**Fees:** £36–45; Second visit: £21–30
East Grinstead RH19,Oxted
RH8,Tonbridge TN10
01342 826374

**Duncan Arnold AACP**
🌿
**Fees:** £26–35; Second visit: £21–30
Haywards Heath RH16
01444 441881

**Belinda M Coppock BAcC**
⊕ 🌸 🌿
**Fees:** £26–35; Second visit: £21–30
Haywards Heath RH16
01444 453813

**Hilke Legenhausen BAcC**
⊕ O ⊕ 🌸 🌿
**Fees:** £36–45; Second visit: £31–40
Haywards Heath RH16,Cuckfield
01444 453182

**Isobel Staynes BAcC**
⊕ ⊕ NHS ⊘ 🌸 🌿
**Fees:** £46–55; Second visit: £31–40
Haywards Heath RH16
01444 441210

**Hillary Copland BAcC**
O 🌸 🌿
**Fees:** £26–35; Second visit: £21–30
Horsham RH13
01403 267352

**Sin Mui Chong-Martin BAcC**
⊕ ⊕ NHS 🌿
**Fees:** £26–35; Second visit: £21–30
Littlehampton BN17
01903 734373

**Louise Baker RCHM**
O ⊘ 🌸 🌿
**Fees:** <£25; Second visit: £21–30
Midhurst GU29
01730 810737

**Usha Stainton BAcC**
⊕ ⓒ 🌸
**Fees:** >£55; Second visit: £31–40
Midhurst GU29,London SW15,Marlow
SL7
01730 810540

**Titus Foster BAcC**
⊕ ⊕ ⊕ 🌿
**Fees:** £26–35; Second visit: £21–30
Pulborough RH20
01903 814489

**Nadia Khalili BMAS**
O ⊘ 🌿
**Fees:** £26–35; Second visit: £21–30
Shoreham-by-Sea BN43
01273 383566

**Nicola Wycherley AACP**
⊕ ⊘ 🌸 🌿
**Fees:** £36–45; Second visit: £41–50
Shoreham-by-Sea BN43
01273 440350

**Sarah Cooper-Olsen BAcC**
⊕ ⊕ 🌸 🌿
**Fees:** £46–55; Second visit: £21–30
Worthing BN11
01903 230066

**Jasper Dicke AACP**
⊕ ⊕ NHS 🌸 🌿
**Fees:** £36–45; Second visit: £41–50
Worthing BN12
01903 242261

**Sally Kenward BAcC**
O ⊕ 🌿
**Fees:** £26–35; Second visit: £21–30
Worthing BN13
01903 262520

**Tim Martin BAcC**
⊕ O ⊕ 🌿
**Fees:** £36–45; Second visit: £21–30
Worthing BN11,Brighton BN1
01903 821248

**Karen Simporis BAcC**
⊕ ⊕ 🌸 🌿
**Fees:** £26–35; Second visit: £21–30
Worthing BN11
01903 232875

## BERKSHIRE

**Alison Harris RSHom**
O 🌐 🎗
Fees: £46–55; Second visit: £31–40
Ascot SL5
01344 626402

**Anthony Dipple RSHom**
⊕ O 🌐 🎗
Fees: £46–55; Second visit: £20–30
Bracknell RG12
01344 646423

**Virginia Campbell RSHom**
O 🌐
Fees: >£55; Second visit: £31–40
Crowthorne RG45
01344 775601

**James Colthurst MFHom**
⊕ 🌐 Ⓔ
Fees: >£55; Second visit: £41–50
Hungerford RG17
01488 684008

**Barbara Johnson RSHom**
O 🌐 Ⓔ 🎗
Fees: £46–55; Second visit: £31–40
Hurst RG10
0118 934 9580

**Adele Miller RSHom**
⊕ 🌐 🎗
Fees: £46–55; Second visit: £20–30
Maidenhead SL6
01628 776407

**Christine Sanders RSHom**
⊕ 🌐 🌐 Ⓔ 🎗
Fees: £46–55; Second visit: £31–40
Maidenhead SL6,Bracknell RG12
01628 638690

**Mary-Jane Whitaker RSHom**
⊕ O 🌐 Ⓔ 🎗
Fees: £46–55; Second visit: £31–40
Maidenhead SL6,London W1
01628 675072

**Dion Tabrett RSHom**
⊕ 🌐 🌐 Ⓔ 🎗
Fees: £46–55; Second visit: £31–40
Newbury RG14
01635 44200

**Brenda Meech RSHom**
O 🌐
Fees: £46–55; Second visit: £20–30
Reading RG10
01628 823177

**Ursula Somers RSHom**
O 🌐 🎗
Fees: £46–55; Second visit: £20–30
Reading RG6
0118 9261183

**Susannah Zys RSHom**
O 🌐 Ⓔ 🎗
Fees: >£55; Second visit: £31–40
Reading RG8
01491 680992

**Trisha Longworth RSHom**
O 🌐 🎗
Fees: £46–55; Second visit: £31–40
Sunninghill SL5
01344 291484

**Anna Foxell RSHom**
O 🌐 Ⓔ 🎗
Fees: £46–55; Second visit: £31–40
Windsor SL4
01753 860539

## BUCKINGHAMSHIRE

**Richard Robinson MFHom**
⊕ 🌐 Ⓔ
Fees: £46–55; Second visit: £31–40
Amersham HP6,Milton Keynes
MK9,London W1U
01494 726228

**Jonathan Hill RSHom**
O 🌐 Ⓔ
Fees: £46–55; Second visit: £31–40
Aylesbury HP20
01296 426470

**Jean Godfrey RSHom**
⊕ O 🌐 🌐 Ⓔ 🎗
Fees: £46–55; Second visit: £31–40
High Wycombe HP10,Princes
Risborough HP27,High Wycombe HP14
01494 565558

# Homeopathy

**Sheila Banks RSHom**
⊕ O ⊕ ⓝ Ⓔ ❀
Fees: £25–35; Second visit: <£20
Marlow SL7
01628 891554

**Elizabeth Courtis RSHom**
⊕ ⓝ Ⓔ ❀
Fees: £46–55; Second visit: £31–40
Marlow SL7,Maidenhead
SL6,Abingdon OX14
01628 476200

**Judith Raeburn RSHom**
ⓝ ❀
Fees: £46–55; Second visit: £20–30
Marlow SL7
01628 476200

**Karen Sternhell RSHom**
⊕ O Ⓔ ❀
Fees: £46–55; Second visit: £31–40
Marlow SL7
01628 476200

**Wendy Stewart RSHom**
ⓝ ⊘
Fees: £46–55; Second visit: £20–30
Princes Risborough HP27
01844 344313

## DORSET

**Marianne Harling FFHom**
⊕ ⊕ ⓝ Ⓔ
Fees: £25–35; Second visit: <£20
Bournemouth BH5
01202 395149

**Martine Dirlik Mercy RSHom**
⊕ ⊕ ⓝ ❀
Fees: £46–55; Second visit: £31–40
Christchurch BH23
01202 484164

**Patricia Partridge RSHom**
⊕ O Ⓔ
Fees: £25–35; Second visit: £20–30
Christchurch BH23
01425 672011

**Jenifer Worden MFHom**
⊕ ⊕ ⊕ ⓝ ⊘ ❀
Fees: >£55; Second visit: £31–40
Christchurch BH23
01425 277505

**Zofia Dymitr RSHom**
O Ⓔ
Fees: £46–55; Second visit: £20–30
Dorchester DT1
01305 265873

**Sheila Ryan RSHom**
O ⓝ Ⓔ
Fees: £46–55; Second visit: £20–30
Dorchester DT5
01305 860428

**Jill Vines MFHom**
O ⓝ ⊘
Fees: £46–55; Second visit: £20–30
Dorchester DT2
01300 320084

**Carole Sanders RSHom**
⊕ O Ⓔ ❀
Fees: £36–45; Second visit: £20–30
Gillingham SP8,Torquay TQ2,East
Molesey KT8
01747 838171

**Angela Young RSHom**
⊕ ⊕ Ⓔ ❀
Fees: <£25; Second visit: <£20
Gillingham SP8
01747 825050

**Erica Douglass MFHom**
⊕ ⊕ ⓝ Ⓔ
Fees: £46–55; Second visit: £20–30
Shaftesbury SP7
01747 856719

## HAMPSHIRE

**Melanie Oxley RSHom**
⊕ ⓝ ❀
Fees: £46–55; Second visit: £31–40
Alresford SO24
01962 773668

**Fiona Hackman FFHom, RSHom**
✚ O ⊕ ©
Fees: £36–45; Second visit: £20–30
Alton GU34,Petersfield GU31,Hook
RG29
01420 511069

**Elizabeth Wills RSHom**
✚ ⊕ 🆖
Fees: >£55; Second visit: £31–40
Alton GU34
01420 544848

**Rachel Lambert MFHom**
O ⊕ ⊕ 🆖 ⊘ © 🐾
Fees: >£55; Second visit: £20–30
Andover SP10
01264 336373

**Gail Loudon MFHom**
O 🆖 ⊘ © 🐾
Fees: £46–55; Second visit: £20–30
Andover SP11
01264 772071

**Sally Carthew RSHom**
✚ ⊕ 🆖 ©
Fees: £46–55; Second visit: £31–40
Fareham PO15
01329 280739

**Susan Willsher RSHom**
✚ O ⊕ 🆖 © 🐾
Fees: £36–45; Second visit: £20–30
Fareham PO14
01329 665871

**Jenny Malyon RSHom**
✚ 🆖 © 🐾
Fees: >£55; Second visit: £31–40
Farnborough GU14
01252 658117

**Jonathan Hardy MFHom**
✚ ⊕ 🆖 ⊘ ©
Fees: >£55; Second visit: £41–50
Havant PO9
02392 471757

**Rachel Chancellor RSHom**
✚ O ⊕ ⊕ 🆖 ⊘ ©
Fees: £46–55; Second visit: £31–40
Horndean PO8
023 9259 9618

**David Lewis RSHom**
✚ O ⊕ 🆖 🐾
Fees: £36–45; Second visit: £20–30
Lymington SO41
01590 670033

**Anthony D Fox MFHom**
✚ O 🆖 ⊘
Fees: £46–55; Second visit: £31–40
New Milton BH25
01425 618801

**Jane Winfield MFHom**
🆖 ⊘ 🐾
Fees: £36–45; Second visit: £20–30
Southsea PO4
023 9273 7373

**Lesley Anne Anderton RSHom**
O 🐾
Fees: £25–35; Second visit: £20–30
Southampton SO31
023 8045 2268

**Michael Clark MFHom**
✚ ⊕ ⊕ 🆖 ⊘
Fees: >£55; Second visit: >£50
Southampton SO15
023 8033 4752

**June Daniels RSHom**
✚ ⊕ 🆖 © 🐾
Fees: £46–55; Second visit: £20–30
Southampton SO17
023 8058 2548

**Caroline Eyles RSHom**
✚ ⊕ 🆖 © 🐾
Fees: £46–55; Second visit: £31–40
Southampton SO15
023 8077 3500

**Rosalind Shapiro RSHom**
✚ O ⊕ 🆖 ⊘ © 🐾
Fees: £46–55; Second visit: £31–40
Southampton SO17
01273 541031

**David Owen And Associates MFHom**
✚ ⊕ ⊕ 🆖 ⊘ ©
Fees: >£55; Second visit: >£50
Winchester SO22
01962 856310

# Homeopathy

## HERTFORDSHIRE

### Carolyn Setterfield RSHom
⊕ O ⊕ ⊛ Ⓔ ❄
**Fees:** £46–55; Second visit: £31–40
Amersham HP6,Aylesbury HP21
01494 431560

### Jayne Wilton RSHom
⊕ ⊕ ⊛
**Fees:** £36–45; Second visit: £20–30
Berkhamsted HP4
01442 866805

### Karin Hirsch RSHom
O ⊛ ❄
**Fees:** £46–55; Second visit: £31–40
Elstree WD6
0208 9534883

### Brigit Crane RSHom
⊕ ⊕ ⊛ ❄
**Fees:** £46–55; Second visit: £31–40
Harpenden AL5,Bedford MK45
01582 713909

### Amanda Bate RSHom
⊕ O ⊕ ⊛ Ⓔ
**Fees:** >£55; Second visit: £31–40
Hemel Hempstead HP1
01923 443240

### Joan Carter RSHom
O ⊛ Ⓔ ❄
**Fees:** >£55; Second visit: £20–30
Hemel Hempstead HP1
01442 261416

### Patricia Darnell RSHom
O ⊛ Ⓔ ❄
**Fees:** £36–45; Second visit: £20–30
Potters Bar EN6
07956 165137

### Joyce Hall RSHom
O ⊛ Ⓔ ❄
**Fees:** £46–55; Second visit: £20–30
Potters Bar EN6
07812 102426

### Vanessa Hope RSHom
⊕ ⊛ Ⓔ ❄
**Fees:** >£55; Second visit: £31–40
St Albans AL9
01707 644309

### Vivienne Newton RSHom
⊕ O ⊕ ⊛
**Fees:** £36–45; Second visit: £20–30
St Albans AL3
01582 841639

### Susan Millican RSHom
O ⊛ Ⓔ ❄
**Fees:** >£55; Second visit: £31–40
Watford WD25
01923 661154

## ISLE OF WIGHT

### Eileen Anne Finch MFHom
⊛ ⊘
**Fees:** £36–45; Second visit: <£20
Cowes PO31
01983 295251

### Hugh Harrison RSHom
⊕ ⊕ ⊛ ⊘ Ⓔ
**Fees:** £36–45; Second visit: £20–30
Newport PO30,Lake PO36
01983 522477

### Jerry Christopher RSHom
⊕ O ⊕ ⊛ Ⓔ ❄
**Fees:** £46–55; Second visit: £20–30
Ryde PO33
01983 551380

## KENT

### Elaine Walker RSHom
⊕ O ⊕ ⊛ Ⓔ ❄
**Fees:** >£55; Second visit: £31–40
Ash CT3
01304 812133

### Martin Miles RSHom
O ⊛ Ⓔ
**Fees:** >£55; Second visit: £20–30
Bexley DA5
01322 520921

### Katya Mons-Rushby RSHom
⊛ ❄
**Fees:** >£55; Second visit: £20–30
Bexley DA5
01322 558334

**Kathryn Vale MFHom**
⊕ 🌐 ⊘
Cranbrook TN18
01580 753211

**Peter A Ustianowski MFHom**
O 🌐 ⊘
Fees: >£55; Second visit: £41–50
Deal CT14
01304 614840

**Lesley Murray RSHom**
⊕ O ⊕ 🌐 © ❀
Fees: £36–45; Second visit: £20–30
Faversham ME13,Herne Bay CT6
01795 537159

**Maryse Summers RSHom**
O 🌐 ❀
Fees: £46–55; Second visit: £31–40
Faversham ME13
01227 751886

**Cornelia Verwijs RSHom**
⊕ 🌐 © ❀
Fees: £36–45; Second visit: £20–30
Faversham ME13
01227 264174

**Giovanna Forrester RSHom**
O ⊕ 🌐 ©
Fees: £46–55; Second visit: £20–30
Gravesend DA12,Canterbury CT1
01474 355204

**Elizabeth Anne Simpson RSHom**
⊕ O ⊕ 🌐 © ❀
Fees: £46–55; Second visit: £20–30
Meopham DA13
01474 815755

**Mark Paine RSHom**
⊕ O 🌐 © ❀
Fees: £36–45; Second visit: £31–40
Rainham ME8
01634 375759

**Jane Sloan RSHom**
O ⊕ 🌐 ©
Fees: £46–55; Second visit: £20–30
Sandhurst TN18
01580 850131

**Katharine Boulderstone RSHom**
⊕ O ⊕ 🌐 © ❀
Fees: £46–55; Second visit: £31–40
Speldhurst TN3
01892 863958

**Jean Osborne MFHom**
⊕ ⊕ ❀
Fees: £46–55; Second visit: £20–30
Tenterden TN30
01580 766424

**Lesley King RSHom**
O ⊕ 🌐 © ❀
Fees: £36–45; Second visit: £20–30
Tonbridge TN37
01424 441397

**Sarah Hemesley RSHom**
⊕ ⊕ © ❀
Fees: £46–55; Second visit: £31–40
Tunbridge Wells TN1
01892 510950

**John Morgan RSHom**
⊕ ⊕ © ❀
Fees: £46–55; Second visit: £20–30
Tunbridge Wells TN1
01892 518663

## NORTHAMPTONSHIRE

**Charlotte (Shusha) Walmsley RSHom**
⊕ O ⊕ ⊕ 🌐 ©
Fees: £36–45; Second visit: £31–40
Kettering NN16,Wellingborough
NN8,Northampton NN1
01536 516220

**Lyn Redman RSHom**
⊕ O ⊕ 🌐
Fees: £46–55; Second visit: £31–40
Northampton NN1,Kettering NN14
01604 624638

## OXFORDSHIRE

**Angela Jones MFHom**
⊕ O ⊕ ⊘
Fees: >£55; Second visit: >£50
Abingdon OX14
01235 848977

# Homeopathy

**Juliet Smith RSHom**
O ⊕ ⊕ ⓝ Ⓔ ✿
**Fees:** £46–55; Second visit: £20–30
Bloxham OX15
01865 331681

**Nick Salzman MFHom**
⊕ ⊕ ⊕ ⊘ ✿
**Fees:** £46–55; Second visit: £20–30
Didcot OX11
01235 511355

**Elizabeth Austin RSHom**
⊕ O ⊕ ⓝ Ⓔ ✿
**Fees:** £46–55; Second visit: £20–30
Oxford OX4
01865 794363

**Steven Cartwright RSHom**
⊕ O ⊕ ⓝ ✿
**Fees:** >£55; Second visit: £20–30
Oxford OX2
01865 558561

**Diana Ferguson MFHom**
⊕ ⊕ ⊘ Ⓔ
**Fees:** >£55; Second visit: £31–40
Oxford OX1
01865 311811

**Jemima Kallas RSHom**
⊕ O ⊕ ⓝ Ⓔ ✿
**Fees:** >£55; Second visit: £31–40
Oxford OX3,London NW6,Oxford OX4
01865 761351

**Katie McLennan RSHom**
O ⓝ
**Fees:** £46–55; Second visit: £20–30
Oxford OX2
01865 556006

**Lucinda Torabi RSHom**
⊕ O ⊕ ⓝ Ⓔ ✿
**Fees:** £46–55; Second visit: £20–30
Oxford OX33
01865 425637

**Margaret Brock RSHom**
⊕ O ⊕ ⓝ ⊘ ✿
**Fees:** £46–55; Second visit: £31–40
Wallingford OX10,Wantage OX12
01491 838246

**Sue Queenborough RSHom**
⊕ O ⊕ ⓝ Ⓔ
**Fees:** £46–55; Second visit: £31–40
Wallingford OX10
01491 824724

## SURREY

**Carolyn Persson RSHom**
⊕ O ⊕ ⊕ ⓝ Ⓔ ✿
Albury GU5,Dorking RH4
01483 203540

**Andrew Ovenden RSHom**
⊕ ⓝ
**Fees:** £46–55; Second visit: £20–30
Camberley GU15
01276 691946

**Mina Weight RSHom**
⊕ ⊕ ⓝ ✿
**Fees:** £46–55; Second visit: £31–40
Cranleigh GU6
01483 274002

**Martine Faure-Alderson RSHom**
O ⊘ Ⓔ ✿
**Fees:** £36–45; Second visit: <£20
East Molesey KT8
020 8398 6943

**Claudia Demire RSHom**
⊕ ⓝ Ⓔ ✿
**Fees:** £46–55; Second visit: £31–40
Farnham GU10
01252 713338

**David T H Williams MFHom**
O ⓝ ⊘
**Fees:** >£55; Second visit: £41–50
Godalming GU8
01428 683136

**Annie Williams RSHom**
⊕ O ⊕ ⓝ Ⓔ ✿
**Fees:** >£55; Second visit: £41–50
Godalming GU7
01483 419478

**Sarah Bogue RSHom**
⊕ O ⊕ ⊕ ⓝ Ⓔ ✿
**Fees:** >£55; Second visit: £20–30
Guildford GU3
01483 812070

**Andrew Lockie MFHom**
Fees: >£55; Second visit: £41–50
Guildford GU1,London W1G
01483 503240

**Ann Thorpe RSHom**
Fees: >£55; Second visit: £31–40
Guildford GU1
01483 300400

**Carolyn Tilson RSHom**
Fees: £46–55; Second visit: £20–30
Haslemere GU27
01428 641664

**Susan Skelcey RSHom**
Fees: £36–45; Second visit: £20–30
Oxted RH8
020 8688 1302

**Catherine Helps RSHom**
Fees: £36–45; Second visit: £20–30
Redhill RH1
01737 762990

**Keith Smeaton RSHom**
Fees: £36–45; Second visit: £20–30
Reigate RH2,Horley RH6,London SW11
01737 243601

**Venita Burnaby RSHom**
Fees: £36–45; Second visit: £20–30
South Croydon CR2
07866 841141

**Caroline Jurdon RSHom**
Fees: £46–55; Second visit: £20–30
South Croydon CR2
020 8654 3700

**Farley R Spink FFHom,**
Fees: >£55; Second visit: £31–40
South Croydon CR2
020 8688 0534

**Marliese Symons RSHom**
Fees: £46–55; Second visit: £31–40
South Croydon CR2
020 8651 6704

**Robert Every RSHom**
Fees: £36–45; Second visit: £31–40
Woking GU22
01483 765288

**Yvonne Stone RSHom**
Fees: £36–45; Second visit: £31–40
Woking GU21
020 8647 2924

## SUSSEX

**Sally Nunn RSHom**
Fees: £25–35; Second visit: £20–30
Arundel BN18
01903 884466

**Pamela Embden RSHom**
Fees: £46–55; Second visit: £31–40
Brighton BN1
01273 509193

**Elizabeth Hemmings RSHom**
Fees: £36–45; Second visit: £31–40
Brighton BN1
01273 324790

**Tricia Taylor RSHom**
Fees: £46–55; Second visit: £31–40
Brighton BN1,Hove BN3
01273 550727

**Jan Mathew RSHom**
Fees: £36–45; Second visit: £20–30
Brighton BN1
01273 388857

**Christian Taylor RSHom**
Fees: £36–45; Second visit: £20–30
Brighton BN1
01273 559823

# Homeopathy

**Jeannette Adair RSHom**
O ⊕ ⓦ Ⓔ ❀
Fees: £36–45; Second visit: £20–30
Brighton BN2
01273 700264

**Sohani Gonzalez RSHom**
O O ⓦ ⓦ ⊘ Ⓔ ❀
Fees: £36–45; Second visit: £31–40
Brighton BN2
01273 689194

**John Kidson RSHom**
O O ⊕ ⓦ Ⓔ ❀
Fees: £36–45; Second visit: <£20
Brighton BN2
01273 307787

**Pema Sanders RSHom**
O O ⊕ ⓦ Ⓔ
Fees: £36–45; Second visit: £31–40
Brighton BN2,Brighton BN1
01273 699775

**Robert Withers RSHom**
O ⊕ ⊕ ⓦ Ⓔ
Fees: £36–45; Second visit: £31–40
Brighton BN2
01273 621841

**Richard Cook RFHom, GCC, BCA**
O ⊕ ⓦ Ⓔ ❀
Fees: >£55; Second visit: £31–40
Chichester PO19
01243 786946

**Christopher Hyslop RSHom**
O ⓦ
Fees: £25–35; Second visit: £20–30
Crawley RH10
01293 533449

**Dee Richards RSHom**
⊕ ⓦ Ⓔ ❀
Fees: £36–45; Second visit: £20–30
Crawley RH10
01293 562601

**Alan Crook RSHom**
O ⓦ
Fees: £36–45; Second visit: £20–30
Crowborough TN6
01892 655217

**Peter Hudson RSHom**
O ⓦ Ⓔ ❀
Fees: £36–45; Second visit: £31–40
Eastbourne BN20
01323 647770

**Susan Josling RSHom**
O ⊕ ⓦ Ⓔ
Fees: £46–55; Second visit: £31–40
Eastbourne BN21
01323 430025

**Jane Montague RSHom**
O O ⓦ ⊘ Ⓔ ❀
Fees: £36–45; Second visit: £20–30
Eastbourne BN20
01323 7208264

**Barbara Turk MFHom**
⊘ ❀
Fees: >£55; Second visit: £20–30
East Grinstead RH19
01342 410606

**Geoffrey Douch FFHom,**
O O ⓦ
Fees: £36–45; Second visit: £20–30
Forest Row RH18
01342 822241

**Llewelyn Ralph Twentyman MFHom**
Forest Row RH18
01342 822151

**Hanna Waldbaum RSHom**
ⓦ Ⓔ ❀
Fees: £36–45; Second visit: £31–40
Forest Row RH18
01342 823714

**Sarah Worne RSHom**
O ⓦ Ⓔ
Fees: £46–55; Second visit: £31–40
Forest Row RH18
01342 826930

**David Fergie-Woods MFHom**
⊕ ⓦ Ⓔ
Fees: £46–55; Second visit: £31–40
Hassocks BN6
01273 832546

**Wanda Whiting RSHom**

O ⊕ 🅜 🅔 ✿

**Fees:** £36–45; Second visit: £20–30
Hastings TN34, St Leonards-on-Sea
TN38
01424 421348

**Margot Barton RSHom**

O 🅜 ✿

**Fees:** >£55; Second visit: £20–30
Haywards Heath RH17
01444 400930

**Philip Edmonds RSHom**

⊕ O 🅖 🅜 🅔 ✿

**Fees:** £36–45; Second visit: £20–30
Haywards Heath RH16
01444 457851

**Mike Andrews RSHom**

⊕ O ⊕ 🅖 🅜 ✿

**Fees:** >£55; Second visit: £31–40
Horsham RH12, London EC3R, London
SW4
01403 754215

**Robin Logan RSHom**

⊕ ⊕ 🅖 🅜 ⊘ ✿

**Fees:** >£55; Second visit: £31–40
Hove BN3, Epsom KT19, London W11
01273 770377

**Jill Wight RSHom**

O 🅜 🅔 ✿

**Fees:** £36–45; Second visit: £31–40
Hove BN3
01273 321250

**Anna Taylor RSHom**

⊕ 🅖 🅜 🅔 ✿

**Fees:** £46–55; Second visit: £31–40
Lewes BN7
01273 486550

**Carolyn Warren RSHom**

⊕ O 🅖 🅜 🅔 ✿

**Fees:** £36–45; Second visit: £20–30
Polegate BN26
01323 811977

**Andrew Sikorski MFHom**

⊕ ⊕ 🅖 🅜 ⊘ ✿

**Fees:** >£55; Second visit: £20–30
Robertsbridge TN32, Tunbridge Wells
TN1
01580 881119

**Michelle Floyd RSHom**

⊕ O 🅖 🅜 🅔

**Fees:** £36–45; Second visit: £20–30
Seaford BN25, Brighton BN1
01323 895088

**William O'Meara RSHom**

O 🅜

**Fees:** £36–45; Second visit: £20–30
Seaford BN25
01323 873617

**Siegfried Trefzer MFHom**

⊕ O 🅖 🅜 ⊘ 🅔

**Fees:** £46–55; Second visit: >£50
Uckfield TN22
07973 702461

**Sarah North RSHom**

⊕ O 🅖 🅜 🅔 ✿

**Fees:** £36–45; Second visit: £31–40
Wadhurst TN5
01580 212775

**Pauline Black RSHom**

⊕ 🅖 🅜

**Fees:** £36–45; Second visit: £20–30
Worthing BN14
01903 208238

# Osteopathy

**M Seatory GOsC, BOA**

⊕ 🅖 🅜 ✿

**Fees:** £26–35; Second visit: £21–30
Ascot SL5
01344 620174

**Michael Smith GOsC, BOA**

⊕ O 🅜 ✿

**Fees:** £26–35; Second visit: £21–30
Ascot SL5
01344 624734

# Osteopathy

**Sarah Shand GOsC**
O ⊛ ❀
**Fees:** £26–35; Second visit: £21–30
Bracknell RG42
01344 301502

**Richard Gulliver GOsC, BOA**
⊕ ⊕ ⊕ ⊛ ⊘ ❀
**Fees:** £36–45; Second visit: £31–40
Bucklebury RG7
01635 865757

**Sophie Parkes GOsC, BOA**
O ⊕ ⊛ ⊘ Ⓔ ❀
**Fees:** £26–35; Second visit: £21–30
Bucklebury RG7
01635 865757

**David Gilhooley GOsC, BOA**
⊕ ⊛ Ⓔ
**Fees:** £36–45; Second visit: £21–30
Maidenhead SL6
01628 620897

**John Qureshi GOsC**
⊕ ⊕ ⊛ ❀
**Fees:** £36–45; Second visit: £31–40
Maidenhead SL6
01753 857095

**Gareth Rogers GOsC**
⊕ ⊛ ❀
**Fees:** £36–45; Second visit: £21–30
Maidenhead SL6
01628 826227

**Sebastian Roles GOsC, BOA**
⊕ ⊛ ❀
**Fees:** £36–45; Second visit: £21–30
Maidenhead SL6
01628 620897

**Karen Withington GOsC, BOA**
⊕ ⊛ ⊘ ❀
**Fees:** <£25; Second visit: £31–40
Maidenhead SL6
01628 624544

**Kim Burnett GOsC, BOA**
⊕ O ⊕ ⊛ Ⓔ ❀
**Fees:** £26–35; Second visit: £21–30
Newbury RG14
01635 580200

**Tim Dennis GOsC**
⊕ ⊕ ⊛ ❀
**Fees:** £36–45; Second visit: £31–40
Newbury RG14
01635 44200

**Kelley Knight GOsC, BOA**
⊕ ⊛ ❀
**Fees:** £26–35; Second visit: £21–30
Newbury RG14
01635 44200

**N Atkinson GOsC, BOA**
O ⊕ ⊕ ⊛ ⊘ ❀
**Fees:** £26–35; Second visit: £21–30
Reading RG10
0118 934 2187

**Frances Aylen GOsC**
⊕ ⊛ ⊘ ❀
**Fees:** £26–35; Second visit: £21–30
Reading RG1
0118 957 3440

**Caroline Baker GOsC, BOA**
⊕ ⊕ ⊛ ⊘ ❀
**Fees:** <£25; Second visit: £21–30
Reading RG12
01344 862646

**Julia Graemer GOsC**
⊕ ⊛ ⊘ Ⓔ
Reading RG1
0118 959 5200

**Melina Harrison GOsC**
⊕ ⊛ ⊘ ❀
**Fees:** £26–35; Second visit: £21–30
Reading RG1
0118 957 3440

**Andrew Jackson GOsC, BOA**
O ⊛ ❀
**Fees:** £26–35; Second visit: £21–30
Reading RG1
0118 957 2882

**Chris Morriss GOsC, BOA**
O ⊛ ❀
**Fees:** £26–35; Second visit: £21–30
Reading RG1
0118 975 3893

**Vian Neville-Towle GOsC**
O ⊕ ⊘ ✿
Fees: £26–35; Second visit: £21–30
Reading RG1
0118 957 3440

**Neil M J Swan GOsC, BOA**
⊕ O ⊕ Ⓔ ✿
Fees: £26–35; Second visit: £21–30
Reading RG8
01491 873874

**Marcus Vaz GOsC, BOA**
⊕ ⊕ Ⓔ ✿
Fees: £26–35; Second visit: £21–30
Reading RG6
0118 961 4072

**Julie Archer GOsC, BOA**
⊕ O ⊕ ✿
Fees: £36–45; Second visit: £21–30
Slough SL3
01753 591622

**Kulwinder Bajwa GOsC**
⊕ ⊕ ⊘ ✿
Fees: £26–35; Second visit: £21–30
Slough SL2
01753 528882

**Mark Bujakowski GOsC**
O ⊕ ⊕ ✿
Fees: <£25; Second visit: £21–30
Slough SL1
01753 576721

**D Jonathan Kanakam GOsC**
⊕ ⊘ ⊕
Fees: <£25; Second visit: £21–30
Slough SL1
01753 552976

**Thais Munro GOsC**
⊕ ⊕ ⊘ ✿
Fees: £46–55; Second visit: £31–40
Slough SL3
01753 593733

**Candida S Smith GOsC, BOA**
⊕ ⊕ ⊘ ✿
Fees: <£25; Second visit: £21–30
Thatcham RG19
01635 871948

**Stephen Baker GOsC**
⊕ O ⊕
Fees: £36–45; Second visit: £21–30
Windsor SL4
01753 850322

**Gareth Butler GOsC, BOA**
⊕ ⊕ ✿
Fees: £36–45; Second visit: £21–30
Windsor SL4
01753 850322

**Matthew Carratu GOsC**
O ⊕ ✿
Fees: <£25; Second visit: £21–30
Windsor SL4
01753 831824

**Hannah Lawrence GOsC, BOA**
⊕ ⊕ ✿
Fees: <£25; Second visit: £41–50
Windsor SL4
01753 831824

**Jon Morton-Bell GOsC, BOA**
⊕ ⊕ ⊕ ✿
Fees: <£25; Second visit: £21–30
Windsor SL4
01344 884799

**Rebecca Day GOsC**
O ⊕ ⊘ ✿
Fees: £36–45; Second visit: £31–40
Wokingham RG41
0118 979 4964

**Michael Relf GOsC, BOA**
O ⊕ ⊘
Fees: £36–45; Second visit: £21–30
Wokingham RG41
0118 989 1226

## BUCKINGHAMSHIRE

**Karen Carroll GOsC, BOA**
⊕ ⊕ Ⓔ ✿
Fees: £26–35; Second visit: £21–30
Amersham HP6
01494 434651

**Simon Chesney GOsC, BOA**
O ⊕ ⊘ ✿
Fees: £36–45; Second visit: £31–40
Amersham HP7
01494 725431

# Osteopathy

**Paul Mitterhuber GOsC, BOA**
✪ Ⓞ ⓜ Ⓞ ✿
**Fees:** £26–35; Second visit: £21–30
Amersham HP6
01494 783962

**Gerhard Stangl GOsC, BOA**
✪ ⊕ ⓜ
**Fees:** £26–35; Second visit: £21–30
Amersham HP6
01494 726228

**Brenda Case GOsC**
✪ Ⓞ ⓜ
**Fees:** <£25; Second visit: £21–30
Aylesbury HP22
01296 622716

**Penny Dathan GOsC, BOA**
⊕ ⓜ Ⓞ ✿
**Fees:** <£25; Second visit: £31–40
Aylesbury HP22
01296 696999

**Harkiran Floura GOsC, BOA**
✪ Ⓞ ⊕ ⓜ ✿
**Fees:** £36–45; Second visit: £31–40
Aylesbury HP21
01296 612361

**Diane Kheir GOsC, BOA**
✪ ⊕ ⊕ ⓜ Ⓞ ✿
**Fees:** <£25; Second visit: £21–30
Beaconsfield HP9
01494 880649

**Damon Peterson GOsC**
✪ Ⓞ ⓜ Ⓞ Ⓔ ✿
**Fees:** £26–35; Second visit: £21–30
Beaconsfield HP9
01494 676821

**Katie Banfield GOsC, BOA**
✪ ⊕ ⊕ ⓜ Ⓔ ✿
**Fees:** £26–35; Second visit: £21–30
Buckingham MK18
01296 714504

**Janet Lawson GOsC, BOA**
✪ ⓜ
**Fees:** £26–35; Second visit: £31–40
Buckingham MK18
01280 823033

**Alan Williams GOsC, BOA**
✪ ⊕ ⊕ ⓜ Ⓞ ✿
**Fees:** <£25; Second visit: £21–30
Buckingham MK18
01280 818600

**Cecilia Williams GOsC, BOA**
✪ Ⓞ ⊕ ⓜ Ⓞ Ⓔ ✿
**Fees:** £26–35; Second visit: £21–30
Buckingham MK18
01280 818600

**Julia Green GOsC, BOA**
Ⓞ ⓜ Ⓞ ✿
**Fees:** £26–35; Second visit: £21–30
Chesham HP5
01442 870733

**Shirley Merrick-Wells GOsC, BOA**
Ⓞ ⓜ Ⓞ Ⓔ
**Fees:** <£25; Second visit: £21–30
Chesham HP5
01494 784309

**David Norton GOsC, BOA**
✪ ⊕ ⓜ
**Fees:** £36–45; Second visit: £21–30
Farnham Common SL2
01753 646381

**Michael Thornton GOsC**
✪ Ⓞ ⓜ ✿
**Fees:** £26–35; Second visit: £21–30
Flackwell Heath HP10
01628 520711

**Karen Goddard GOsC, BOA**
✪ ⊕ ⓜ ✿
**Fees:** £26–35; Second visit: £21–30
Gerrards Cross SL9
01753 887855

**Charles Hunt GOsC**
Ⓞ ✿
**Fees:** £26–35; Second visit: £21–30
Gerrards Cross SL9
01753 887855

**John Armitstead GOsC,**
✪ ⊕ ⓜ
**Fees:** <£25; Second visit: £21–30
High Wycombe HP13
01494 529769

**Susan P Clark GOsC, BOA**
O ⊕ 🔵 🄔 ✿
Fees: £36–45; Second visit: £31–40
High Wycombe HP14
01494 883970

**Mark Holtom GOsC**
⊕ O 🔵 ✿
Fees: <£25; Second visit: £21–30
High Wycombe HP10
01494 471264

**Miranda Souter GOsC, BOA**
O 🔵 ✿
Fees: £26–35; Second visit: £21–30
High Wycombe HP10
01494 814723

**Steven Butcher GOsC**
⊕ ⊕ 🔵 ✿
Fees: £26–35; Second visit: £21–30
Iver SL0
01753 630871

**Tracey Hou GOsC**
⊕ ⊕ 🔵 ✿
Fees: £26–35; Second visit: £21–30
Iver Heath SL0
01753 630871

**David Hou GOsC**
⊕ ⊕ 🔵 ✿
Fees: £26–35; Second visit: £21–30
Iver Heath SL0
01753 630871

**Barry Harker GOsC, BOA**
⊕ ⊕ ⊕ 🔵 🄔
Fees: <£25; Second visit: £21–30
Marlow SL7
01628 479965

**Helen Johnson GOsC**
O 🔵 ✿
Fees: <£25; Second visit: £21–30
Marlow SL7
01628 477779

**Deborah Rogers GOsC, BOA**
⊕ 🔵 ⊘ 🄔 ✿
Fees: £26–35; Second visit: £21–30
Marlow SL7
01628 477466

**Christine Langley GOsC, BOA**
⊕ ⊕ 🔵
Fees: £26–35; Second visit: £21–30
Princes Risborough HP27
01844 275055

**Ian Luxton GOsC**
⊕ O ⊕ 🔵 ✿
Fees: £26–35; Second visit: £21–30
Princes Risborough HP27
01844 275055

**Oliver Vass GOsC, BOA**
⊕ O ⊕ ⊕ 🔵 ✿
Fees: £36–45; Second visit: £21–30
Princes Risborough HP27
01844 261467

**Russell May GOsC**
⊕ ⊕ 🔵 ✿
Fees: £26–35; Second visit: £31–40
Stoke Mandeville HP21
01296 612361

## CHANNEL ISLANDS

**Guy Wildy GOsC, BOA,**
⊕ ⊕ 🔵 ⊘ ✿
Fees: <£25; Second visit: £31–40
Jersey JE2
01534 728777

**Jeff Harris GOsC**
⊕ ⊕ 🔵 ⊘ ✿
Fees: £46–55; Second visit: £41–50
Guernsey GY4
01481 232900

**Christine Budd GOsC,**
⊕ ⊘
Fees: £26–35; Second visit: <£20
Jersey JE2
01534 735419

## DORSET

**Adrian Culling GOsC**
O ⊕ 🔵 ✿
Fees: £36–45; Second visit: £21–30
Bournemouth BH4,Wareham BH20
01202 769976

# Osteopathy

**Rebecca Evans GOsC**
⊕ ⓝ ✿
**Fees:** £26–35; Second visit: £21–30
Bournemouth BH6
01202 417656

**Nigel Graham GOsC, BOA**
⊕ ⓝ ✿
**Fees:** £46–55; Second visit: £21–30
Bournemouth BH6
01202 770007

**Dustie Houchin GOsC, BOA**
⊕ O ⊕ ⓝ Ⓔ ✿
**Fees:** <£25; Second visit: £21–30
Bournemouth BH7
01202 417600

**Steve Hussey GOsC, BOA**
⊕ ⊕ ✿
**Fees:** £26–35; Second visit: £21–30
Bournemouth BH1
01202 554098

**Edward Kennedy GOsC, BOA**
⊕ O ⊕ ⓝ ⊘ Ⓔ ✿
**Fees:** £36–45; Second visit: £21–30
Bournemouth BH8
01202 304382

**Laurence Andrew McCaffery GOsC**
⊕ O ⓝ
**Fees:** <£25; Second visit: £21–30
Bournemouth BH9
01202 527719

**Deirdre Rowell GOsC, BOA**
⊕ O ⊕ Ⓔ ✿
**Fees:** £36–45; Second visit: £21–30
Bournemouth BH8
01202 777998

**David J Allen GOsC**
⊕ ⊕ ⊕ ⓝ ✿
**Fees:** <£25; Second visit: £21–30
Broadstone BH18
01202 692493

**Fiona Terry GOsC, BOA**
⊕ ⊕ ⓝ ⊘ ✿
**Fees:** <£25; Second visit: £21–30
Christchurch BH23
01425 672741

**Tamara De Bardi GOsC**
⊕ O ⊕ ⓝ
**Fees:** <£25; Second visit: £21–30
Dorchester DT1
01305 266887

**Kathrine Read GOsC, BOA**
O ⓝ
**Fees:** £26–35; Second visit: £21–30
Dorchester DT1, Frome BA11
01305 267052

**Graeme Saxby GOsC**
⊕ ⓝ ✿
**Fees:** <£25; Second visit: £21–30
Poole BH12
01202 743333

**H Neeshe Annauth GOsC, BOA**
⊕ ⊕ Ⓔ ✿
**Fees:** £26–35; Second visit: £21–30
Poole BH14
01202 743100

**Richard Bazalgette GOsC, BOA**
O ⓝ
**Fees:** <£25; Second visit: <£20
Poole BH14
01202 744090

**Carolyn Chamberlain GOsC**
ⓝ
**Fees:** £26–35; Second visit: £21–30
Poole BH12
01202 743333

**Christopher Galloway GOsC**
⊕ ⊕ ⓝ ✿
**Fees:** Second visit: £21–30
Poole BH15, Southampton SO40
01202 661966

**Emma Childs GOsC**
⊕ ⊕ ⓝ ✿
**Fees:** £26–35; Second visit: £21–30
Shaftesbury SP7
01747 851726

**Richard Gribble GOsC, BOA,**
⊕ ⊕ ⊕ ⓝ ⊘ ✿
**Fees:** £36–45; Second visit: £31–40
Shaftesbury SP7
01747 856719

**Alexander C Gibbs GOsC, BOA**
Fees: <£25; Second visit: £31–40
Sherborne DT9
01935 817442

**Anita Hegerty GOsC, BOA**
Fees: £26–35; Second visit: £21–30
Sherborne DT9
01935 817442

**Ian J Lever GOsC**
Fees: <£25; Second visit: <£20
Weymouth DT3
01305 786893

**Michael Talbot GOsC, BOA**
Fees: £26–35; Second visit: £21–30
Weymouth DT3
01305 833800

## HAMPSHIRE

**Christine Clements GOsC**
Fees: £36–45; Second visit: £21–30
Aldershot GU11
01252 322419

**Catherine Mary Garside GOsC**
Fees: <£25; Second visit: £21–30
Aldershot GU11
01252 324048

**Jennifer Gove GOsC, BOA**
Fees: <£25; Second visit: £21–30
Alton GU34
01420 544408

**J Sexton GOsC**
Fees: £36–45; Second visit: £21–30
Alverstoke PO12
023 9251 1107

**Alan Lloyd Davies GOsC,**
Fees: £36–45; Second visit: £21–30
Andover SP10
01264 352983

**Ian Harrison GOsC**
Fees: £36–45; Second visit: £31–40
Basingstoke RG24
01256 357111

**Darcy Jones GOsC**
Fees: £36–45; Second visit: £21–30
Basingstoke RG21
01256 352241

**Richenda Power GOsC, BOA**
Fees: £36–45; Second visit: £31–40
Basingstoke RG23
01256 322959

**Yvonne D Ridguard GOsC**
Fees: £26–35; Second visit: £21–30
Basingstoke RG21
01256 325560

**Robert Cartwright GOsC**
Fees: £26–35; Second visit: £21–30
Eastleigh SO50
023 8061 2166

**Laurent Heib GOsC, BOA**
Fees: <£25; Second visit: £31–40
Eastleigh SO53
023 8026 9809

**Philip Hull GOsC**
Fees: £26–35; Second visit: £21–30
Eastleigh SO50
023 8061 2166

**Stanley MacLeod GOsC**
Fees: £26–35; Second visit: £21–30
Eastleigh SO50
023 8060 1119

**Nicholas Cowx GOsC**
Fees: <£25; Second visit: £21–30
Emsworth PO10
01243 375112

# Osteopathy

**Kim Prichard GOsC**
✪ ⊕ ⊕ ⊕
**Fees:** £26–35; Second visit: £21–30
Emsworth PO10
01243 372623

**T D Alldridge GOsC**
✪ O ⊕ ⊕ ⊘ ✿
**Fees:** <£25; Second visit: £21–30
Fareham PO15
01329 232213

**Michael Spenceley GOsC**
✪ O ⊕
**Fees:** <£25; Second visit: £21–30
Fareham PO15
01329 822657

**Simon Griffiths GOsC**
✪ O ⊕ ⊘ ✿
**Fees:** £26–35; Second visit: £21–30
Fleet GU13, Sevenoaks TN14
01252 622530

**Philip Gamble GOsC**
O ⊕ ⊘ ✿
**Fees:** <£25; Second visit: <£20
Gosport PO12
023 9252 1531

**Lyn Samler GOsC, BOA**
O ⊕ ✿
**Fees:** £26–35
Gosport PO13
01329 827739

**Gabriel Konrad GOsC**
✪ ⊕ ⊕ ✿
**Fees:** <£25; Second visit: £21–30
Havant PO9
023 9248 6957

**Isabelle Bras GOsC**
✪ O ⊕ ✿
**Fees:** <£25; Second visit: £21–30
Lymington SO41
01590 670706

**Gavin Gobell GOsC**
✪ ✿
**Fees:** <£25; Second visit: >£50
Lymington SO41
01590 670706

**Louise Sanders GOsC**
✪ ⊕ ⊘ ✿
**Fees:** £26–35; Second visit: £21–30
Odiham RG29
01256 702371

**Christopher Grey GOsC**
✪ ⓔ
**Fees:** £36–45; Second visit: £31–40
Petersfield GU31
01730 233802

**Carina Petter GOsC**
✪ ⊕ ✿
**Fees:** £26–35; Second visit: £31–40
Petersfield GU32
01732 231655

**Anne-Marie Sivyer GOsC, BOA**
✪ ⊕ ⊕
**Fees:** £26–35; Second visit: £21–30
Petersfield GU32
01730 267423

**N John Parry GOsC, BOA**
✪ O ⊕ ⊕
**Fees:** <£25; Second visit: £31–40
Ringwood BH24
01425 476930

**Paul Vickerman GOsC**
✪ O ⊕ ⊕ ⓔ ✿
**Fees:** £26–35; Second visit: £21–30
Romsey SO51
01794 517688

**Catherine Welsh GOsC**
O ⊕
**Fees:** £26–35; Second visit: £21–30
Romsey SO51
01794 523371

**Peter Das GOsC,**
O ⊕ ⊘ ✿
**Fees:** £26–35; Second visit: £21–30
Southampton SO16
023 8047 2126

**P Franckeiss GOsC, BOA**
✪ ⊕ ✿
**Fees:** <£25; Second visit: £31–40
Southampton SO32
01489 891880

**Jane Horton GOsC, BOA**
O ⊛
**Fees:** <£25; Second visit: £31–40
Southampton SO31
01489 573184

**P Robin Husband GOsC, BOA,**
⊕ O ⊕ ⊘ Ⓔ ❅
**Fees:** £26–35; Second visit: £21–30
Southampton SO45
023 8089 2579

**Steven Orton GOsC, BOA**
⊕ ⊕ ⊛ ⊘ ❅
**Fees:** £26–35; Second visit: £31–40
Southampton SO45
023 8084 0411

**Alan Reynolds GOsC, BOA**
O ⊛ Ⓔ ❅
**Fees:** £26–35; Second visit: £21–30
Southampton SO45,
North Somerset BS23
023 8084 1148

**Jonathan Le Bon GOsC**
⊕ ⊕ ⊛ ⊘ ❅
**Fees:** £36–45; Second visit: £31–40
Southampton SO19
023 8044 8901

**Roy Smith GOsC, BOA**
⊕ ⊛ Ⓔ ❅
**Fees:** £26–35; Second visit: £21–30
Southampton SO19
023 8043 1776

**Ross Valentine GOsC, BOA**
⊕ ⊕ ⊛ ❅
**Fees:** <£25; Second visit: £31–40
Southampton SO17
023 8055 4076

**Anna Stainer GOsC, BOA**
⊕ ⊕ ⊛ ❅
**Fees:** £26–35; Second visit: £21–30
Southsea PO4
023 9273 4815

**D N H Harding GOsC**
⊕ ⊛ ⊘ ❅
**Fees:** £26–35; Second visit: £21–30
Winchester SO22
01962 867196

**Sarah Moore GOsC**
⊕ O ⊕ ⊛ ❅
**Fees:** £26–35; Second visit: £21–30
Winchester SO22
01962 849247

**Daniel Nelson GOsC**
O ⊕ ⊛ ❅
**Fees:** £26–35; Second visit: £21–30
Winchester SO23
01962 866329

**Heidi Stubbs GOsC**
⊕ ⊕ ⊛
**Fees:** £26–35; Second visit: £21–30
Winchester SO23
01962 866903

**Emma Wightman GOsC, BOA**
⊕ ⊕ ⊛ Ⓔ ❅
**Fees:** £46–55; Second visit: £21–30
Winchester SO22
01962 856310

## HERTFORDSHIRE

**Edward C Buckwald GOsC, BOA**
⊕ O ⊕ ⊕ ⊛ ⊘ ❅
**Fees:** <£25; Second visit: £21–30
Abbots Langley WD5
01923 268787

**Timothy Moynihan GOsC, BOA**
⊕ O ⊕ ⊕ ⊛ ⊘ ❅
**Fees:** £26–35; Second visit: £21–30
Baldock SG7
01462 742942

**Christopher Evans GOsC, BOA**
⊕ ⊕ ⊛ ⊘ ❅
**Fees:** £26–35; Second visit: £21–30
Barnet EN4
020 8449 7754

**Professor Laurie Hartman GOsC, BOA**
⊕ O ⊛ ⊘
**Fees:** £46–55; Second visit: £41–50
Barnet EN4
020 8441 2876

**Sarah Rosewarne GOsC, BOA**
⊕ O ⊛ ❅
**Fees:** <£25; Second visit: £21–30
Barnet EN5
020 8441 8726

# Osteopathy

**Juliet Hanwell GOsC**
⊕ ⊕ ⊛ ❄
Fees: £26–35; Second visit: £21–30
Berkhamsted HP4
01442 878900

**Tim Hanwell GOsC**
⊕ ⊛ ❄
Fees: £26–35; Second visit: £21–30
Berkhamsted HP4
01442 878900

**Christian Scharsach GOsC**
O ⊛ ❄
Fees: £26–35; Second visit: £21–30
Berkhamsted HP4
01442 871551

**Vicki Aldridge GOsC**
⊕ ⊛ Ⓔ ❄
Fees: £26–35; Second visit: £21–30
Bishop's Stortford CM23
01279 464504

**Kamila Jakubowska-Barry GOsC, BOA**
⊕ ⊕ ⊛ ❄
Fees: £36–45; Second visit: £21–30
Bishop's Stortford CM23
01279 655052

**Helen Neary GOsC, BOA**
⊕ ⊕ ⊛ ❄
Fees: £36–45; Second visit: £21–30
Bishop's Stortford CM23
01279 655052

**Hazel Williams GOsC, BOA**
⊕ O ⊕ ⊕ ⊛ ❄
Fees: £36–45; Second visit: £21–30
Bishop's Stortford CM23
01279 504787

**Kim Millhouse GOsC**
⊕ O ⊛ ❄
Fees: £26–35; Second visit: £21–30
Broxbourne EN10
01992 443026

**Karen Prince GOsC**
⊕ ⊕ ⊛ ❄
Fees: £26–35; Second visit: £21–30
Buntingford SG9
01763 274760

**Michael Morton GOsC, BOA**
⊕ ⊛ Ⓔ ❄
Fees: £26–35; Second visit: £21–30
Bushey WD23
020 8950 8886

**Marc Czerwinski GOsC, BOA**
⊕ ⊛ ❄
Fees: £26–35; Second visit: £21–30
Cheshunt EN8
01992 634105

**Christophe Becquereau GOsC, BOA**
⊕ ⊕ ⊛ ⊘ ❄
Fees: <£25; Second visit: £21–30
Harpenden AL5
01582 765900

**Peter Colvin GOsC, BOA**
⊕ ⊕ ⊛ ⊘
Fees: £36–45; Second visit: £21–30
Harpenden AL5
01582 713648

**Christopher Eke GOsC, BOA**
⊕ ⊛ ⊘ ❄
Fees: £26–35; Second visit: £21–30
Harpenden AL5
07973 882387

**Catherine Hamilton-Plant GOsC, BOA**
⊕ ⊕ ⊛ ⊘
Fees: <£25; Second visit: £21–30
Harpenden AL5
01582 713648

**Mackenzie Lacey GOsC, BOA**
⊕ ⊕ ⊛ ⊘ ❄
Fees: £26–35; Second visit: £21–30
Harpenden AL5
01582 765900

**Kenneth McLean GOsC, BOA**
⊕ O ⊛
Fees: £26–35; Second visit: £21–30
Hatfield AL10
01707 274148

**Ian Norman GOsC**
⊕ ⊕ ⊕ ⊛ ⊘ ❄
Fees: <£25
Hatfield AL10
01707 888229

**Caroline Penn GOsC**
Fees: <£25; Second visit: £21–30
Hatfield AL10
01707 274148

**Nikki Walker GOsC, BOA**
Fees: <£25; Second visit: £21–30
Hatfield AL9
01707 664321

**Sharon Winkler GOsC, BOA**
Fees: <£25; Second visit: £21–30
Hatfield AL10
01707 274148

**Amanda Evans GOsC**
Fees: <£25; Second visit: £21–30
Hemel Hempstead HP3
01442 236227

**Brian Lewis GOsC**
Fees: £36–45; Second visit: £21–30
Hemel Hempstead HP2
01442 211223

**Samantha Sullivan GOsC, BOA**
Fees: £26–35; Second visit: £21–30
Hemel Hempstead HP2
01442 236939

**Christopher Sullivan GOsC**
Fees: £26–35; Second visit: £21–30
Hemel Hempstead HP2
01442 236939

**Julia Buckwald GOsC**
Fees: £36–45; Second visit: £31–40
Henfield WD3
020 8449 9996

**Joanna Walsh GOsC, BOA**
Fees: <£25; Second visit: £21–30
Hertford SG14
01992 516704

**Mathew Cousins GOsC, BOA**
Fees: <£25; Second visit: £31–40
Hitchin SG5
01462 713031

**Ahmed El-Sayed GOsC, BOA**
Fees: £26–35; Second visit: £21–30
Hitchin SG5
01462 452929

**Tiffany Kirby GOsC, BOA**
Fees: <£25; Second visit: £21–30
Hitchin SG5
01462 436881

**Linda Premadasa GOsC, BOA**
Fees: £26–35; Second visit: £21–30
Hitchin SG5
01462 452929

**Paul Culverhouse GOsC, BOA**
Fees: <£25; Second visit: £21–30
Hoddesdon EN11
01992 460669

**Paul Summers GOsC**
Fees: £26–35; Second visit: £21–30
Kings Langley WD4
01923 260535

**Cindy McIntyre GOsC**
Fees: £26–35; Second visit: £21–30
Letchworth SG6
01462 674438

**Elaine Everitt GOsC, BOA**
Fees: <£25; Second visit: £41–50
Potters Bar EN6
01707 661411

**Barry L Jacobs GOsC, BOA**
Fees: <£25; Second visit: £21–30
Radlett WD7
01923 855884

# Osteopathy

### Clare Richmond GOsC, BOA
⊕ ⓝ ⓢ
**Fees:** £36–45; Second visit: £21–30
Radlett WD7
01923 855884

### Philip Aarons GOsC
⊕ ⓐ ⊘ ⓢ ⓛ
Rickmansworth WD3
01923 896655

### Charles Bennett GOsC, BOA
⊕ ⓝ ⓢ
**Fees:** £36–45; Second visit: £21–30
Rickmansworth WD3
01923 773337

### Natalie Cartwright-Adams GOsC, BOA
⊕ ⓝ ⊘ ⓢ
**Fees:** <£25; Second visit: £21–30
Rickmansworth WD3
01923 712171

### Tsenka Mack GOsC
○ ⓝ ⓢ
**Fees:** £36–45; Second visit: £31–40
Rickmansworth WD3
01923 493517

### Ian Collinge GOsC, BOA
⊕ ○ ⓐ ⓝ ⊘
**Fees:** <£25; Second visit: £21–30
Royston SG8
01763 246782

### Neil Mellerick GOsC
⊕ ⓝ ⓢ
**Fees:** <£25; Second visit: £21–30
Sawbridgeworth CM21
01279 723790

### Meraz Ahmed GOsC, BOA
⊕ ⓐ ⓝ ⓢ
**Fees:** <£25; Second visit: £21–30
St Albans AL1
01727 857704

### Emma Bailey GOsC
⊕ ⓝ ⓒ ⓢ
**Fees:** £36–45; Second visit: £21–30
St Albans AL1
01727 834038

### Nicholas Coe GOsC, BOA
⊕ ⓝ ⊘ ⓢ
**Fees:** £26–35; Second visit: £31–40
St Albans AL3
01727 832359

### Trevor Cox GOsC, BOA
⊕ ⓐ ⓜ ⊘ ⓢ
**Fees:** <£25; Second visit: £31–40
St Albans AL4
01582 834004

### Karine Joelle Leostic GOsC, BOA
⊕ ⓝ ⊘ ⓢ
**Fees:** <£25; Second visit: £21–30
St Albans AL1
020 8208 8147

### Claire Merriweather GOsC, BOA
⊕ ⓝ ⊘
**Fees:** £36–45; Second visit: £21–30
St Albans AL1
01727 834038

### Caroline Quigley GOsC, BOA
⊕ ○ ⓝ ⊘ ⓢ
**Fees:** <£25; Second visit: £21–30
St Albans AL3
01727 840682

### Mark Rush GOsC, BOA
⊕ ⓝ ⊘ ⓢ
**Fees:** £36–45; Second visit: £21–30
St Albans AL1
01727 834038

### Mark Thompson GOsC
⊕ ⓝ ⓢ
**Fees:** £46–55; Second visit: £41–50
St Albans AL4
01727 838032

### Matthew Tant GOsC
⊕ ⊕ ⓒ ⓢ
**Fees:** £26–35; Second visit: £31–40
St Albans AL5
01582 622000

### Vincent Cullen GOsC
ⓝ
**Fees:** £26–35; Second visit: £21–30
Stevenage SG1
01438 242652

**Hannah-Jane Setchell GOsC, BOA**
✛ ⊕ 🔵 ⊘ ❀
Fees: <£25; Second visit: £21–30
Stevenage SG1
01438 351400

**Graham Gard GOsC**
✛ 🔵 Ⓔ ❀
Fees: £26–35; Second visit: £21–30
Ware SG12
01920 465345

**Jane Honeyman GOsC, BOA**
✛ ⊕
Fees: £36–45; Second visit: £21–30
Ware SG12
01920 885010

**K Goddard GOsC, BOA**
✛ ⊕ ⊕ 🔵 ❀
Fees: <£25; Second visit: £21–30
Watford WD1
01923 241188

**Elizabeth Huzzey GOsC**
✛ 🔵
Fees: <£25; Second visit: £21–30
Watford WD17
01923 241188

**Martin Tunmore GOsC, BOA**
✛ ⊕ ⊕ 🔵 ⊘ ❀
Fees: £26–35; Second visit: £21–30
Watford WD18
01923 221303

**Stephen Perry GOsC, BOA**
✛ 🔵 ⊘ ❀
Fees: <£25; Second visit: £31–40
Welwyn Garden City AL8
01707 334902

## ISLE OF WIGHT

**Peter Gillett GOsC**
✛ 🔵
Fees: £36–45; Second visit: £21–30
Newport PO30
01983 822313

**Stephen Milton GOsC**
❀
Fees: £26–35; Second visit: £21–30
Newport PO30
01983 528149

**Clare Noiret GOsC**
O 🔵
Fees: £26–35; Second visit: £21–30
Newport PO30
01983 740678

**Simon Poulter GOsC**
✛ 🔵 ❀
Fees: £26–35; Second visit: £21–30
Newport PO30
01983 855203

**Nicholas Saunders GOsC, BOA**
O 🔵 ⊘ ❀
Fees: £26–35; Second visit: £21–30
Newport PO30
01983 721442

**David Barton GOsC, BOA**
✛ ⊕ ⊘ Ⓔ ❀
Fees: £26–35; Second visit: £21–30
Ryde PO33
01983 614777

**Brian G Howard GOsC, BOA**
✛ ⊕ 🔵 Ⓔ ❀
Fees: £26–35; Second visit: £21–30
Sandown PO36
01983 408833

## KENT

**Andrew Greig GOsC, BOA**
✛ O ⊕ 🔵 Ⓔ ❀
Fees: <£25; Second visit: £21–30
Ashford TN26
01233 860153

**Desmond Henley GOsC**
✛ ⊕ 🔵 Ⓔ ❀
Fees: <£25; Second visit: £21–30
Ashford TN24
01233 660882

**Mark Hutchin GOsC**
✛ 🔵
Fees: £26–35; Second visit: <£20
Ashford TN26
01233 820008

**Alison Ley GOsC**
✛ ⊕ 🔵 ⊘
Fees: <£25; Second visit: £21–30
Canterbury CT1
01227 451317

# Osteopathy

**Caroline Turck GOsC**
⊕ ⊕ ⊕ ⊘ ⊛
**Fees:** <£25; Second visit: £21–30
Ashford TN27
01622 892266

**Zara Van-Herbert GOsC**
⊕ ⊕ ⊛
**Fees:** <£25; Second visit: £21–30
Ashford TN23
01233 662929

**P Austin GOsC, BOA**
⊕ ⊕ ⊘ ⊛
**Fees:** <£25; Second visit: £21–30
Aylesford ME20
01622 718084

**Paul Gould GOsC**
⊕ ⊕ ⊕ ⊘ ⊛
**Fees:** £26–35; Second visit: £21–30
Aylesford ME20
01622 710536

**Caryn Lewis GOsC**
⊕ O ⊕ ⊛
**Fees:** £26–35; Second visit: £21–30
Aylesford ME20
01732 844441

**A Kennett-Brown GOsC**
⊕ O ⊕ ⊕ ©
**Fees:** <£25; Second visit: £21–30
Beckenham BR3
020 8650 3414

**A Lebret GOsC**
⊕ O ⊛
**Fees:** <£25; Second visit: >£50
Beckenham BR3
020 8658 0404

**Christopher Leighton GOsC, BOA**
⊕ ⊕ ⊕ ⊛
**Fees:** £26–35; Second visit: £21–30
Bexleyheath DA6
020 8303 3726

**Bernard Kingston GOsC**
O ⊕
**Fees:** £26–35; Second visit: £21–30
Biddenden TN27
01580 292744

**Sharon Dempster GOsC, BOA**
⊕ ⊕ ⊕ ⊛
**Fees:** <£25; Second visit: £21–30
Bromley BR1,Southend SS1
020 8467 4451

**Andreas Jochim GOsC, BOA**
O ⊕ ⊕ ⊘ ⊛
**Fees:** £26–35; Second visit: £21–30
Bromley BR2
020 8650 0509

**B Judge GOsC**
O ⊕ ⊛
**Fees:** £26–35; Second visit: £21–30
Bromley BR1
020 8464 1129

**D Frances Lumley GOsC, BOA**
⊕ O ⊕ ⊛
**Fees:** <£25; Second visit: £21–30
Bromley BR2
020 8462 8027

**Tanya Newman GOsC, BOA**
⊕ O ⊕ ⊕ ⊕ © ⊛
**Fees:** <£25; Second visit: £21–30
Bromley BR1
020 8460 1646

**Tom Greenfield GOsC, BOA**
⊕ ⊕ ⊕ ⊛
**Fees:** <£25; Second visit: £21–30
Canterbury CT1
01227 454848

**K Sean McLean GOsC, BOA**
⊕ O ⊕ ⊕ ⊕ ⊛
**Fees:** £26–35; Second visit: £21–30
Canterbury CT3
01227 860573

**Allison Roberts GOsC, BOA**
⊕ ⊕
**Fees:** <£25; Second visit: £21–30
Canterbury CT1
01227 462152

**Stephen Smith GOsC, BOA**
⊕ ⊕ ⊛
**Fees:** £26–35; Second visit: £21–30
Canterbury CT2
01227 458430

**Jonathan Davies GOsC**
Fees: £26–35; Second visit: £21–30
Charing TN27
01233 714700

**Jean Hopkins GOsC**
Fees: <£25; Second visit: £21–30
Chatham ME5
01634 681138

**Graham Mason GOsC**
Fees: <£25; Second visit: £21–30
Chatham ME4
01634 842583

**Philip A Williamson GOsC, BOA**
Fees: £26–35; Second visit: £31–40
Cranbrook TN18
01580 753526

**Nigel Herterich GOsC**
Fees: £26–35; Second visit: £21–30
Dartford DA1
01322 279248

**Ajit Patel GOsC, BOA**
Fees: £26–35; Second visit: £21–30
Sidcup DA14
020 8302 2624

**Stephen Comfort GOsC, BOA**
Fees: £26–35; Second visit: £31–40
Deal CT14
01304 375658

**Susan Fairley GOsC, BOA**
Fees: £46–55; Second visit: £21–30
Deal CT14
01304 364879

**Pauline Morgan GOsC**
Fees: <£25; Second visit: £21–30
Dover CT16
01304 202352

**Paul Strutt GOsC**
Fees: £26–35; Second visit: £21–30
Dover CT16
01304 214686

**Robert McCoy GOsC, BOA**
Fees: £26–35; Second visit: £21–30
Edenbridge TN8
01732 865444

**Susan M Smith GOsC, BOA**
Fees: <£25; Second visit: £21–30
Faversham ME13
01795 537832

**Julian Drion GOsC**
Fees: £36–45; Second visit: £31–40
Folkestone CT20
01303 850077

**Thomas Drion GOsC, BOA**
Fees: £36–45; Second visit: £31–40
Folkestone CT20
01303 850077

**Peter George Smith GOsC**
Fees: <£25; Second visit: £21–30
Folkestone CT19
01303 278188

**Lucinda Bensted GOsC, BOA**
Fees: <£25; Second visit: £21–30
Gillingham ME7
01634 850500

**Emma Crosby GOsC, BOA**
Fees: <£25; Second visit: £21–30
Gillingham ME7
01634 281388

**Jon H Leigh GOsC, BOA**
Fees: <£25; Second visit: £21–30
Gillingham ME7
01634 576292

# Osteopathy

**Brian Wren GOsC**
⊕ ⊕ ⊛ ❈
**Fees:** £26–35; Second visit: £21–30
Headcorn TN27
01622 890803

**Jonathan Davies GOsC**
⊕ ⊕ ⊘ ❈
**Fees:** £26–35; Second visit: £21–30
Herne Bay CT6
01227 370067

**Jennifer Couling GOsC, BOA**
O ⊕ ⊛ ❈
**Fees:** £26–35; Second visit: £21–30
Hextable BR8
01322 665166

**Jean Draisey GOsC**
⊕ ⊛
**Fees:** £26–35; Second visit: £21–30
Hildenborough TN11
01732 832713

**Deborah Doole GOsC, BOA**
⊕ ⊛ ❈
**Fees:** £26–35; Second visit: £21–30
Maidstone ME18
01622 618637

**Bruce M Leiper GOsC**
⊕ ⊕ ⊛ Ⓔ ❈
**Fees:** £26–35; Second visit: £21–30
Maidstone ME14
01622 735568

**Annette Pantall GOsC**
⊕ ⊕ ⊛ ❈
**Fees:** <£25; Second visit: £21–30
Maidstone ME16
01622 674656

**Shireen Sherif GOsC**
⊕ O ⊛ Ⓔ ❈
**Fees:** £26–35; Second visit: £21–30
Maidstone ME14
01622 679990

**Kathryn Arnold GOsC, BOA**
⊕ ⊛ ⊘ ❈
**Fees:** £26–35; Second visit: £21–30
Margate CT9
01843 295863

**Matthew Green GOsC, BOA**
⊕ ⊕ ⊛ ❈
**Fees:** <£25; Second visit: £21–30
Margate CT9
01843 292056

**Gayle Shearer GOsC, BOA**
⊕ ⊕ ⊛ Ⓔ
**Fees:** £26–35; Second visit: £21–30
Margate CT9
01843 292056

**Kerry Willgoss GOsC**
⊕ O ⊕ ⊕ ❈
**Fees:** £26–35; Second visit: <£20
Margate CT9
01843 292056

**Anne Leigh GOsC**
⊕ ⊛ ⊘ Ⓔ
**Fees:** £26–35; Second visit: £21–30
Medway ME7
01634 576292

**Kate Miles GOsC, BOA**
⊕ ⊛ ❈
**Fees:** £26–35; Second visit: £21–30
New Romney TN28
01797 361111

**Jonathan Daniells GOsC, BOA**
⊕ ⊕ ⊛ ⊘ ❈
**Fees:** £26–35; Second visit: £21–30
Orpington BR6
01689 877500

**Robert Burge GOsC, BOA**
O ⊛ ⊘ ❈
**Fees:** <£25; Second visit: <£20
Rochester ME2
01634 710051

**Mark Smith GOsC**
⊕ ⊛ ❈
**Fees:** <£25; Second visit: £21–30
Rochester ME1
01634 880202

**E M Baker GOsC, BOA**
⊕ O ⊕ ⊕ ⊛ ❈
**Fees:** <£25; Second visit: £21–30
Sandwich CT13
01304 620061

### Piers Chandler GOsC
**O** ⊕ ⓜ Ⓞ Ⓔ ✿
**Fees:** £26–35; Second visit: £21–30
Sevenoaks TN13
01732 452886

### Daniel Graham GOsC
**O** ⊕ ⓜ ✿
**Fees:** £26–35; Second visit: £21–30
Sevenoaks TN13
01732 452886

### Jacqueline Hayes GOsC, BOA
⊕ **O** ⊕ ⓜ ✿
**Fees:** <£25; Second visit: £21–30
Sevenoaks TN14
01959 532714

### Jonathan Hoggard GOsC, BOA
**O** ⓜ Ⓞ ✿
**Fees:** £26–35; Second visit: £21–30
Sevenoaks TN13
01732 842091

### Jill Mew GOsC, BOA
⊕ ⓜ
**Fees:** <£25; Second visit: £21–30
Sevenoaks TN13
01732 450979

### Mark Pitcairn-Knowles GOsC
⊕ ⊕ ⓜ Ⓔ ✿
**Fees:** £26–35; Second visit: £21–30
Sevenoaks TN13
01732 453956

### Christakis Georgiou GOsC
⊕ ✿
**Fees:** <£25; Second visit: <£20
Sittingbourne ME10
01795 428817

### Andrew Hills GOsC
⊕ ⓜ ✿
**Fees:** <£25; Second visit: <£20
Sittingbourne ME10
01795 477264

### Rossana de Sousa GOsC
⊕ ⓜ
**Fees:** <£25; Second visit: <£20
Sittingbourne ME10
01795 477264

### Lindley Horner GOsC
⊕ ⓜ ✿
**Fees:** £26–35; Second visit: £21–30
Sutton at Hone DA4
01322 860544

### Daniel Savage GOsC
⊕ ⊕ ⓜ ✿
**Fees:** £26–35; Second visit: £21–30
Sutton at Hone DA4
01322 860544

### Graham Smith GOsC, BOA
ⓜ Ⓞ ✿
**Fees:** £26–35; Second visit: £21–30
Swanley BR8
01322 660923

### Lizzie Spring GOsC, BOA
⊕ ⊕ ⓜ
**Fees:** £26–35; Second visit: £21–30
Tenterden TN30
01580 766424

### Ivo Van Gils GOsC
⊕ ⊕ ✿
**Fees:** £26–35; Second visit: £21–30
Tenterden TN30
01622 201881

### J West GOsC
⊕ ⊕ ⓜ Ⓔ ✿
**Fees:** £26–35; Second visit: £21–30
Tenterden TN30
01580 764434

### Chris Bowman GOsC,
⊕ ⓜ Ⓞ ✿
**Fees:** £26–35; Second visit: £21–30
Tonbridge
01732 350255

### Maurice Hills GOsC
**O** ⓜ ✿
**Fees:** £26–35
Tonbridge TN2
01892 529730

### Margaret Hills GOsC
**O** ⓜ Ⓞ ✿
**Fees:** £26–35; Second visit: £21–30
Tonbridge TN2
01892 529730

# Osteopathy

**Christine Huggett GOsC**
➕ ➐
**Fees:** £26–35; Second visit: £21–30
Tonbridge TN1
01892 514112

**Louise James GOsC, BOA**
➕ ⭕ ❄
**Fees:** <£25; Second visit: £21–30
Tonbridge TN12
01622 873481

**Shirley Kay GOsC, BOA**
➕ 🅝 ❄
**Fees:** £26–35; Second visit: £21–30
Tonbridge TN4
01892 521134

**Stuart Korth GOsC, BOA**
➕ 🅝
**Fees:** >£55; Second visit: £41–50
Tonbridge TN4
01892 521134

**Randall Lederman GOsC, BOA**
➕ ❄
**Fees:** £26–35; Second visit: £21–30
Tonbridge TN1
01892 535858

**Judith McCreath GOsC, BOA**
➕ ➐ 🅝 ❄
**Fees:** £26–35; Second visit: £21–30
Tonbridge TN4
01892 543033

**Carolyn McGregor GOsC, BOA**
➕ 🅝 ⊘ ❄
**Fees:** £26–35; Second visit: £21–30
Tonbridge TN4
01892 521134

**Susan Morton GOsC, BOA**
➕ ⭕ 🅝 ❄
**Fees:** <£25; Second visit: £21–30
Tonbridge TN9
01732 783522

**Timothy Nelson GOsC**
❄
**Fees:** £26–35; Second visit: £21–30
Tonbridge TN12
01892 833914

**Hannelie (Yem) Nusselein GOsC, BOA**
➕ 🅝 ❄
**Fees:** <£25; Second visit: £21–30
Tonbridge TN11
01732 834713

**Susan Rayner GOsC**
➕ ⭕ 🅝 ❄
**Fees:** <£25; Second visit: £21–30
Tonbridge TN11
01732 850836

**Robert Thomas GOsC**
➕ ⭕ 🅝 ❄
**Fees:** <£25; Second visit: £21–30
Tonbridge TN11
01732 851016

**Geoffrey Montague-Smith GOsC, BOA**
➕ ⊕ ➐ 🅝 ⊘ ❄
**Fees:** £36–45; Second visit: £21–30
Tunbridge Wells TN1
01892 544783

**Helen Crook GOsC**
➕ ➐ 🅝 ❄
**Fees:** <£25; Second visit: £21–30
West Malling ME19
01732 873114

**Pierrick Morlet GOsC**
➕ 🅝 ❄
**Fees:** £36–45; Second visit: £21–30
Westerham TN16
01959 562111

**Daniel Brown GOsC, BOA**
➕ 🅝 ❄
**Fees:** £26–35; Second visit: £21–30
Whitstable CT5
01227 264044

**W Neil Wayman GOsC**
➕ 🅝 ⊘ ❄
**Fees:** <£25; Second visit: £31–40
Whitstable CT5
01227 264044

## MILTON KEYNES

**Elizabeth Walker GOsC, BOA**
➕ ⊕ ➐ 🅝 🄲
**Fees:** £26–35; Second visit: £21–30
Milton Keynes MK7
01908 604666

**Simon Petrides GOsC, BOA,**
Fees: <£25; Second visit: £31–40
Milton Keynes MK7
01908 604666

**Mark Booth GOsC, BOA**
Fees: <£25; Second visit: £21–30
Newport Pagnell MK16
01908 615045

**Fiona Cockings-Mason GOsC, BOA**
Fees: £26–35; Second visit: £21–30
Olney MK46
01234 711344

## NORTHAMPTONSHIRE

**Jo Clarkson GOsC**
Fees: £26–35; Second visit: £21–30
Kettering NN15,Oundle PE8
01536 512927

**Rachel Davies GOsC, BOA**
Fees: £26–35; Second visit: £21–30
Kettering NN16
01536 414567

**Jody Grace GOsC**
Fees: £26–35; Second visit: £21–30
Kettering NN15
01536 512927

**Jane Bellingham GOsC, BOA**
Fees: <£25; Second visit: £31–40
Northampton NN1
01604 632232

**Jillian Forsyth GOsC**
Fees: <£25; Second visit: £21–30
Northampton NN3
01604 714821

**Elizabeth Walker GOsC, BOA**
Fees: <£25; Second visit: £21–30
Northampton NN1
01604 632232

**Edward Triance GOsC**
Fees: £26–35; Second visit: £21–30
Rushden NN10
01933 355230

**Robert McGregor GOsC**
Fees: £26–35; Second visit: £21–30
Wellingborough NN8
01933 278391

## OXFORDSHIRE

**Michael Davis GOsC, BOA**
Fees: £26–35; Second visit: £21–30
Abingdon OX14,Newbury RG14
01235 531021

**Natalie Shinh GOsC**
Fees: £26–35; Second visit: £21–30
Abingdon OX14
01235 531021

**Philippa Rayne GOsC**
Fees: <£25; Second visit: £21–30
Bampton OX18
01993 851359

**Robert Marriott GOsC, BOA**
Fees: £26–35; Second visit: £21–30
Banbury OX16
01295 272903

**H Wells GOsC, BOA**
Fees: <£25; Second visit: £41–50
Banbury OX16
01295 265267

**Angela Stevenson GOsC, BOA**
Fees: £26–35; Second visit: £21–30
Carterton OX18
01993 843466

**Susan Chambers GOsC, BOA**
Fees: <£25; Second visit: £21–30
Henley-on-Thames RG9
01491 641610

# Osteopathy

### Kim Rolshoven GOsC, BOA
✛ ⓝⓗⓢ Ⓔ ❋
**Fees:** £36–45; Second visit: £21–30
Henley-on-Thames RG9
01491 641610

### John Leaman GOsC
✛ ⓝⓗⓢ ❋
**Fees:** £26–35
Kidlington OX5
01865 378808

### Clive Power GOsC
Ⓞ ⓝⓗⓢ ❋
**Fees:** £26–35; Second visit: £21–30
Minster Lovell OX29
01993 776225

### Tom Bedford GOsC
✛ ⊕ ⓝⓗⓢ Ⓔ ❋
**Fees:** £26–35; Second visit: £31–40
Oxford OX4
01865 200678

### Duncan Cameron-Mitchell GOsC
✛ ⓝⓗⓢ ⊘
**Fees:** £36–45; Second visit: £21–30
Oxford OX2
01865 558561

### Kelston Chorley GOsC, BOA
✛ ⊕ ⓝⓗⓢ Ⓔ ❋
**Fees:** £36–45; Second visit: £31–40
Oxford OX4
01865 790235

### Rukmani Day GOsC
Ⓞ ⓝⓗⓢ ❋
**Fees:** £26–35; Second visit: £21–30
Oxford OX17
01295 768488

### Jorge Esteves GOsC, BOA
✛ ⊕ ⓝⓗⓢ ⊘ Ⓔ ❋
**Fees:** £26–35; Second visit: £21–30
Oxford OX3
01865 484157-8

### Richard Ferguson GOsC, BOA
Ⓞ Ⓔ
**Fees:** £26–35; Second visit: £21–30
Oxford OX1
01865 791274

### Rodney Hobbs GOsC, BOA
✛ ⓝⓗⓢ Ⓔ ❋
**Fees:** £26–35; Second visit: £21–30
Oxford OX15
01869 338078

### Clive Lindley-Jones GOsC, BOA
✛ ⓝⓗⓢ Ⓔ ❋
**Fees:** >£55; Second visit: £31–40
Oxford OX4
01885 243351

### Nina Manston GOsC
Ⓞ ⊕ ⓝⓗⓢ ⊘ Ⓔ ❋
**Fees:** £36–45; Second visit: £31–40
Oxford OX33
01865 875854

### John O'Brien GOsC
✛ ⓝⓗⓢ ⓖⓞⓢⓟ
**Fees:** <£25; Second visit: £21–30
Oxford OX2
01865 556954

### David Ruddick GOsC
✛ ⓝⓗⓢ
**Fees:** £36–45; Second visit: £31–40
Oxford OX2
01865 558561

### Oonagh Ruddick GOsC, BOA
✛ ⊕ ⓝⓗⓢ
**Fees:** £36–45; Second visit: £31–40
Oxford OX2
01865 558561

### Lisa Thomas GOsC
✛ ⓝⓗⓢ ⊘ ❋
**Fees:** <£25; Second visit: £21–30
Oxford OX2
01865 556954

### Kieren Spencer GOsC, BOA
✛ ⊕ ⓝⓗⓢ ⊘ Ⓔ ❋
**Fees:** £36–45; Second visit: £21–30
Thame OX9
01844 215555

### Rohan Iswariah GOsC
✛ Ⓞ ⊕ ⓝⓗⓢ ❋
**Fees:** £36–45; Second visit: £31–40
Wallingford OX10
01491 838866

**Gitte Pedersen GOsC**
⊕ O ⊕ ⊕ € ❀
Fees: £26–35; Second visit: £31–40
Wallingford OX10
01491 824724

**Caroline Abrams GOsC**
⊕ ⊕ ⊕ ⊘ € ❀
Fees: £26–35; Second visit: £21–30
Wantage OX12
01235 760079

**Katherine Jane Harris GOsC, BOA**
⊕ ⊕ ❀
Fees: £26–35; Second visit: £21–30
Wantage OX12
01235 768748

## SURREY

**Donna Fox GOsC, BOA**
⊕ ⊕ ⊕ € ❀
Fees: £36–45; Second visit: £21–30
Addlestone KT15
01932 351120

**Maria Buckley-Garnham GOsC**
⊕ ⊕ ⊕ € ❀
Fees: £26–35; Second visit: £21–30
Ashford TW15
01784 255535

**Ivan Christiny GOsC**
⊕ ⊕ ⊕ ❀
Fees: £26–35; Second visit: £21–30
Ashtead KT21
01372 277311

**Lisa Eicke GOsC, BOA**
⊕ ⊕ ⊕
Fees: £26–35; Second visit: £21–30
Ashtead KT21
01372 277311

**Helen Stevens GOsC**
⊕ ⊕ ⊕ ❀
Fees: £26–35; Second visit: £21–30
Banstead SM7
01737 373684

**Lise Court GOsC, BOA**
⊕ ⊘ ❀
Fees: <£25
Betchworth RH3
01737 843516

**Katharine Benstead GOsC, BOA**
⊕ ⊕ ⊕ € ❀
Fees: £26–35; Second visit: £21–30
Camberley GU17
01276 36475

**Stephen Green GOsC**
⊕ ⊕ ❀
Fees: <£25; Second visit: £21–30
Camberley GU15
01276 20411

**Helen Robinson GOsC**
⊕ ⊕ ❀
Fees: £26–35; Second visit: £21–30
Camberley GU15
01276 20411

**Alex Watson GOsC, BOA**
O € ❀
Fees: £36–45; Second visit: £21–30
Camberley GU16
01276 708954

**Suzanne Jackson GOsC**
⊕ ⊕ ❀
Fees: £26–35; Second visit: £21–30
Caterham-on-the Hill CR3
01883 344301

**Gary Riley GOsC**
⊕ ⊕ ❀
Fees: £26–35; Second visit: £21–30
Caterham-on-the Hill CR3
01883 344301

**John Bayliss GOsC**
O ⊕ ⊕ ❀
Fees: £26–35; Second visit: £21–30
Chessington KT9
020 8397 3802

**Richard Mays GOsC**
⊕ ⊕ ❀
Fees: £26–35; Second visit: £21–30
Chessington KT9
020 8397 8629

**Matthew Davies GOsC, BOA**
⊕ ⊕ ⊘
Fees: £26–35; Second visit: £31–40
Cobham KT11
01932 866852

# Osteopathy

**David Reynolds GOsC**
⊕ ⊕ ⊘ ❀
**Fees:** £26–35; Second visit: £31–40
Cranleigh GU6
01483 275500

**Annabelle Mundy GOsC, BOA**
⊕ ⛎ ❀
**Fees:** <£25; Second visit: £21–30
Croyden CR2
020 8651 3315

**Raymond Hallam GOsC**
◐ ⛎ ❀
**Fees:** £26–35; Second visit: £21–30
Dorking RH4,Newport NP9
01306 884097

**Liz Simons GOsC**
⊕ ⛎ ❀
**Fees:** <£25; Second visit: £31–40
Dorking RH4
01306 741152

**Samantha Taylor GOsC, BOA**
⊕ ⊕ ⛎ ❀
**Fees:** £26–35; Second visit: £21–30
Dorking RH4
01306 741152

**Joanna Wyatt GOsC**
❀
Dorking RH4
01306 881249

**Martine Faure-Alderson GOsC, BOA**
⊕ ◐ ⊕ ⛎ ⊘ ❀
**Fees:** £36–45
East Molesey KT8
020 8398 6943

**Sophie Dhenin GOsC, BOA**
⊕ ◐ ⊕ ⛎ ⊘ ❀
**Fees:** <£25; Second visit: £31–40
Egham TW20
01784 433973

**Jonathan Eyres GOsC, BOA**
⊕ ◐ ⊕ ⊕ ⛎ ❀
Egham TW20
01784 433973

**Helena Greenwood GOsC, BOA**
⊕ ◐ ⊕ ⊕ ⛎ ❀
**Fees:** <£25; Second visit: £21–30
Egham TW20
01784 437219

**Janice Moss GOsC, BOA**
⊕ ⛎ ⊘ ❀
**Fees:** £36–45; Second visit: £21–30
Egham TW20
01784 220990

**Morag Christie GOsC**
⊕ ◐ ⊕ ⛎ ❀
**Fees:** £26–35; Second visit: £21–30
Epsom KT17
01372 803604

**Mark Dare GOsC, BOA**
⊕ ⛎ ❀
**Fees:** <£25; Second visit: £21–30
Epsom KT18
01737 353660

**R Ganpatsingh GOsC, BOA**
⊕ ⊕ ⛎ ❀
**Fees:** <£25; Second visit: £21–30
Epsom KT17
020 8393 3038

**David Owen Jenkins GOsC, BOA**
⊕ ◐ ⛎
**Fees:** £26–35; Second visit: £21–30
Epsom KT17
01372 726080

**R Katesmark GOsC**
⊕ ⊕ ⛎ ⊘ ❀
**Fees:** £36–45; Second visit: £31–40
Epsom KT17
020 8393 3038

**Carolynn Milton GOsC, BOA**
⊕ ⊕ ⛎ ❀
**Fees:** <£25; Second visit: £21–30
Epsom KT18
01737 353660

**Simeon Milton GOsC**
⊕ ⊕ ⛎ ⊘ ❀
**Fees:** <£25; Second visit: £21–30
Epsom KT18
01737 353660

# Osteopathy

**Jane Pettifer GOsC, BOA**
O 🔵 🔷
Fees: <£25; Second visit: £21–30
Epsom KT19
020 8393 2050

**Nigel Gates Stevens GOsC, BOA**
O 🔷
Fees: £26–35; Second visit: £21–30
Epsom KT17
020 8393 9736

**Simon Tang GOsC, BOA**
O 🔵 🔷
Fees: £26–35; Second visit: £21–30
Epsom KT19
01372 728533

**Fiona Hendry GOsC, BOA**
🔵 O 🔵 ⊘ 🔷
Fees: <£25; Second visit: £31–40
Esher KT10
01372 460738

**Anna-Maria Peacock GOsC**
🔵 O 🔵 🔷
Fees: £26–35; Second visit: £21–30
Ewell KT19
020 8393 1477

**Taylor Desmond GOsC, BOA**
O 🔵 ⊘ 🔷
Fees: £26–35; Second visit: £21–30
Farnham GU9
01252 714514

**Saffron Ray GOsC, BOA**
🔵 🔵 © 🔷
Fees: £26–35; Second visit: £21–30
Farnham GU10
01252 672265

**Clare Badrick GOsC**
🔵 🔵
Fees: £36–45; Second visit: £31–40
Godalming GU7
01483 418103

**Kharis Fausset GOsC, BOA**
🔵 🔵
Fees: £26–35; Second visit: £21–30
Godalming GU7
01483 418103

**David Frankcom GOsC, BOA**
🔵 🔵 🔵 🔵 ⊘ 🔷
Fees: <£25; Second visit: £21–30
Guildford GU1
01483 576438

**Andrew Peters GOsC, BOA**
🔵 🔵 ⊘
Fees: £26–35; Second visit: £31–40
Guildford GU1
01483 570921

**Donna Watson GOsC**
🔵 🔵 🔵 🔵 ⊘ 🔷
Fees: £26–35; Second visit: £21–30
Guildford GU3
01483 594250

**Mark Arrindell GOsC**
🔵 🔵 🔷
Fees: <£25; Second visit: £21–30
Haslemere GU27
01428 651067

**Greg Barker GOsC**
🔵 🔵 🔷
Fees: £36–45; Second visit: £21–30
Haslemere GU27
01428 661933

**Martin Coleman GOsC**
🔵 🔷
Fees: £26–35; Second visit: £21–30
Haslemere GU27
01428 651067

**Kurt Jager GOsC**
🔵 🔵 ⊘ 🔷
Fees: >£55; Second visit: £21–30
Haslemere GU27
01428 651067

**Jager Kurt GOsC**
🔵 🔵 ⊘ 🔷
Fees: <£25; Second visit: £21–30
Haslemere GU27
01428 651067

**Elaine Seymour GOsC**
🔵 🔵 🔵 🔵 🔷
Fees: £36–45; Second visit: £31–40
Haslemere GU27
01428 661933

# Osteopathy

**Andrew Wilson-Smith GOsC**
⊕ 🌐 ❄
**Fees:** £26–35; Second visit: £21–30
Haslemere GU27
01428 651067

**Mario-Paul Cassar GOsC**
○ 🌐 ⊘ ❄
**Fees:** <£25; Second visit: £21–30
Horley RH6
01293 775467

**Jonathan D Cove GOsC, BOA**
⊕ ⊕ 🌐 🌐 ⊘ ⓔ ❄
**Fees:** £26–35; Second visit: £21–30
Horley RH6
01293 784200

**Timothy Payne GOsC, BOA**
⊕ ⊕ 🌐 🌐 ⊘ ❄
**Fees:** <£25; Second visit: <£20
Horley RH6
01293 784200

**Trevor Strutt GOsC, BOA**
⊕ 🌐 🌐 ❄
**Fees:** £26–35; Second visit: £21–30
Horley RH6
01342 842939

**Karim Boukhalfa GOsC**
⊕ ❄
**Fees:** £26–35; Second visit: £21–30
Kingston Upon Thames KT2
020 8546 8314

**Beate Guenther GOsC, BOA**
○ 🌐 ❄
**Fees:** £26–35; Second visit: £21–30
Kingston Upon Thames KT2
020 8541 5566

**Philippa Guildford GOsC, BOA**
⊕ 🌐 ❄
**Fees:** £26–35; Second visit: £21–30
Kingston Upon Thames KT2
020 8546 5995

**Carragh McAree GOsC, BOA**
⊕ ⊕ 🌐 ❄
**Fees:** £26–35; Second visit: £21–30
Kingston-on-Thames KT1
07957 348513

**Alison van der Molen GOsC**
⊕ ○ 🌐 🌐 ❄
**Fees:** £26–35; Second visit: £21–30
Kingston-on-Thames KT17
01737 359835

**Rebecca Morrison GOsC**
⊕ 🌐 ⊘ ⓔ ❄
**Fees:** £26–35; Second visit: £21–30
Kingston-on-Thames KT2
020 8546 5995

**Christina Hood GOsC, BOA**
⊕ 🌐 ❄
**Fees:** £26–35; Second visit: £21–30
Kingswood KT20,Odiham RG29
01737 355114

**Josephine Luard GOsC, BOA**
⊕ 🌐 🌐 ❄
**Fees:** £26–35; Second visit: £21–30
Kingswood KT20
01737 355114

**Matthew Wallden GOsC, BOA**
⊕ 🌐 🌐 ❄
**Fees:** £26–35; Second visit: £31–40
Leatherhead KT22
01372 374530

**Nick Woolley GOsC**
⊕ ○ 🌐 ❄
**Fees:** £26–35; Second visit: £21–30
Leatherhead KT18
01372 379270

**Elizabeth Brennan-Jesson GOsC**
⊕ ⊕ 🌐 🌐 ❄
**Fees:** £26–35; Second visit: £21–30
Lingfield RH7
01342 833844

**Sally Gardner GOsC, BOA**
⊕ ○ ❄
**Fees:** <£25; Second visit: £31–40
Oxted RH8
01883 723345

**Paul Moody GOsC**
⊕ 🌐 🌐 ❄
**Fees:** £26–35; Second visit: £21–30
Oxted RH8
01883 717277

# Osteopathy

**Andrew Bushe GOsC, BOA**
⊕ ⊕ 🌑 ❄
**Fees:** £26–35; Second visit: £21–30
Redhill RH1
01737 767070

**Nigel Kettle GOsC, BOA**
⊕ 🌑 ❄
**Fees:** £26–35; Second visit: £21–30
Redhill RH1
01737 760276

**Mark Piraino GOsC, BOA**
⊕ ⊕ ⊕ 🌑 ⊘ € ❄
**Fees:** £26–35; Second visit: £21–30
Redhill RH1
01737 766659

**Carole Smith GOsC**
⊕ O ⊕ 🌑 ❄
**Fees:** £26–35; Second visit: £21–30
Redhill RH1
01737 218251

**Amanda Begg GOsC, BOA**
⊕ ⊕ 🌑 ❄
**Fees:** <£25; Second visit: £21–30
Reigate RH2
01737 240791

**Lesley Griggs GOsC, BOA**
⊕ ⊕ 🌑 ❄
**Fees:** £26–35; Second visit: £21–30
Reigate RH2
01737 224488

**B Unwin Lambert GOsC**
⊕ O 🌑 ⊘
**Fees:** <£25; Second visit: £31–40
Reigate RH2
01737 245041

**Andrew James Olorenshaw GOsC**
⊕ 🌑
**Fees:** <£25; Second visit: £21–30
Reigate RH2
01737 245041

**Christopher Williams GOsC, BOA**
⊕ O ⊕ 🌑 ❄
**Fees:** <£25; Second visit: £21–30
Reigate RH2
01737 763626

**Robin Jackson GOsC, BOA**
⊕ 🌑 € ❄
**Fees:** £26–35; Second visit: £31–40
Richmond TW10
020 8943 0371

**David Millard GOsC**
⊕ ⊕ 🌑 ⊘ ❄
**Fees:** £26–35; Second visit: £21–30
Richmond TW9
020 8940 2336

**J N Walters GOsC, BOA,**
O 🌑 ⊘ ❄
**Fees:** <£25; Second visit: £31–40
Shepperton TW17
01932 231003

**Jane Griffith-Ward GOsC, BOA**
O ⊕ 🌑
**Fees:** £36–45; Second visit: £21–30
Staines TW18
01784 450042

**Sarah Boswall GOsC**
⊕ ⊕ 🌑 ❄
**Fees:** £26–35; Second visit: £21–30
Surbiton KT6
020 8399 2772

**Philip McNulty GOsC**
⊕ O ⊕ 🌑 ❄
**Fees:** £26–35; Second visit: £21–30
Sutton SM3
020 8644 8317

**Peter D Midgley GOsC, BOA**
⊕ 🌑
**Fees:** £26–35; Second visit: £21–30
Sutton SM1
020 8643 3990

**David John Midgley GOsC, BOA**
O 🌑 ❄
**Fees:** £26–35; Second visit: £21–30
Sutton SM1
020 8643 3990

**Katie Nunn GOsC**
⊕ ⊕ 🌑 ⊘ ❄
**Fees:** <£25; Second visit: £31–40
Sutton SM1
020 8643 0251

# Osteopathy

**Nadine Hobson GOsC, BOA**
✪ O ✛ ⊞ ⓝ ⊘
Fees: £26–35; Second visit: £31–40
Virginia Water GU25
01344 845444

**Christopher Mason GOsC, BOA**
✪ O ✛ ⊞ ⓝ ⊘ ✿
Fees: £26–35; Second visit: £21–30
Virginia Water GU25
01344 845801

**Tracy Lomax GOsC**
✪ ⓝ ⊘ ✿ ⊜
Fees: £36–45; Second visit: £21–30
Walton-on-Thames KT12
01932 227360

**Nicola Sammut GOsC, BOA**
O ⓝ ⊘
Fees: £26–35; Second visit: £21–30
Walton-on-Thames KT12
01932 245801

**Adrian Barnes GOsC**
O ⓝ ✿
Fees: £26–35; Second visit: £21–30
Weybridge KT13
01932 225288

**Deborah English GOsC**
O ⓝ ⊘ ✿
Fees: £26–35; Second visit: £21–30
Weybridge KT13
01932 820208

**Caroline Schofield GOsC**
O ⓝ ⓔ ✿
Fees: £26–35; Second visit: £21–30
Weybridge KT13
01932 852944

**Jane Wheeler GOsC, BOA**
✪ O ⓝ ✿
Fees: <£25; Second visit: £21–30
Weybridge KT13
01932 887111

**Michelle Henfrey GOsC, BOA**
✪ ⊞ ⓝ ✿
Fees: £36–45; Second visit: £21–30
Woking GU22
01483 769509

**Suzanne Hoddinott GOsC, BOA**
O ⊞ ⓝ ⊘ ✿
Fees: <£25; Second visit: £21–30
Woking GU22
01483 764582

**Laurens Holve GOsC, BOA**
✪ ⊞ ⓝ ✿
Fees: £36–45; Second visit: £21–30
Woking GU22
01483 720464

**Joanna Kolker GOsC, BOA**
O ⓝ ✿
Fees: £26–35; Second visit: £21–30
Woking GU22
01483 755597

**Ivan Lawler GOsC**
✪ ⓝ ✿
Fees: £36–45; Second visit: £21–30
Woking GU22
01483 770529

**Lisa Lindsay GOsC, BOA**
O ⓝ ✿
Fees: <£25; Second visit: £21–30
Woking GU21
01483 489501

**Andrea Rasmussen GOsC**
✪ ⓝ ✿
Fees: £26–35; Second visit: £21–30
Woking GU22
01483 768810

## SUSSEX

**Angela Gadd GOsC**
✪ ⊞ ⊘ ⊜
Fees: £26–35; Second visit: £21–30
Arundel BN18
01903 882200

**Jamie Taylor GOsC**
✪ ⓝ ⊘
Fees: <£25; Second visit: £21–30
Battle TN33
01424 772435

**Jitendra Vara GOsC**
✪ ⓝ ✿
Fees: £26–35; Second visit: £21–30
Brighton BN25
01323 892002

# Osteopathy

**Mark Andrews GOsC, BOA**
✛ ⊕ ⊕ ⊛ ✿
Fees: <£25; Second visit: £21–30
Brighton BN2
07973 404885

**Duncan Barrow GOsC, BOA**
✛ ⊕ ✿
Fees: <£25; Second visit: £21–30
Brighton BN2
01273 666426

**Maxine Brooks GOsC**
✛ O ⊕ ⊛ £ ✿
Fees: <£25; Second visit: £21–30
Brighton BN2
01273 699620

**Jasmina Cordal GOsC, BOA**
✛ ⊕ ⊛ ⊘ £ ✿
Fees: £26–35; Second visit: £21–30
Brighton BN1
01273 696295

**Sue Van Emden GOsC**
✛ ⊕ ⊛ ✿
Fees: £26–35; Second visit: £21–30
Brighton BN1
01273 550727

**Virginia Keefe GOsC, BOA**
✛ ⊕ ⊛ £ ✿
Fees: £26–35; Second visit: £21–30
Brighton BN1
01273 550727

**Nicholas Mitchell GOsC**
✛ ⊛ ✿
Fees: <£25; Second visit: £21–30
Brighton BN1
01273 566172

**Richard Pointon GOsC, BOA**
✛ ⊛
Fees: <£25; Second visit: £21–30
Brighton BN1
01273 326622

**Carl Surridge GOsC, BOA**
✛ ⊕ ⊛ £ ✿
Fees: £26–35; Second visit: £21–30
Brighton BN1
01273 324790

**Rick Webbe GOsC, BOA**
✛ ✿
Fees: £26–35; Second visit: £21–30
Brighton BN1
01273 273005

**Andrew Bellamy GOsC**
✛ ⊕ ⊛ ✿
Fees: £26–35; Second visit: £21–30
Brighton BN43
01273 464900

**John Laundon GOsC, BOA**
✛ ⊕ ⊛ ⊘ ✿
Fees: £26–35; Second visit: £21–30
Brighton BN15
01903 750770

**Michaela Kullack GOsC**
✛ ⊕ ⊛ £
Fees: £26–35; Second visit: £21–30
Brighton BN3
01273 324420

**Meta Pike GOsC**
O ⊕ ⊛ ✿
Fees: £26–35; Second visit: £21–30
Brighton BN3
01273 552425

**Nicholas Tuckley GOsC**
✛ ⊕ ⊛
Fees: £26–35; Second visit: £21–30
Brighton BN3
01273 326777

**Phillip Skates GOsC, BOA**
✛ ⊕ ⊛ ⊘
Fees: £26–35; Second visit: £21–30
Bognor Regis PO21
01243 870678

**Karen Smallcorn GOsC**
✛ ⊛ ⊘ ✿
Fees: £26–35; Second visit: £21–30
Bognor Regis PO21
01243 862832

**Lachlan Beveridge GOsC**
✛ O ✿
Fees: £26–35; Second visit: £21–30
Burgess Hill RH15
01444 870473

# Osteopathy

**Jonathan Horton GOsC, BOA**
❶ ⊕ ⊕ ⬤ ❋
Fees: £26–35; Second visit: £21–30
Chichester PO19
01243 786356

**Gayle Palmer GOsC, BOA**
❶ ❶ ⬤ ⊘ Ⓔ ❋
Fees: £26–35; Second visit: £21–30
Chichester PO20
01243 512522

**Elaine Sturgess GOsC, BOA**
❶ ⬤ Ⓔ ❋
Fees: £26–35; Second visit: £21–30
Chichester PO20
01243 545200

**John Tanner GOsC,**
❶ ⊕ ⊕ ⬤ ⊘ Ⓔ ❋
Fees: >£55; Second visit: >£50
Chichester PO20
01243 773167

**Sherilyn Bungay GOsC**
❶ ⬤ ❋
Fees: £26–35; Second visit: £21–30
Crawley RH10
01293 888600

**Suzanna Frisby GOsC**
❶ ⊕ ⬤ ❋
Fees: £26–35; Second visit: £21–30
Crawley RH10
01293 562601

**Leslie Jennings GOsC**
❶ ❶ ⬤ ❋
Fees: £26–35; Second visit: £21–30
Crawley RH10
01306 880446

**Marc Jones GOsC**
❶ ❋
Fees: £26–35; Second visit: £21–30
Crawley RH10
01342 712266

**S R Palmer GOsC, BOA**
❶ ⬤ Ⓔ ❋
Fees: <£25; Second visit: £31–40
Crawley RH10
01293 533082

**Jeffrey Richards GOsC**
❶ ⊕ ⬤ ❋
Fees: £26–35; Second visit: £21–30
Crawley RH10
01293 562601

**Karen Pelling GOsC**
❶ ⬤ ⊘ Ⓔ ❋
Fees: £26–35; Second visit: £21–30
Crawley Down RH10
01342 712764

**Paula Humphries GOsC**
❶ ⬤
Fees: £26–35; Second visit: £21–30
Crowborough TN6
01892 654605

**Sheelagh Pluckrose GOsC, BOA**
❶ ⬤ ❋
Fees: <£25; Second visit: £21–30
Crowborough TN6
01892 665291

**Nicolas Tanguy GOsC, BOA**
❶ ⊕ ⬤ ⊘ ❋
Fees: <£25; Second visit: £41–50
Crowborough TN6
01892 654978

**John Barkworth GOsC**
⊕ ⬤ ⊘
Fees: £26–35; Second visit: £21–30
Eastbourne BN21
01323 638606

**Philippa A Barnett GOsC, BOA**
❶ ⬤ ❋
Fees: <£25; Second visit: £21–30
Eastbourne BN21
01323 723887

**G J Cudlipp GOsC, BOA**
❶ ⬤ ❋
Fees: £26–35; Second visit: £21–30
Eastbourne BN20
01323 733539

**Elizabeth Davenport GOsC**
❶ ⊕ ⊕ ⬤ ⊘
Fees: £26–35; Second visit: £21–30
Eastbourne BN21
01323 638606

**Mark J Walsh GOsC**

Fees: <£25; Second visit: £31–40
Eastbourne BN21
01323 723887

**Tari Martin MacDonald GOsC**
Fees: £36–45; Second visit: £21–30
East Grinstead RH19
01342 324375

**Christopher Self GOsC**
Fees: £26–35; Second visit: £21–30
East Grinstead RH19
01342 410606

**Marina Urquhart-Pullen GOsC, BOA**
Fees: £26–35; Second visit: £21–30
East Grinstead RH19
01342 326708

**Sabine White GOsC**
Fees: £26–35; Second visit: £21–30
East Grinstead RH10
01342 712764

**Graham Ganson GOsC, BOA**
Fees: £26–35; Second visit: £21–30
Forest Row RH18
01342 823722

**Sasha Matthews GOsC, BOA**
Fees: £26–35; Second visit: £21–30
Forest Row RH18
01342 823722

**Carole Meredith GOsC**
Fees: £26–35; Second visit: £21–30
Hailsham BN27
01323 832395

**Nigel Bassett GOsC, BOA**
Fees: <£25; Second visit: £21–30
Hastings TN35,Rye TN31
01424 433991

**Miriam Eastaugh GOsC, BOA**
Fees: <£25; Second visit: £21–30
Hastings TN34
01424 719455

**June Leech GOsC, BOA**
Fees: <£25; Second visit: £21–30
Hastings TN34
01424 719455

**Paul Teale GOsC**
Fees: <£25; Second visit: <£20
Hastings TN34
01424 428754

**Paul Heeler GOsC, BOA**
Fees: £26–35; Second visit: £21–30
Hassocks BN6
01273 843780

**Susan Holliday GOsC, BOA**
Fees: £26–35; Second visit: £21–30
Hassocks BN6
01273 556823

**Jamie Parker-Smith GOsC**
Fees: £26–35; Second visit: £21–30
Hassocks BN6
01273 843780

**Emma Ross GOsC, BOA**
Fees: £26–35; Second visit: £21–30
Hassocks BN6
01273 843380

**Christian Bates GOsC**
Fees: £26–35; Second visit: £21–30
Haywards Heath RH16
01444 410944

**Julia Brooks GOsC**
Fees: £26–35; Second visit: £21–30
Haywards Heath RH17
01444 831576

# Osteopathy

**Amanda Jane Brown GOsC, BOA**
➕ 🆘 ∅ 🏀
**Fees:** <£25; Second visit: £21–30
Horsham RH12
01403 276272

**Nicholas Emens GOsC, BOA**
➕ 🅾 🈺 🏀
**Fees:** £26–35; Second visit: £21–30
Horsham RH12
01403 272144

**Tracy Gates GOsC, BOA**
➕ 🈺 🆘 🏀
**Fees:** £46–55; Second visit: £31–40
Horsham RH13
01403 734321

**Henry Lee GOsC**
➕ 🆘 🏀
**Fees:** £26–35; Second visit: £21–30
Horsham RH13
01306 742150

**Alexander Milne GOsC**
➕ 🈺 🆘 🏀
**Fees:** <£25; Second visit: £21–30
Horsham RH13
01403 272788

**Ian Pothecary GOsC,**
🅾 🆘 🏀
**Fees:** £26–35; Second visit: £21–30
Horsham RH12
01403 253146

**Christopher Wilson GOsC**
🅾 🆘 ∅ 🏀
**Fees:** £36–45; Second visit: £21–30
Horsham RH12
01403 252228

**Jonathan Hearsey GOsC**
➕ ➕ 🆘 🏀
**Fees:** £26–35; Second visit: £21–30
Hove BN3
01273 241949

**Clare Hearsey GOsC**
🅾 🈺 🆘 ∅ ⓔ 🏀
**Fees:** £26–35; Second visit: £21–30
Hove BN3
01273 241949

**Lisa Richter GOsC**
➕ 🈺 🆘 ⓔ 🏀
**Fees:** £36–45; Second visit: £21–30
Hove BN3
01273 770377

**Philip Russell GOsC, BOA**
➕ ➕ 🈺 🆘 ⓔ 🏀
**Fees:** £26–35; Second visit: £21–30
Hove BN3
01273 203820

**Sonia D Welbourne GOsC**
🅾 🆘 🏀
**Fees:** <£25; Second visit: £21–30
Hove BN3
01273 722518

**Rex Brangwyn & Associates GOsC**
➕ ➕ 🈺 🆘
**Fees:** <£25; Second visit: £21–30
Hove BN3
01273 775559

**Jeremy A Buck GOsC, BOA**
➕ ➕ 🈺 🆘 ∅ ⓔ 🏀
**Fees:** £26–35; Second visit: £21–30
Hove BN3
01273 203820

**Sara Pope GOsC, BOA**
🆘 ∅ 🏀
**Fees:** £36–45; Second visit: £31–40
Hove BN3
01273 208410

**Bee Musson GOsC**
➕ 🆘
**Fees:** £26–35; Second visit: £21–30
Lancing BN15
01903 761596

**Jonathan Curtis-Lake GOsC**
➕ 🈺 🆘 ∅
**Fees:** £36–45; Second visit: £21–30
Lewes BN7
01273 474428

**Simon Murray GOsC**
➕ 🈺 🆘
**Fees:** £26–35; Second visit: £21–30
Lewes BN7
01273 488547

**Lin Peters GOsC**
✚ 🅞 🅐 🅝 ✿
**Fees:** £26–35; Second visit: £21–30
Lewes BN7
01273 476371

**Nigel Jones GOsC**
✚ 🅐 🅝 ✿
**Fees:** <£25; Second visit: £21–30
Littlehampton BN17
01903 734373

**T W Peters GOsC, BOA,**
✚ 🅝 🅐 🅔
**Fees:** £26–35; Second visit: £21–30
Littlehampton BN17
01903 843600

**Ben Cull GOsC**
✚ 🅐 🅝 ✿
**Fees:** £26–35; Second visit: £21–30
Peacehaven BN10
01273 580370

**Michael J Wickham GOsC**
🅞 🅝 ✿
**Fees:** <£25; Second visit: £21–30
Peacehaven BN10
01273 585444

**Robert Sadler GOsC, BOA**
✚ 🅞 🅝 🅐 ✿
**Fees:** £26–35; Second visit: £21–30
Pulborough RH20
01798 874736

**Rachel Pointon GOsC, BOA**
✚ ⊕ 🅝 ✿
**Fees:** <£25; Second visit: £21–30
Shoreham-by-Sea BN43
01273 453594

**Simon Allison GOsC**
✚ 🅐 ✿
**Fees:** £26–35; Second visit: £31–40
Southwater RH13
01403 734321

**Matthew Bourne GOsC, BOA**
✚ 🅐 ✿
**Fees:** £26–35; Second visit: £21–30
Steyning BN44
01903 201447

**Geoff Green GOsC**
🅞 🅝 🅔 ✿
**Fees:** <£25; Second visit: £31–40
Steyning BN44
01903 812458

**Claire Piper GOsC, BOA**
✚ 🅐 🅝 🅐 🅔
**Fees:** <£25; Second visit: <£20
St Leonards-on-Sea TN37
01424 440898

**Diane P Chrismas GOsC**
🅞 🅝 🅐
**Fees:** <£25; Second visit: £21–30
Uckfield TN22
01825 733766

**Carl Humphries GOsC, BOA**
✚ 🅝 ✿
**Fees:** <£25; Second visit: £21–30
Uckfield TN22
01825 762657

**John Taberman-Pichler GOsC**
🅞 🅝 ✿
**Fees:** £26–35; Second visit: £21–30
Uckfield TN22
01825 760264

**Fred Taylor GOsC, BOA**
✚ 🅝 ✿
**Fees:** <£25; Second visit: £31–40
Uckfield SK7
01825 749474

**Timothy Fermor GOsC**
✚ ⊕ 🅐 🅝 ✿
**Fees:** £26–35; Second visit: £21–30
Wadhurst TN5
01892 784633

**Sacha Babbage-Clark GOsC, BOA**
🅞 🅝 ✿
**Fees:** <£25; Second visit: £21–30
Worthing BN11
01903 235018

**Alan D F Webb GOsC, BOA**
✚ ⊕ 🅐 🅝 ✿
**Fees:** <£25; Second visit: £21–30
Whitstable CT5
01227 264655

# Osteopathy

**Susan Bunce GOsC, BOA**
➕ ➕ 🆖 ✳
**Fees:** <£25; Second visit: £21–30
Worthing BN14,Hove BN3
01903 820206

**Christopher D Dyer GOsC, BOA**
➕ ➕ 🆖 ∅
**Fees:** <£25; Second visit: £21–30
Worthing BN11
01903 200748

**Michael Morris GOsC, BOA**
➕ ⊕ ➕ 🆖 ∅
**Fees:** £26–35; Second visit: £21–30
Worthing BN14
01903 820206

**Michael Tyrie GOsC, BOA**
➕ O 🆖 ∅
**Fees:** <£25; Second visit: £21–30
Worthing BN14
01903 235360

# Chiropractic

**Emma Roberts GCC, BAAC**
O 🆖 ✳
**Fees:** £26–35; Second visit: £21–30
Bracknell RG42
01344 482851

**Ann Galpin GCC, MCA**
➕ O 🆖 ✳
**Fees:** £46–55; Second visit: £31–40
Cookham SL6
01628 532163

**Matthew D Holmes GCC, BCA**
➕ ⊕
Reading RG18
01635 868691

**Melanie D'avigdor-Hamilton GCC, M**
➕ ➕ 🆖 ✳
**Fees:** £36–45; Second visit: £21–30
Reading RG20
01635 278636

**Vera Christensen GCC, BCA**
➕ 🆖 ∅ ✳ 🔵
**Fees:** £36–45; Second visit: £21–30
Reading RG21
01256 328128

**Felicia Kilner GCC, BCA**
➕ 🆖 ∅ ✳
**Fees:** £36–45; Second visit: £21–30
Reading RG1
0118 926 7438

**Gill Lewis GCC, MCA**
O ➕ 🆖 © ✳
**Fees:** £36–45; Second visit: £21–30
Reading RG8
0118 984 3473

**April Rose GCC, MCA**
O ∅ ✳
**Fees:** £36–45; Second visit: £21–30
Reading RG7
0118 988 5422

**Katherine Ryan GCC, MCA**
O 🆖 ∅ ✳
**Fees:** £36–45; Second visit: £21–30
Reading RG31
0118 942 6192

**Annette Storm Williams GCC, BCA**
➕ 🆖 ∅ © ✳ 🔵
**Fees:** £36–45; Second visit: £21–30
Reading RG21
01256 328128

**Ray Swaine GCC, MCA**
➕ O ➕ 🆖 ∅ © ✳
**Fees:** £26–35; Second visit: £21–30
Reading RG5
0118 969 7769

**Anna Maynard GCC, BCA**
➕ 🆖 ∅ ✳
**Fees:** £36–45; Second visit: £21–30
Reading RG40
0118 978 7466

### Henry Butterfield GCC, BCA
**Fees:** £36–45; Second visit: £21–30
Reading RG40, Wokingham RG40
0118 978 7466

### Dominic Bostock GCC, MCA
**Fees:** £26–35; Second visit: £21–30
Slough SL1
01753 740769

### Martin R Storr GCC, BCA
**Fees:** £36–45; Second visit: £21–30
Slough SL1, Reigate RH2
01628 669117

### Russell M Dean GCC, BCA
**Fees:** £46–55; Second visit: £31–40
Windsor SL4
01753 833299

## BUCKINGHAMSHIRE

### Jatinder Benepal GCC, BCA
**Fees:** £36–45; Second visit: £21–30
Aylesbury HP20
01296 489231

### Kathie Harkness Lait GCC, MCA
**Fees:** £26–35; Second visit: £21–30
Bierton HP22
01296 482980

### Karen Jarman GCC, MCA
**Fees:** £26–35; Second visit: £21–30
Buckingham MK18
01280 816623

### Anne Mette Marup GCC, BCA
**Fees:** £26–35; Second visit: £21–30
High Wycombe HP11
01494 524194

### Belinda Randall GCC, MCA
**Fees:** £36–45; Second visit: £21–30
Marlow SL7
01628 488988

### Juliet Lock GCC, BAAC
**Fees:** <£25; Second visit: £21–30
Shabbington HP18, Thame OX9
01844 201560

### Christopher Turner GCC, BCA
**Fees:** £36–45; Second visit: £21–30
Slough SL6
01628 629236

### Helen Tweedale GCC, BCA
**Fees:** £26–35; Second visit: £21–30
Slough SL3
01753 545805

### Sean O'Gorman GCC, MCA
**Fees:** £36–45; Second visit: £21–30
Wendover HP22
01296 622286

## DORSET

### Ruth Otter GCC, BCA
**Fees:** £26–35; Second visit: <£20
Broadstone BH18
01202 694159

### Rosamund Drake GCC, BCA
**Fees:** >£55; Second visit: £21–30
Bournemouth BH21
01202 880136

### Amritam Mills GCC, MCA
**Fees:** £26–35; Second visit: £21–30
Bournemouth BH21
01725 517508

### Jamie Fraser-Nash GCC, BCA
**Fees:** £36–45; Second visit: £21–30
Bournemouth BH17
01202 699581

### Gilbert Meal GCC, BCA
**Fees:** £46–55; Second visit: £21–30
Bournemouth BH23
01202 483281

# Chiropractic

**David Fleetwood GCC, BCA**
🔘 🔘 ⊘ 🔘 🔘
**Fees:** £36–45; Second visit: £21–30
Blandford Forum DT11,
New Milton BH25
01258 455214

**Louis Alicea GCC, BCA**
🔘 🔘
**Fees:** >£55; Second visit: £31–40
Bournemouth BH4
01202 768508

**Simon Austin GCC, BCA**
🔘 🔘 ⊘ 🔘
**Fees:** £36–45; Second visit: £21–30
Bournemouth BH5
01202 436222

**Sheila Breeze GCC, BCA**
🔘 🔘 🔘
**Fees:** £26–35; Second visit: £21–30
Bournemouth BH9
01202 519138

**Marianne Cook GCC, BCA**
🔘 🔘 ⊘ 🔘 🔘
**Fees:** £36–45; Second visit: £21–30
Bournemouth BH5
01202 936200

**Janis Duff GCC, BCA**
🔘 🔘 🔘 🔘 ⊘ 🔘
**Fees:** £26–35; Second visit: £21–30
Bournemouth BH6
01202 424833

**Marjorie Furniss GCC, MCA**
🔘 🔘 ⊘
**Fees:** <£25; Second visit: <£20
Bournemouth BH6
01202 425433

**Guy Gosselin GCC, BCA**
🔘 🔘 🔘
**Fees:** £36–45; Second visit: £21–30
Bournemouth BH5
01202 436200

**S C Hudson-Cook GCC, BCA**
🔘 🔘 🔘
**Fees:** £36–45; Second visit: £21–30
Bournemouth BH3
01202 769100

**Martin Krir GCC, MCA**
🔘 🔘 ⊘ Ⓔ 🔘
**Fees:** £26–35; Second visit: £21–30
Bournemouth BH8
01202 296756

**Balbir K Singh GCC, BCA**
🔘 🔘 ⊘ 🔘
**Fees:** £26–35; Second visit: £21–30
Bournemouth BH5
01202 394526

**Haymo Thiel GCC, BCA**
🔘 🔘 🔘 ⊘ Ⓔ 🔘
**Fees:** £26–35; Second visit: £21–30
Bournemouth BH5
01202 346317

**Francis J H Wilson GCC, BCA**
🔘 ⊘ 🔘
**Fees:** £36–45; Second visit: £21–30
Bournemouth BH5
01202 436200

**Travis E Webb GCC**
🔘 🔘 ⊘ 🔘 🔘
**Fees:** £46–55; Second visit: £21–30
Christchurch BH23
01202 471481

**Tony Gilmore GCC, MCA**
🔘 🔘 🔘
**Fees:** £26–35; Second visit: £31–40
Corfe Castle BH20
01929 480332

**Susan Hill GCC, BCA**
🔘 🔘 🔘 ⊘ 🔘 🔘
**Fees:** £36–45; Second visit: £21–30
Dorchester DT1
01305 263048

**Jocelyn Medley GCC, BCA**
🔘 🔘 🔘 🔘 🔘
**Fees:** £26–35; Second visit: £21–30
Dorchester DT1
01305 250700

**Paul Miller GCC, MCA**
🔘 🔘 ⊘ 🔘
**Fees:** £26–35; Second visit: £21–30
Dorchester DT1, Weymouth DT4
01305 263678

# Chiropractic

**Quentin Standish-Hayes GCC, BCA**
🔵 ⚫ 🔵 🔵
**Fees:** £36–45; Second visit: £21–30
Dorchester DT1
01305 263048

**Helga Hopkins GCC, BCA**
🔵 ⚪ ⊕ 🔵 🔵 ⊘
**Fees:** £36–45; Second visit: £21–30
Ferndown BH22
01202 870852

**David Allen GCC, BCA**
🔵 🔵 Ⓔ 🔵
**Fees:** £46–55; Second visit: £21–30
Christchurch BH23
01425 277866

**Carolyn Smyth GCC, BCA**
⊕ 🔵 ⊘ 🔵
**Fees:** £26–35; Second visit: £21–30
Parkstone BH14
01202 741345

**Steven Oldale GCC, BCA**
🔵 🔵 ⊘ 🔵
**Fees:** £26–35; Second visit: £21–30
Poole BH15
01202 649900

**Zoe Heritage GCC, MCA**
🔵 ⚪ ⊕ 🔵 ⊘
**Fees:** £26–35; Second visit: £21–30
Shaftesbury SP7,
Sturminster Newton DT10
01747 851503

**Tracy White GCC, MCA**
🔵 ⊕ 🔵 🔵
**Fees:** £26–35; Second visit: £21–30
Sturminster Newton DT10
01258 473109

**Jonathan Sharp GCC, BCA**
🔵 ⊕ 🔵 ⊘
**Fees:** £36–45; Second visit: £21–30
Verwood BH31
01202 827609

**Heidemarie Underwood GCC, BCA**
🔵 ⚪ 🔵
**Fees:** £26–35; Second visit: £21–30
Weymouth DT3
01305 768393

**Ann-Britt Nilsson GCC, BCA**
🔵 ⚪ ⊕ 🔵 🔵
**Fees:** £26–35; Second visit: £21–30
Weymouth DT4
01202 761507

## HAMPSHIRE

**Lisa Morley GCC, MCA**
🔵 🔵 🔵
**Fees:** £36–45; Second visit: £21–30
Andover SP11
01264 710811

**Nicholas Richmond GCC, MCA**
🔵 ⊕ 🔵 ⊘ 🔵
**Fees:** £36–45; Second visit: £21–30
Andover SP11
01264 361060

**Heather Ryman GCC, BCA**
🔵 🔵 🔵
**Fees:** £36–45; Second visit: £21–30
Andover SP10
01264 337133

**Rachael Stopps GCC, BCA**
🔵 ⊘ 🔵
**Fees:** £36–45; Second visit: £21–30
Basingstoke RG21
01256 326590

**Jonathan Melhuish GCC, BCA**
🔵 ⊕ 🔵 🔵
**Fees:** £26–35; Second visit: £21–30
Bournemouth BH25
01425 620222

**R J Cole GCC, BCA**
🔵 🔵 🔵 🔵
**Fees:** £36–45; Second visit: £21–30
Eastleigh SO50
023 8061 6069

**Elaine Cooke GCC, BCA**
🔵 ⊕ 🔵 🔵 🔵
**Fees:** £26–35; Second visit: £21–30
Fareham PO16
01329 280283

**Stephen Booty GCC, MCA**
⚪ 🔵
**Fees:** £26–35; Second visit: £21–30
Farnborough GU14
01252 510284

# Chiropractic

**Stephen Brown GCC, BCA**
⊕ ⓝ ⓖ
**Fees:** £26–35; Second visit: £21–30
Fleet GU51
01252 616511

**Madeleine Jefferies GCC, MCA**
⊕ ⊕ ⓝ ⊘
**Fees:** £26–35; Second visit: £21–30
Fleet GU51
01252 614818

**Nicola Eldridge GCC, MCA**
⊕ ⊕ ⊕ ⓝ ✿
**Fees:** £26–35; Second visit: £21–30
Fleet GU51
01252 614818

**Martin Laking GCC, BCA**
⊕ ⓝ ⊘ ✿ ⓔ
**Fees:** £26–35; Second visit: £21–30
Fordingbridge SP6
01425 652951

**Keith Johnson GCC, BCA**
⊕ ⊕ ⓝ ✿
**Fees:** £26–35; Second visit: <£20
Havant PO9
023 92 471757

**Emma Kinch GCC, BCA**
⊕ ⊕ ⊕ ⓝ ⊘ ✿
**Fees:** £46–55; Second visit: £21–30
Havant PO9
023 9245 5025

**Gail Benes GCC**
⊕ ⊕ ⓝ ✿
**Fees:** £36–45; Second visit: £21–30
Lymington SO41
01590 642749

**Wendy Johnson GCC, MCA**
⊕ ⊕ ⊕ ⓝ ✿
**Fees:** £36–45; Second visit: £41–50
Lymington SO41,Daventry
NN11,Southampton SO17
01425 620177

**Morten Westergaard GCC, BCA**
⊕ ⓝ ✿ ⓔ
**Fees:** £26–35; Second visit: £21–30
New Milton BH25
01425 628844

**Jonathan Field GCC, BCA**
⊕ ⊕ ⓝ ⊘ ✿ ⓖ
**Fees:** £26–35; Second visit: £21–30
Petersfield GU32
01730 267423

**Guy Blomfield GCC, BCA**
⊕ ⓝ
**Fees:** £26–35; Second visit: £21–30
Portsmouth PO41
01983 761100

**Stuart Herbert GCC, BCA**
⊕ ○ ⓝ ⊘ ⓔ ✿
**Fees:** £26–35; Second visit: £21–30
Portsmouth PO4
023 9287 0110

**Richard Hope GCC, BCA**
⊕ ⊕ ⓝ
**Fees:** £46–55; Second visit: £21–30
Portsmouth PO33
01983 563539

**Clare Horsfield GCC, BCA**
⊕ ⓝ ⊘ ✿
**Fees:** £26–35; Second visit: £21–30
Portsmouth PO2
023 9265 4758

**Sheila Stakim GCC**
⊕ ⓝ ⊘ ⓔ ✿ ⓔ
**Fees:** £26–35; Second visit: £21–30
Portsmouth PO4
023 9287 0707

**Meg Crafer GCC, MCA**
⊕ ⓝ ⓔ ✿
**Fees:** £26–35; Second visit: £21–30
Ringwood BH24
01202 871545

**Susan Claire Waller GCC, MCA**
⊕ ○ ✿
**Fees:** £36–45; Second visit: £21–30
Romsey SO51
01794 517141

**Stephen Williams GCC, BCA**
⊕ ⊕ ⓝ ✿ ⓔ
**Fees:** >£55; Second visit: £21–30
Shirley SO16
023 8078 8111

**Erik Holm GCC, BCA**
Fees: £46–55; Second visit: £21–30
Southampton SO15
023 8022 7200

**Janet Krir GCC, BCA**
Fees: £36–45; Second visit: £21–30
Southampton SO15
023 8033 0090

**R A Pauc GCC, BCA**
Fees: £36–45; Second visit: £21–30
Southampton SO15, Brockenhurst
SO42, Andover SP10
023 8033 0090

**Christopher Webb GCC, BCA**
Fees: £26–35; Second visit: £21–30
Southampton SO16
023 8078 3321

**Pam Elkins GCC, BCA**
Fees: £46–55; Second visit: £21–30
Southampton SO30
01489 787170

**Martine Huisman GCC, BCA**
Fees: £26–35; Second visit: £21–30
Southampton SO45
023 8020 7826

**Jane Rowley GCC, MCA**
Fees: £46–55; Second visit: £31–40
Southampton SO40
023 8066 7205

**Paul Godwin GCC, BAAC, MCA**
Fees: £26–35; Second visit: £21–30
Stockbridge SO20
01264 860269

**Vanessa Churchill GCC, MCA**
Fees: £46–55; Second visit: £31–40
Totton SO40
023 8060 7205

**Glo Becvar GCC, BCA**
Fees: £26–35; Second visit: £21–30
Waterlooville PO7
025 9223 1501

**Maxwell Atkinson GCC, BCA**
Fees: >£55; Second visit: £21–30
Winchester SO23
01962 861188

**R Michael Hutchinson GCC, BCA**
Fees: £36–45; Second visit: £21–30
Winchester SO23
01962 853984

**Mark Kennedy GCC, BCA**
Fees: £46–55; Second visit: £21–30
Winchester SO23
01962 843242

## HERTFORDSHIRE

**Margie Craib GCC, MCA**
Fees: £36–45; Second visit: £21–30
Berkhamsted HP4
01442 842729

**William Tomlin GCC, BCA**
Fees: >£55; Second visit: £21–30
Berkhamsted HP4
01442 863800

**D L Tribe GCC, BCA**
Fees: £26–35; Second visit: £21–30
Berkhamsted HP4
01442 863800

**Amanda Jones-Harris GCC, BCA**
Fees: £26–35; Second visit: £21–30
Buntingford SG9, Huntingdon
PE28, Colchester CO3
01763 274646

# Chiropractic

**Tracy Morgan GCC, MCA**
⊕ O ⊘ ✿
**Fees:** £26–35; Second visit: £21–30
Bushey WD23
01923 250605

**Lise Rose GCC, MCA**
⊕ O ⬤ ✿
**Fees:** £46–55; Second visit: £31–40
Harpenden AL5
01582 713464

**Michael B Gould GCC, BCA**
⊕ O ⬤ ⊘ ✿
**Fees:** £36–45; Second visit: £21–30
Hemel Hempstead HP7
01494 434366

**Avtar Bhamber GCC, BCA**
⊕ ⬤ ⊘ ✿ ⬤
**Fees:** £26–35; Second visit: £21–30
Hemel Hempstead HP11
01494 558061

**Glenda Lenton GCC, BAAC**
⊕ O ⊕ ⬤ ⊘ ✿
**Fees:** £36–45; Second visit: £21–30
Hemel Hempstead HP3
01442 267858

**Paul Trusty GCC, BAAC**
⊕ ⊘ ✿ ⬤
**Fees:** £26–35; Second visit: £21–30
Rickmansworth WD3
01923 773060

**Michael Bassett GCC, BCA**
⊕ O ⊕ ⬤ ⊘ ✿
**Fees:** £46–55; Second visit: £31–40
St Albans AL3
01727 856687

**Karen Flintoff GCC, MCA**
O ⊕ ⬤ ⬤ © ✿
**Fees:** £26–35; Second visit: £21–30
Stevenage SG18
01462 700183

**Ray Tant GCC, MCA**
⊕ ⊕ ⬤ ✿
**Fees:** £36–45; Second visit: £21–30
St Albans AL4
01582 768247

## ISLE OF WIGHT

**Anna Sherwell GCC, MCA**
O ⬤ ⊘ ✿
**Fees:** £26–35; Second visit: £21–30
Cowes PO31
01983 298205

**Rebecca Taylor GCC, MCA**
⊕ ⬤ ⊘ ✿
**Fees:** £26–35; Second visit: £21–30
Cowes PO31
01983 298205

**Martin Scotcher GCC, MCA**
⊕ ⊕ ⊕ ⬤ © ✿
**Fees:** £26–35; Second visit: £21–30
Newport PO30, Freshwater PO40,
Totland Bay PO39
01983 522477

**Mhairi Simon GCC, MCA**
⊕ ⊕ ⬤ ✿
**Fees:** £26–35; Second visit: £21–30
Ryde PO33
01983 566009

**Keith Saunders GCC, MCA**
⊕ ⬤ ✿
**Fees:** £26–35; Second visit: £21–30
Shanklin PO37
01983 866514

## KENT

**Christopher Foley GCC, BCA**
⊕ ⬤ ⊘ ✿ ⬤
**Fees:** £26–35; Second visit: £21–30
Bidborough TN3
01892 870587

**Daniel GH Sparks GCC, BCA**
⊕ ⬤ ⊘ ✿
**Fees:** £36–45; Second visit: £21–30
Birchington CT7
01843 841508

**Trevor Francis-Jones GCC, BCA**
⊕ ⬤ © ✿ ⬤
**Fees:** £36–45; Second visit: £21–30
Bromley BR6
01689 890894

**Victoria Jackson GCC, BCA**

Fees: £26–35; Second visit: £21–30
Canterbury CT1
01227 769998

**Lucy Woodcock GCC, BCA**

Fees: £36–45; Second visit: £21–30
Canterbury CT10
01843 601631

**Alyson Wreford GCC, BCA**

Fees: £26–35; Second visit: £21–30
Canterbury CT5
01227 273821

**Deborah Cain GCC, MCA**

Fees: £26–35; Second visit: £21–30
Deal CT14
01304 379598

**David Hipkiss GCC, BAAC**

Fees: £26–35; Second visit: £21–30
Deal CT14
01304 381831

**Alasdair Smith GCC, MCA**

Fees: £26–35; Second visit: £21–30
Maidstone ME17
01622 745178

**Farid Moshtael GCC, BCA**

Fees: £26–35; Second visit: £21–30
Maidstone ME2
01634 710980

**Jesper Dahl GCC, BCA**

Fees: £36–45; Second visit: £21–30
Maidstone ME14
01622 661883

**Lene Feldborg GCC, BCA**

Fees: £36–45; Second visit: £21–30
Maidstone ME14
01622 661883

**Sian Forrest GCC, MCA**

Fees: £26–35; Second visit: £21–30
Maidstone ME16
01622 726626

**Alan T Plenty GCC, BCA**

Fees: £26–35; Second visit: £21–30
Ramsgate CT11
01843 599366

**Gillian Mauger GCC, MCA**

Fees: £36–45; Second visit: £21–30
Sevenoaks TN13
01732 465266

**Katie Boughton GCC, MCA**

Fees: £46–55; Second visit: £21–30
Tenterden TN30
01580 766153

**Penny Brignall GCC, MCA**

Fees: £26–35; Second visit: £21–30
Tonbridge TN6,Crowborough TN6
01892 610022

**Paul Dupker GCC, MCA**

Fees: £26–35; Second visit: £21–30
Tonbridge TN39
01424 842098

**Kevin Murphy GCC, MCA**

Fees: £26–35; Second visit: £21–30
Tonbridge TN34
01424 465050

**Janet Adams GCC, MCA**

Fees: £26–35; Second visit: £21–30
Tonbridge TN11
01732 850695

**Belinda Ambrose GCC, BCA**

Fees: £36–45; Second visit: £21–30
Tonbridge TN24
01233 640047

# Chiropractic

**Claire Amos GCC, MCA**
⊕ ○ ⊕ ❀ ⊜
**Fees:** £26–35; Second visit: £21–30
Tonbridge TN6
01892 668852

**Susan Court GCC, MCA**
○ ❀
**Fees:** £26–35; Second visit: £21–30
Tonbridge TN9,Orpington BR5
01732 366543

**Simon Hobbs GCC, BCA**
⊕ ⊜ ⊘ ❀ ⊜
**Fees:** £26–35; Second visit: £21–30
Tonbridge TN34,Bexhill-on-Sea TN40
01424 429042

**Paul Gibby GCC, MCA**
⊕ ⊕ ❀
**Fees:** £26–35; Second visit: £21–30
Tonbridge TN2
01892 523879

**Simon Green GCC, MCA**
○ ⊜
Tonbridge TN1
01892 520636

**Jacqueline O'Donnell GCC, MCA**
○ ⊕ ❀
**Fees:** £26–35; Second visit: £21–30
Tonbridge TN4
01892 544343

**Deirdre Palmer GCC, MCA**
○ ❀
**Fees:** £26–35; Second visit: £21–30
Tonbridge TN4
01892 522755

## MILTON KEYNES

**Fiona Dowdell GCC, MCA**
⊕ ○ ⊕ ⊜ ⊘ ❀
**Fees:** £26–35; Second visit: £21–30
Milton Keynes MK17
01296 720695

**Jane E A Halford GCC, BAAC, MCA**
○ ⊜ ❀
**Fees:** £36–45; Second visit: £21–30
Newport Pagnell MK16
01908 610545

**Heather Wright GCC, MCA**
⊕ ⊕ ⊕ ⊘ ❀
**Fees:** £36–45; Second visit: £21–30
Newport Pagnell MK16
01908 614051

**Per Kleberg GCC, BCA**
⊕ ⊜ ⊘ ❀ ⊜
**Fees:** £26–35; Second visit: £21–30
Shenley Church End
MK5,Northampton NN1
01908 506154

## NORTHAMPTONSHIRE

**Dana Green GCC, MCA**
⊕ ○ ⊕ ⊜ ❀
**Fees:** £26–35; Second visit: £21–30
Abingdon NN1
01604 231088

**Patricia Griffiths GCC, BAAC**
⊕ ○ ⊕ ❀
**Fees:** £36–45; Second visit: £21–30
Brackley NN13,Towcester NN12
07974 118475

**Liz Linford GCC, BAAC, BCA**
⊕ ⊜ ⊘ ❀
**Fees:** £36–45; Second visit: £31–40
Brackley NN13
07767 658743

**Arthur Redrup GCC, MCA**
⊕ ○ ⊕ ⊜ ⊘ ❀
**Fees:** £26–35; Second visit: £21–30
Brackley NN13
01295 711089

**Jennifer Leighton GCC, BAAC**
⊕ ❀
**Fees:** £26–35; Second visit: £21–30
Daventry NN11
01295 760374

**Michael Oliff GCC, MCA**
⊕ ⊕ ⊜ ⊘ ❀
**Fees:** £26–35; Second visit: £21–30
Daventry NN11
01327 877010

**Philippa Throssell GCC, MCA**
Fees: £26–35; Second visit: £21–30
Daventry NN11
01327 261011

**Clifford Thompson GCC, BCA**
Fees: £26–35; Second visit: £21–30
Duddington PE9
01780 444651

**Zafar Iqbal GCC, BCA**
Fees: £26–35; Second visit: £21–30
Kettering NN14
01536 510998

**Ann Farmer GCC, BAAC, MCA**
Fees: £26–35; Second visit: £21–30
Long Buckby NN6
01327 844291

**Maxine Chimes GCC, MCA**
Fees: £36–45; Second visit: £21–30
Northampton NN3
01604 645533

**Sunil Solanki GCC, BCA**
Fees: £26–35; Second visit: £21–30
Northampton NN1
01604 460200

## OXFORDSHIRE

**John Bradford GCC, BCA**
Fees: £26–35; Second visit: £21–30
Abingdon OX14
07968 162654

**Holly Burgess GCC, MCA**
Fees: £36–45; Second visit: £21–30
Abingdon OX13
01865 820708

**Andrew Rowe GCC, BCA**
Fees: £26–35; Second visit: £21–30
Abingdon OX14
01235 554435

**Dee Craven GCC, MCA**
Fees: £36–45; Second visit: £21–30
Banbury OX16
01295 253386

**Barbara Minter GCC, MCA**
Fees: £36–45; Second visit: £21–30
Banbury OX17
01295 811947

**Ian Spiers GCC, MCA**
Fees: £26–35; Second visit: £31–40
Banbury OX17
01295 690394

**Graham Wilkins GCC, MCA**
Fees: <£25; Second visit: £21–30
Banbury OX16
01295 264332

**Peter Bennett GCC, MCA**
Fees: £36–45; Second visit: £21–30
Bicester OX6,Brackley NN13
01869 322516

**Elizabeth Hearle GCC, MCA**
Fees: £36–45; Second visit: £21–30
Bloxham OX15
01295 721735

**Leigh Miller GCC, MCA**
Fees: £26–35; Second visit: £21–30
Burford OX18
01451 844684

**Nicola Morgan GCC, MCA**
Fees: <£25; Second visit: £21–30
Charlbury OX7
01608 811673

**Shelagh James-Hudson GCC, BAAC**
Fees: £36–45; Second visit: £21–30
Chipping Norton OX7
01608 643704

# Chiropractic

## Alan Craft GCC, MCA
✛ 🔘 ⦸ ❋
**Fees:** £26–35; Second visit: £21–30
Eynsham OX29
01865 882992

## Imelda Twine GCC, MCA
✛ 🔾 ⊕ 🔘 ⦸ ❋
**Fees:** £26–35; Second visit: £21–30
Faringdon SN7, Wantage OX12
01367 240473

## Christopher Perkins GCC, BAAC
✛ 🔘 ❋
**Fees:** £26–35; Second visit: £21–30
Kidlington OX5
01865 376555

## Stuart Rynsburger GCC
✛ 🔘 ❋
**Fees:** £26–35; Second visit: £21–30
Kidlington OX5
01865 377877

## Raymond Broome GCC, BCA
✛ 🔾 🔘 ⦸ 🔘
**Fees:** £36–45; Second visit: £21–30
Oxford OX2
01865 204246

## Sally Evans GCC, BAAC
✛ ⊕ 🔘 ❋
**Fees:** £36–45; Second visit: £31–40
Oxford OX2
01865 513 388

## Dawn Akers GCC, MCA
✛ ⊕ 🔘 ⦸ ❋
**Fees:** £36–45; Second visit: £21–30
Oxford OX2
01865 250200

## Fatima Alcantara GCC, BAAC
✛ 🔾 ⊕ ❋
**Fees:** £26–35; Second visit: £21–30
Oxford OX4
01865 249062

## Amanda Brooks GCC, BAAC
✛ 🔾 ⊕ 🔘 ❋
**Fees:** £26–35; Second visit: £21–30
Oxford OX2
01865 721064

## Lynne Davies GCC, MCA
✛ ⊕ 🔘 ❋
**Fees:** £36–45; Second visit: £21–30
Oxford OX4
01865 715615

## Debbie Edens GCC, BAAC
🔾
**Fees:** <£25; Second visit: £21–30
Oxford OX5
01865 370777

## Stan Harding GCC, MCA
✛ 🔾 🔘 ⦸ ❋
**Fees:** £46–55; Second visit: £21–30
Oxford OX2
01865 200489

## Jonathan M P Howat GCC, BCA
✛ ⊕ 🔘 🔘
**Fees:** >£55; Second visit: £41–50
Oxford OX3
01865 761802

## Anthony Larcombe GCC, BCA
✛ 🔘 Ⓔ ❋ 🔘
**Fees:** £36–45; Second visit: £21–30
Oxford OX2
01865 204246

## Rupert Molloy GCC, BCA
✛ 🔘 Ⓔ ❋
**Fees:** £36–45; Second visit: £21–30
Oxford OX20
01993 811815

## Lorna Walton GCC, MCA
🔾 🔘 ❋
**Fees:** £36–45; Second visit: £21–30
Oxford OX11
01235 821858

## Joanna Harrison GCC, BAAC, MCA
✛ ⊕ Ⓔ ❋
**Fees:** £26–35; Second visit: £21–30
Oxford OX2
07970 876656

## Nicola Plested GCC, BAAC
✛ ⊕ 🔘 ❋
**Fees:** £36–45; Second visit: £31–40
Oxford OX4
01865 790235

**Suzanne Bird GCC, BAAC**
○ ⊛
**Fees:** £26–35; Second visit: £21–30
Thame OX9
01844 216878

**William Rees Lewis GCC, MCA**
○ ⊕ ⊕ ⊛ ⊘ ❀
**Fees:** £26–35; Second visit: £21–30
Wallingford OX10
01491 651806

**Christina Cunliffe GCC, MCA**
⊕ ○ ⊕ ⊛ ⊘ ❀
**Fees:** £46–55; Second visit: <£20
Wheatley OX33
01865 876900

**Mark Anderson GCC, BAAC**
⊕ ⊕ ⊛ Ⓔ ❀
**Fees:** £26–35; Second visit: £21–30
Witney OX8
01993 708583

**R Nicholson GCC, BAAC**
⊕ ⊕ ⊛ ❀
**Fees:** £26–35; Second visit: £21–30
Witney OX28
01993 774418

**Carol Conner GCC, MCA**
○ ⊛ ⊘
**Fees:** £36–45; Second visit: £21–30
Woodstock OX20
01993 811120

### SURREY

**Clare E Hyland GCC, BCA**
⊕ ⊛ ⊘ ❀
**Fees:** £46–55; Second visit: £21–30
Ashtead KT21
01372 271970

**Rosanne Heagerty GCC, MCA**
⊕ ○ ⊛ ⊘ ❀
**Fees:** £36–45; Second visit: £21–30
Bletchingley RH1,Hassocks BN6
01883 743355

**Marisa Pinnock GCC, MCA**
⊕ ⊛ ⊘ ❀
**Fees:** £36–45; Second visit: £21–30
Bletchingley RH1
01883 743355

**Tanja Brandt GCC, MCA**
○ ⊛ ❀
**Fees:** £36–45; Second visit: £21–30
Camberley GU17
01276 34181

**Terry Murphy GCC, MCA**
○ ⊛ ❀
**Fees:** £36–45; Second visit: £21–30
Camberley GU17
01276 34181

**Christopher Walker GCC, BCA**
⊕ ⊕ ⊛ ❀ ⊛
**Fees:** £36–45; Second visit: £21–30
Camberley GU15
01276 21637

**Maria Kinderas GCC, BCA**
⊕ ⊛ ❀ ⊛
**Fees:** £26–35; Second visit: £21–30
Farnham GU9
01252 710549

**J P Weston GCC, BCA**
⊕ ○ ⊕
**Fees:** Second visit: £21–30
Farnham GU9
01252 734670

**David B Young GCC, BCA**
⊕ ⊕ ⊛ ⊛
**Fees:** £26–35; Second visit: £21–30
Farnham GU9
01252 710549

**Anna Franklin GCC, BCA**
⊕ ⊛ ⊘ ❀ ⊛
**Fees:** £46–55; Second visit: £21–30
Godalming GU7
01483 419538

**Tone Tellefsen GCC, BCA**
⊕ ⊛ ⊘ ⊛
**Fees:** £46–55; Second visit: £21–30
Guildford GU7
01483 419538

**William Beckinsale GCC, BCA**
⊕ ⊕ ⊛ ⊛
**Fees:** £26–35; Second visit: £21–30
Guildford GU13
01252 616511

# Chiropractic

**Jeremy Spanton GCC**
Fees: £36–45; Second visit: £21–30
Guildford GU21
01483 723688

**Ailsa Barrett GCC, BCA**
Fees: £46–55; Second visit: £21–30
Godalming GU7
01483 419538

**Robert Brock GCC, BAAC, MCA**
Fees: £26–35; Second visit: £21–30
Guildford GU9,Guildford GU1
01252 728252

**Alain Michelotti GCC, BCA**
Fees: £36–45; Second visit: £21–30
Guildford GU1
01483 562830

**Cherye Roche GCC, BCA**
Fees: >£55; Second visit: £21–30
Guildford GU2
01483 306722

**Robert La Touche GCC, MCA**
Fees: £26–35; Second visit: £21–30
Guildford GU1
01483 827039

**Penelope Edwards-Moss GCC, BCA**
Fees: £36–45; Second visit: £21–30
Guildford GU6
01483 274002

**Andrew Thoma GCC, MCA**
Fees: <£25; Second visit: £21–30
Guildford GU33
01730 893740

**Michelle Carrington GCC, BCA**
Fees: £26–35; Second visit: £21–30
Haslemere GU27
01428 642778

**Richard Lanigan GCC, BAAC, BCA**
Fees: £26–35; Second visit: £21–30
Kingston Upon Thames KT2
020 82862606

**M Boles GCC, BCA**
Fees: £36–45; Second visit: £21–30
Leatherhead KT22,East Molesey KT8
01372 374443

**Tracey Hutchings GCC**
Fees: £26–35; Second visit: £21–30
Mytchett GU16
01252 404240

**Robert Scott GCC, BCA**
Fees: £26–35; Second visit: £21–30
Mytchett GU16
01252 404240

**Gerald Chambers GCC, MCA**
Fees: £36–45; Second visit: £21–30
Redhill RH15
01444 257444

**Aaron Farber GCC, BCA**
Fees: £26–35; Second visit: £21–30
Redhill RH17
01444 452220

**Peter Westergaard GCC, BCA**
Fees: £26–35; Second visit: £21–30
Redhill RH12
01403 275000

**Christopher Hamp GCC, BAAC**
Fees: £26–35; Second visit: £21–30
Redhill RH2
01737 247171

**Nicholas Oram GCC, BCA**
Fees: £26–35; Second visit: £21–30
Shepperton TW17
01932 429584

**Artur Mazur GCC, BCA**
Fees: £26–35; Second visit: £21–30
Weybridge KT13
01932 859006

**Stephanie Glen GCC, BCA**
Fees: £36–45; Second visit: £21–30
Woking GU22
01483 831396

## SUSSEX

**Jon Mason GCC, MCA**
Fees: £36–45; Second visit: £31–40
Ashington RH20
01903 892171

**Nicola Jempson GCC, MCA**
Fees: £26–35; Second visit: £21–30
Battle TN33
01424 777391

**Christopher Garland GCC, MCA**
Fees: £26–35; Second visit: £21–30
Brighton BN2,Brighton BN2,Brighton BN1
01273 622301

**Graham Roberts GCC, BCA**
Fees: £26–35; Second visit: £21–30
Brighton BN20
01323 734664

**Sheila Ruth Urbanowicz GCC, MCA**
Fees: £26–35; Second visit: £21–30
Brighton BN2
01273 628221

**Matthew Bennett GCC, BCA**
Fees: £36–45; Second visit: £21–30
Brighton BN1
01273 774114

**Madeleine Brzeski GCC, MCA**
Fees: £36–45; Second visit: £21–30
Brighton BN14
01903 217160

**Simon Edwards GCC, BAAC**
Fees: <£25; Second visit: £21–30
Brighton BN16
01903 859525

**Paul Harris GCC, BCA**
Fees: £36–45; Second visit: £21–30
Brighton BN3,Worthing BN11
01273 733469

**Helle Henriksen GCC, BCA**
Fees: £26–35; Second visit: £21–30
Brighton BN7
01273 477535

**Jacqueline Holden GCC, MCA**
Fees: £26–35; Second visit: £21–30
Brighton BN1
01273 271831

**Jeffrey McTavish GCC, BCA**
Fees: £36–45; Second visit: £21–30
Brighton BN1,Worthing BN14
01273 774114

**Bill Chambers GCC, MCA**
Fees: £36–45; Second visit: £21–30
Burgess Hill RH15
01444 257444

**Hanne Krogsgaard-Neilsen GCC, BCA**
Fees: £36–45; Second visit: £21–30
Burgess Hill RH15,High Wycombe HP11
01444 235021

**Roger S White GCC, BCA**
Fees: £26–35; Second visit: £21–30
Burgess Hill RH15
01444 257555

# Chiropractic

**John Springard GCC, BCA**
⊕ ⓜ Ⓔ ✿ ⓖ
**Fees:** £36–45; Second visit: £21–30
Chichester PO19
01243 774336

**Susan Drew GCC, MCA**
⊕ O ⓜ ✿
**Fees:** £26–35; Second visit: £21–30
Crowborough TN6
01892 853512

**Robert Ions GCC, MCA**
⊕ ⊕ ⓜ ✿
**Fees:** £46–55; Second visit: £21–30;
Second visit: £41–50
Eastbourne BN21, GY2
01323 410050

**Hilton Kelly GCC, BCA**
⊕ ⓜ ✿ ⓖ
**Fees:** £36–45; Second visit: £21–30
Eastbourne BN21
01323 733361

**Alan Smith GCC, MCA**
⊕ ✿
East Grinstead RH19
01342 313396

**David Thomas GCC, MCA**
⊕ ⊕ Ⓔ
**Fees:** >£55; Second visit: £41–50
Forest Row RH18
01342 822802

**Tony Dawson GCC, MCA**
⊕ ⊕ ✿
**Fees:** £36–45; Second visit: £21–30
Haywards Heath RH16
01444 440857

**Stephen Minter GCC, MCA**
O ⓜ ⊘ ✿
**Fees:** £36–45; Second visit: £21–30
Haywards Heath RH17
01444 831005

**Sue Minter GCC, MCA**
O ⓜ ⊘ ✿
**Fees:** £36–45; Second visit: £21–30
Haywards Heath RH17
01444 831005

**Carolyn Marshall-Hall GCC, BCA**
⊕ ⊕ ⓜ ⊘ Ⓔ ✿ ⓖ
**Fees:** £36–45; Second visit: £21–30
Hove BN3,Hove BN3
01273 206868

**Philip Curtis GCC, BCA**
⊕ ⓜ ⊘ ✿ ⓖ
**Fees:** <£25; Second visit: £21–30
Littlehampton BN16
01903 775577

**Patrick Layen GCC, MCA**
⊕ O ⊕ ⊕ ⓜ ⊘
**Fees:** £36–45; Second visit: £21–30
Maresfield TN22
01825 761768

**Adrian Cobb GCC, BCA**
⊕ ⊕ ⓦ ⊘ Ⓔ ✿
**Fees:** <£25; Second visit: £21–30
Nyetimber PO21
01243 268787

**Duncan Frewen GCC, BCA**
⊕ O ⊕ Ⓔ ✿
**Fees:** £26–35; Second visit: <£20
Rye TN31,Cranbrook TN17
01797 252123

**Steve Rudd GCC, BCA**
⊕ O ⊕ ⓜ ⊘ ✿
**Fees:** £46–55; Second visit: £31–40
Uckfield TN22
01825 713457

**Bernadette Martin GCC, BAAC**
O ⓜ ⊘ ✿
**Fees:** <£25; Second visit: <£20
Worthing BN11
01903 520050

**Jan Nymark Olsen GCC, BCA**
⊕ ⊕ ⓜ ⊘ Ⓔ ✿
**Fees:** £46–55; Second visit: £21–30
Worthing BN11
01903 230066

## BERKSHIRE

**L Wood MNIMH**
⊕ O ⊕
**Fees:** £36–45; Second visit: £21–30
Ascot SL5
020 8446 6320

**M U Adejumo MNIMH**
O
**Fees:** £26–35; Second visit: <£20
Maidenhead SL6
01628 778121

**Christine J Alder MNIMH**
O ⊕ ❀
**Fees:** £26–35; Second visit: £21–30
Reading RG7
0118 971 3009

**David Potterton MNIMH**
O ⊕
**Fees:** £26–35; Second visit: £21–30
Reading RG31
0118 945 4040

**L Bostock MNIMH**
O ⊕ ⊕ ❀
**Fees:** <£25; Second visit: <£20
Slough SL1
01753 791566

## BUCKINGHAMSHIRE

**S K Bradshaw MNIMH**
⊕ ⊕ ⊕ ❀
**Fees:** £26–35; Second visit: £21–30
Aylesbury HP21
01296 425363

**Daniel Coaten MNIMH**
⊕ ⊕ ❀
**Fees:** £26–35; Second visit: <£20
Aylesbury HP22
01296 614163

**Susan T Jamieson IRCH**
⊕ ⊕ ⊕ ⊕ ⊘ ❀
**Fees:** £26–35; Second visit: £21–30
Buckingham MK18,
Barton Hartshome
01280 816397

## DORSET

**S J Fursey MNIMH**
⊕ O ⊕ ⊕ ❀
**Fees:** £36–45; Second visit: £21–30
Bournemouth BH10, Bournemouth
BH5, Lymington SO41
01202 531501

**E Gallia MNIMH**
O ⊕ ❀
Dorchester DT2
01300 341750

**F H James MNIMH,**
⊕ ⊕ ⊘ ❀
**Fees:** £46–55; Second visit: £21–30
Dorchester DT1
01305 262626

**C Reynolds MNIMH**
O ⊕ ⊘
**Fees:** £26–35; Second visit: <£20
Lyme Regis DT7
01297 443814

**A Cowling MNIMH**
O ⊕ Ⓔ ❀
**Fees:** £26–35; Second visit: <£20
Portland DT5,Hailsham BN27
01305 860611

**S Nelson MNIMH**
O ⊕
Sherborne DT9
01963 220172

**Linda Harrold IRCH**
⊕ ⊕ ❀
**Fees:** £36–45; Second visit: <£20
Wimborne BH21
01202 888272

## HAMPSHIRE

**S Startup MNIMH**
O ⊕ Ⓔ
**Fees:** £26–35; Second visit: <£20
Andover SP11,Hailsham BN27
01264 771212

**S Mariscotti MNIMH**
O ❀
**Fees:** £26–35; Second visit: £21–30
Bordon GU35
01420 475872

# Western Herbal Medicine

**S J L Taylor MNIMH**
⊕ ⊕ ⊛ Ⓔ
**Fees:** £26–35; Second visit: £21–30
Emsworth PO10
01243 378555

**L Bird MNIMH**
Fareham PO15
01329 822657

**D N Oliver MNIMH**
O ⊛ Ⓔ ❀
**Fees:** £26–35; Second visit: £21–30
Fleet GU52
01252 626427

**Sandra Hillawi AMH**
⊕ O ⊛ ❀
**Fees:** £26–35; Second visit: £21–30
Gosport PO12,Winchester SO23
023 9243 3928

**Mahmood D Chaudhry IRCH**
⊕ O ⊛ ⊘ ❀
**Fees:** £46–55; Second visit: <£20
Havant PO9
023 9247 1781

**A Armstrong MNIMH**
⊕ O ⊕ ❀
**Fees:** £26–35; Second visit: <£20
Overton RG25
01256 773155

**I S Johnstone MNIMH**
⊕
**Fees:** £26–35; Second visit: £21–30
Winchester SO23
01962 851951

**D Leibbrandt MNIMH**
⊕ ⊛ Ⓔ ❀
**Fees:** £26–35; Second visit: <£20
Winchester SO23,Hailsham BN27
01962 851951

## HERTFORDSHIRE

**Melanie Cardwell AMH**
⊕ O ❀
Bishops Stortford CM23, London W13,
Bishop's Stortford CM23
07947 381520

**Ian Coughlin MNIMH**
O ⊛ Ⓔ ❀
**Fees:** £36–45; Second visit: £31–40
Hitchin SG5
01462 457551

**L Duffy MNIMH**
O ⊘ Ⓔ ❀
**Fees:** £36–45; Second visit: £21–30
Potters Bar EN6
01707 850176

**K Watson MNIMH**
O ⊕ ⊛ Ⓔ ❀
**Fees:** £36–45; Second visit: £21–30
Rickmansworth WD3
01923 772060

**G Wright MNIMH**
❀
**Fees:** £26–35; Second visit: £21–30
St Albans AL1,Near Polegate
01727 858243

**A Haldeos MNIMH**
⊕ O ❀
**Fees:** £26–35; Second visit: <£20
Waltham Cross EN8
01992 301470

**M Barton MNIMH**
O ⊛ ⊘ ❀
**Fees:** £26–35; Second visit: £21–30
Welwyn AL6
01438 716733

## KENT

**P Evans MNIMH**
⊕ ⊕ ⊛ Ⓔ ❀
**Fees:** £36–45; Second visit: £21–30
Canterbury CT1,Folkestone CT20
01227 471771

**M A Muirhead MNIMH**
O ⊕ ❀
**Fees:** £26–35; Second visit: <£20
Canterbury CT3
01227 720971

**V Ridley MNIMH**
⊕ ⊕ ⊛ ⊘ Ⓔ ❀
**Fees:** £26–35; Second visit: <£20
Canterbury CT4
01227 720952

**Amanda Oliver MNIMH**
✚ ⊕ ✿
Fees: £26–35; Second visit: <£20
Faversham ME13
01795 591337

**S J Entwisle MNIMH**
O Ⓔ ✿
Fees: £36–45; Second visit: £21–30
Maidstone ME14
01622 762003

**M C Wagner MNIMH**
✚ ⊕ ⊘
Fees: £26–35; Second visit: £21–30
Tonbridge TN38, Surbiton KT6
01424 422011

**D Benjamin MNIMH**
✚ O ⊕ Ⓔ
Fees: £26–35
Tonbridge TN10, Exeter EX4
01732 355868

**L Kimber MNIMH**
O ⊕ ⓝ ✿
Fees: £26–35; Second visit: <£20
Tonbridge TN11
01732 352206

**M Bergmann MNIMH,**
⊕ ⓝ ⊘ Ⓔ ✿
Fees: >£55; Second visit: £31–40
Tunbridge Wells TN2
01892 552940

**P Conway MNIMH**
✚ ⊕ ⓝ ⊘ ✿
Fees: £36–45; Second visit: £31–40
Tunbridge Wells TN1
01892 544783

**S E Tosoni MNIMH**
✚ ⊕ ✿
Fees: £36–45; Second visit: £21–30
Tunbridge Wells TN1
01892 510950

**Anita Ralph MNIMH**
✚ ⊕ ⓝ ✿
Fees: £36–45; Second visit: £21–30
West Malling ME19, Canterbury CT1
01732 871818

**C Wasik MNIMH**
✚ ⊕ ⓝ Ⓔ ✿
Fees: £36–45; Second visit: £21–30
West Malling ME19
01732 871818

**Graeme J Litchfield IRCH**
O ⓝ ✿
Fees: £46–55; Second visit: £21–30
Westerham TN16
01959 577240

**B A Murray MNIMH**
✚ O ⊕
Fees: £26–35; Second visit: <£20
Whitstable CT5
01227 772918

## NORTHAMPTONSHIRE

**R M Barnes MNIMH**
O ✿
Fees: <£25; Second visit: <£20
Northampton NN1
01604 231735

## OXFORDSHIRE

**K Mehrabi MNIMH**
✚ ⊕ ⊘ Ⓔ ✿
Fees: £36–45; Second visit: £21–30
Abingdon OX14
01235 523336

**R Evans MNIMH**
✚ ⊕ ⓝ ✿
Fees: £26–35; Second visit: <£20
Banbury OX16
01295 265293

**F Taylor MNIMH**
✚ ⊕ ⊕ ⓝ
Fees: £36–45; Second visit: £31–40
Banbury OX15
01295 738609

**S M Strachan MNIMH**
O ⓝ Ⓔ ✿
Fees: £26–35; Second visit: £21–30
Charlbury OX7, Hailsham BN27
01608 811185

# Western Herbal Medicine

**L Derrington MNIMH**
⊕ ⊕ ⊛ ⊘ Ⓔ
**Fees:** £26–35; Second visit: <£20
Oxford OX3,Reading RG1
01865 768156

**N Manston MNIMH**
O ⊕ ❀
**Fees:** £36–45; Second visit: £21–30
Oxford OX33
01865 875854

**A McIntyre MNIMH**
⊕
**Fees:** £36–45; Second visit: £21–30
Oxford OX7
01993 830419

**R C Young MNIMH**
⊕ ⊕ Ⓔ ❀
**Fees:** £26–35; Second visit: £21–30
Oxford OX2
01865 200365

## SURREY

**Binh Thien Phung MNIMH**
O ⊕
**Fees:** <£25; Second visit: <£20
Farnham GU9
01252 726868

**C Galloway MNIMH**
⊕ ⊕ ⊛ Ⓔ ❀
**Fees:** £26–35; Second visit: £21–30
Godalming GU7,Enfield EN3
01483 428537

**N Harding MNIMH**
⊕ ⊛
**Fees:** £36–45; Second visit: £21–30
Godalming GU7
01483 418103

**I Mirza MNIMH**
⊕ O ⊕ ❀
**Fees:** £36–45; Second visit: <£20
Guildford GU22
01483 771821

**E L Shannon MNIMH**
⊛ ❀
Malden KT3
020 8715 4749

**C Getty MNIMH**
⊕
**Fees:** £26–35; Second visit: £21–30
Stoneleigh KT17
020 8646 4024

**J Wharam MNIMH**
O ⊛ ❀
**Fees:** £36–45; Second visit: £31–40
Woking GU21
01483 721355

## SUSSEX

**J Behrens MNIMH**
⊕ O ⊕
**Fees:** £26–35; Second visit: £21–30
Brighton BN2
01273 600143

**J J White MNIMH**
⊕ O ⊕ ❀
**Fees:** £26–35; Second visit: <£20
Battle TN33
01424 777151

**F M Campbell-Atkinson MNIMH**
⊕ ⊕ ⊕ ⊘ ❀
**Fees:** £26–35; Second visit: £21–30
Bexhill-on-Sea TN40
01424 210237

**J Bowerman MNIMH**
⊕ ⊕ ⊛ ⊘
**Fees:** £46–55; Second visit: £31–40
Brighton BN1
01273 324790

**Hera Jonas MNIMH**
⊕ O ⊕ ⊕ ❀
**Fees:** £26–35; Second visit: <£20
Brighton BN1
01273 516456

**A Wright MNIMH**
O ⊕ ⊕ ⊛ ❀
**Fees:** £26–35; Second visit: <£20
Burwash TN19
01435 882751

**Afifah Hamilton MNIMH**
O ⊛ Ⓔ ❀
**Fees:** £26–35; Second visit: <£20
Chichester PO19, Hailsham BN27
01243 776555

**Gina Carrington AMH**
O 🔵 ⊘
**Fees:** £26–35; Second visit: <£20
Chichester PO20
01243 641145

**D B Caudwell MNIMH**
🟢 🔵 🟤
**Fees:** £26–35; Second visit: £21–30
Durgates, Wadhurst TN5
01892 783027

**H C Boys MNIMH**
🟢 🔵 🔵 ⓒ 🟤
**Fees:** £36–45; Second visit: <£20
Eastbourne BN20
01323 734664

**Kelly Holden AMH**
🟢 🔵 🔵 🟤
**Fees:** >£55; Second visit: £31–40
Forest Row RH18
01342 826899

**J Postlethwaite MNIMH**
🟢 O 🔵 🔵 🟤
**Fees:** £26–35; Second visit: £21–30
Hastings TN34
01424 465050

**Samantha Stille MNIMH**
🟢 🔵 🟤
**Fees:** £26–35; Second visit: £21–30
Haywards Heath RH16
01444 456699

**Toria Horner MNIMH**
🟢 ⓒ
**Fees:** £26–35; Second visit: <£20
Herstmonceux BN27
01323 832426

**A J Spicer MNIMH**
🟢
**Fees:** £26–35; Second visit: <£20
Herstmonceux BN27
01323 832426

**Julian Barker MNIMH**
🟢 🔵 🔵 🟤
**Fees:** £26–35; Second visit: <£20
Hove BN3
01273 324420

**Diana Mantripp MNIMH**
🟢 🔵
**Fees:** £26–35; Second visit: £21–30
Hove BN3
01273 324420

**K Murden MNIMH**
🟢 🔵
**Fees:** £26–35; Second visit: £21–30
Lewes BN7,Hove BN3
01273 474428

**Frances B Hambly MNIMH**
🟢 🔵 🔵 🟤
**Fees:** £36–45; Second visit: £21–30
Wadhurst TN5
01727 852992

**D L Jones MNIMH**
🟢 O 🔵 🟤
**Fees:** £26–35; Second visit: £21–30
Wadhurst TN5
01892 783027

## Chinese Herbal Medicine

**BERKSHIRE**

**Katie Scampton RCHM**
🟢 O 🔵 🟤
**Fees:** £36–45; Second visit: £31–40
Ascot SL5,London SE14
01344 620174

**Judith Clark RCHM**
🟢 O 🔵
**Fees:** £36–45; Second visit: <£20
Reading RG1
0118 950 8880

# Chinese Herbal Medicine

**John Hicks RCHM**
✪ ✪
**Fees:** £26–35; Second visit: £21–30
Reading RG1
0118 950 8880

## BUCKINGHAMSHIRE

**David Reynolds RCHM**
✪ ✪ ⊛ ⊘ ✿
**Fees:** £36–45; Second visit: <£20
Marlow SL7
01628 476443

## DORSET

**Frances Mason RCHM**
✪ ✪ ✪ ⊛ ⊘ ✿
**Fees:** £36–45; Second visit: £21–30
Broadstone BH18
01202 692493

**Dianne Stewart RCHM**
✪ ✪ © ✿
**Fees:** £26–35; Second visit: £21–30
Canterbury CT1, Hythe CT21,
Ashford TN24
01227 454404

**Anthony Booker RCHM**
✪ ✪ ✿
**Fees:** £36–45; Second visit: £21–30
Dartford DA2
07966 474722

**Renate Blacker RCHM**
✪ ✪ ⊛ ✿
**Fees:** £26–35; Second visit: £21–30
Gravesend DA13
01474 812135

**John Gavin RCHM**
✪ ✪ ✪ ⊛ ✿
**Fees:** £26–35; Second visit: £21–30
Maidstone ME18
01622 812736

**Gillian Allsop RCHM**
✪ O ✪
**Fees:** £26–35; Second visit: £21–30
Sevenoaks TN14
01959 525995

**Yanhua Yin RCHM**
✪ ⊛ ✿
**Fees:** £26–35; Second visit: £21–30
Sevenoaks TN13,Orpington BR6
01732 458810

**Andrew Gordon RCHM**
✪ O ✪ ✪ ⊛ ✿
**Fees:** £26–35; Second visit: £31–40
Tonbridge TN2

**Deirdre Parrinder RCHM**
✪ O ✪ © ✿
**Fees:**  Second visit: £21–30
Tonbridge TN19,London SE14
01580 861269

**Terry Simou RCHM**
✪ O ✪ ⊛ ✿
**Fees:** £46–55; Second visit: >£50
Tonbridge TN19
01580 860234

**Ulla Johari RCHM**
O ✿
**Fees:** £26–35; Second visit: £21–30
Wareham BH20
01929 400 581**KENT**

## HAMPSHIRE

**Caroline Mountford RCHM**
✪ ✪ ⊛ ✿
**Fees:** £46–55; Second visit: £21–30
Basingstoke RG21
01256 479500

**Hua Shang RCHM**
✪ ✪ ⊛ ✿
**Fees:** <£25; Second visit: <£20
Portsmouth PO2, Southampton SO14
023 9267 0800

**Xiao Yang Zhang RCHM**
✪ ✪ ⊛ ✿
**Fees:** £36–45; Second visit: £31–40
Southampton SO15
023 8022 2214

**Qing Zhang RCHM**
✪ ✪ ⊛ ⊘ ✿
**Fees:** <£25
Southampton SO15
023 8022 2214

**Ruolin Sun RCHM**
🜨 ⊕ ⊕ 🌑 ⊘ ❖
Fees: £46–55; Second visit: £31–40
Winchester SO22
01962 856310

### HERTFORDSHIRE

**Melvyn Epstein RCHM**
🜨 O ⊕ 🌑 ❖
Fees: £36–45; Second visit: £31–40
Berkhamsted HP4
01442 863430

**Martin Silliton RCHM**
🜨 ⊕ 🌑 ⊘ ❖
Fees: £26–35; Second visit: £21–30
Hemel Hempstead HP1
01442 249080

**Ming Xie RCHM**
🜨 ❖
Hertford SG14
01992 536888

**Helen Thomas RCHM**
🜨 O ⊕ 🌑 ❖
Fees: £26–35; Second visit: £21–30
St Albans AL1
01727 860737

**Jethro Rowland RCHM**
🜨 O ⊕ ❖
Fees: £26–35; Second visit: £21–30
Stevenage SG4
01462 440762

### ISLE OF WIGHT

**Thierry March MNIMH, RCHM**
🜨 ⊕ ❖
Fees: £26–35; Second visit: £21–30
Ryde PO33
01983 812711

### MILTON KEYNES

**Maxwell Naiken RCHM**
🜨 ⊕ ⊘ ❖
Fees: £26–35; Second visit: £21–30
Milton Keynes MK3, Bedford MK40,
Southall UB1
01908 366957

### NORTHAMPTONSHIRE

**Stephen Lee RCHM**
O 🌑 ❖
Fees: £26–35; Second visit: <£20
Northampton NN1
01604 717585

### OXFORDSHIRE

**A Lyon MNIMH, RCHM**
🜨 ⊕
Fees: £26–35; Second visit: <£20
Oxford OX4
07968 339032

**Louanne Richards RCHM**
O
Fees: £26–35; Second visit: £21–30
Oxford OX1
01865 727671

### SURREY

**Soui King Lau RCHM**
🜨 O ⊕ 🌑 ⊘ ❖
Fees: Second visit: £21–30
Camberley GU15
01276 469888

**M Faure-Alderson MNIMH, RCHM**
O ⊕ 🌑 ⊘ ❖
Fees: £36–45; Second visit: £31–40
East Molesey KT8
020 8398 6942

**Louise Baker RCHM**
O ⊘ ❖
Fees: £26–35; Second visit: <£20
Guildford GU29
01730 810737

**Richard Cross RCHM**
🜨 🌑 ❖
Fees: £26–35; Second visit: £21–30
Oxted RH8
01883 714036

**Andrew Sordyl RCHM**
🜨 O ⊕ 🌑 ❖
Fees: £36–45; Second visit: £31–40
Dorking RH4, Leatherhead KT24,
Walton-on-Thames KT12
01306 742150

# Chinese Herbal Medicine

## SUSSEX

### Mei Rong Chen RCHM
⊕ ⓝ ✿
**Fees:** <£25; Second visit: <£20
Brighton BN2
01273 699852

### Timothy Martin RCHM
⊕ ○ ⊕ ⓝ
**Fees:** £36–45; Second visit: £21–30
Brighton BN11
01903 821248

### Guo Yao Yu RCHM
⊕ ⓝ ✿
**Fees:** <£25; Second visit: <£20
Eastbourne BN21
01323 727238

### Francesca Diebschlag RCHM
○
**Fees:** £46–55; Second visit: £31–40
East Grinstead RH19
01342 313973

### Tim Haines RCHM
⊕
**Fees:** £36–45; Second visit: £21–30
East Grinstead RH18
01342 823053

### Isobel Staynes RCHM
⊕ ⊕ ✿
**Fees:** £46–55; Second visit: £31–40
Haywards Heath RH16
01444 441210

### Mazin Al-Khafaji RCHM
⊕ ⊕ ⊕ ⓝ
**Fees:** £26–35; Second visit: <£20
Hove BN3
01273 776499

### Deborah Ridley RCHM
⊕ ○ ⊕ ⓝ ✿
**Fees:** £26–35; Second visit: £21–30
Southwick BN42,Horsham
RH12,Horsham RH13
01273 596560

# South West

Bristol
Cornwall
Devon
Gloucestershire
Somerset
Wiltshire

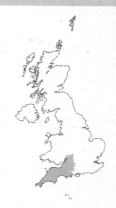

## Acupuncture

### BRISTOL

**Karen Alexander BAcC**
⊙ 🌐 ✱ 🔵
Fees: £26–35; Second visit: £21–30
Bristol BS40
01761 462022

**Lynne Cornelius BAcC**
⊙ ✱ 🔵
Fees: >£55; Second visit: £31–40
Bristol BS6
0117 942 3813

**Louise Dodds AACP**
⊕ ⊘ 🔵
Fees: £26–35; Second visit: £31–40
Bristol BS32
01454 618525

**Kangnian Dong BAcC**
⊙ ⊕ 🌐 ✱ 🔵
Fees: £36–45; Second visit: £31–40
Bristol BS8
0117 973 4594

**M J Downs-Wheeler AACP**
⊕ ⊕ ✱ 🔵
Fees: £26–35; Second visit: £21–30
Bristol BS16
0117 975 3858

**Heather Falconer BAcC**
⊙ ⊕ 🌐
Fees: <£25; Second visit: £21–30
Bristol BS5
0117 965 8694

**Helen Fielding BAcC**
⊕ ⊕ 🌐 ✱ 🔵
Fees: £36–45; Second visit: £21–30
Bristol BS8,London SE1,Bristol BS6
0117 946 6035

**David Gaunt BAcC**
⊙ ⊕ ⊕ Ⓔ ✱ 🔵
Fees: £26–35; Second visit: £21–30
Bristol BS3,Bristol BS16
0117 9774853

**Richard Gibbons BAcC**
⊙ ⊕ ⊕ ✱ 🔵
Fees: £26–35; Second visit: £21–30
Bristol BS7
0117 944 4448

**Suzanne Gibson AACP**
⊕ ⊕ ⊘ ✱ 🔵
Fees: £36–45; Second visit: £21–30
Bristol BS6
0117 9804022

# Acupuncture

Anthony Harcourt BAcC
⊕ ⊘
**Fees:** £26–35; Second visit: £21–30
Bristol BS37
01454 326256

Anthony Harrison BAcC
⊕ ⊕ 🌸 😊
**Fees:** £26–35; Second visit: £21–30
Bristol BS6
0117 974 1199

Martin Harvey BAcC
O 🌐 🌸 😊
**Fees:** £36–45; Second visit: £21–30
Bristol BS7
0117 908 7250

Kate Henderson BAcC
O 🌸 😊
**Fees:** £26–35; Second visit: £21–30
Bristol BS3
0117 963 5676

Qiuyu Huang BAcC
O 🌐 ⊘ 🌸 😊
**Fees:** <£25; Second visit: <£20
Bristol BS6
0117 942 7467

Avis Lane-Willaw BAcC
⊕ ⊕ 🌸 😊
**Fees:** £26–35; Second visit: £21–30
Bristol BS7
0117 944 4448

Brendagh O'Sullivan BAcC
⊕ O ⊕ 🌸 😊
**Fees:** £36–45; Second visit: £21–30
Bristol BS41,Bristol BS6
01275 394425

Alan Papier BAcC
O ⊕ 🌸 😊
**Fees:** £26–35; Second visit: £21–30
Bristol BS6
0117 907 7737

Annie D V Plessis BAcC
⊕ ⊕ 🌸 😊
**Fees:** £36–45; Second visit: £21–30
Bristol BS6
0117 974 1199

Lynne Pretty BAcC
⊕ 😊
**Fees:** >£55; Second visit: £21–30
Bristol BS6
0117 924 1727

Malai Sontheimer BAcC
O 😊
**Fees:** £26–35; Second visit: £21–30
Bristol BS3
0117 953 7219

Caroline Williams BAcC
⊕ 🌸 😊
**Fees:** £26–35; Second visit: £21–30
Bristol BS7
0117 944 3173

Li Jing Zhou BAcC
⊕ 🌸 😊
**Fees:** £26–35; Second visit: £21–30
Bristol BS1
0117 929 8588

Zara Ford GOsC, BOA
⊕ ⊕ 😊 ⊘ ⓒ 🌸
**Fees:** £26–35; Second visit: £31–40
Bristol BS20
01275 818303

## CORNWALL

Sally Ann Patterson AACP
O 😊 ⊘ 😊
**Fees:** £36–45; Second visit: £21–30
Liskeard PL14
07890 152939

Peter Hall BAcC
⊕ O ⊕ 😊 🌸 😊
**Fees:** £26–35; Second visit: <£20
Penryn TR10
01209 861511

Kate Wilson BAcC
⊕ O ⊕ 😊
**Fees:** £36–45; Second visit: £21–30
Penzance TR19
01736 810394

Steve Todd BAcC
⊕ O ⊕ 🌸 😊
**Fees:** £26–35; Second visit: £21–30
Perranporth TR6
01872 573123

**Claire Berncastle AACP**

Fees: £36–45; Second visit: £31–40
Torpoint PL11
01503 240622

**Reg D'souza BAcC, AACP**

Fees: £46–55; Second visit: £21–30
Truro TR1
01872 241882

**Candy McLeavy BAcC**

Fees: £36–45; Second visit: £21–30
Truro TR1
01872 263163

---

**DEVON**

**Nigel De Salengre BAcC**

Fees: £36–45; Second visit: £21–30
Barnstaple EX31
01271 373346

**Christine Haines BAcC**

Fees: £26–35; Second visit: £21–30
Barnstaple
01271 373346

**R MacDonald BAcC**

Fees: <£25; Second visit: <£20
Bideford EX39
01237 475023

**Peter Hands BAcC**

Fees: <£25; Second visit: <£20
Dawlish EX7
01626 863256

**Robin Costello BAcC**

Fees: £26–35; Second visit: £21–30
Exeter EX4,Ascot SL5
01392 424276

**Jennie Dallas BAcC**

Fees: £26–35; Second visit: £21–30
Exeter EX4
01392 217422

**Simon King BAcC**

Fees: £26–35; Second visit: £21–30
Exeter EX4
01392 217422

**Catherine Mudge BAcC**

Fees: £26–35; Second visit: £21–30
Exeter EX2
01392 832956

**Iris Robinson BAcC**

Fees: £26–35; Second visit: £21–30
Exeter EX2
01392 433365

**Richard Walters BAcC**

Fees: £36–45; Second visit: £21–30
Exeter EX1
01392 499364

**Fiona Matthews BAcC**

Fees: £26–35; Second visit: £21–30
Ivybridge PL21
01752 895401

**John Dice BAcC**

Fees: £26–35; Second visit: £21–30
Newton Abbot TQ12
01626 334433

**Kim Maidment BAcC**

Fees: £26–35; Second visit: £21–30
Paignton TQ3
01803 525019

**Michael Clements BAcC**

Fees: £36–45; Second visit: £21–30
Plymouth PL4
01752 672709

**Kim Lay Im BAcC**

Fees: <£25; Second visit: <£20
Plymouth PL4
01752 227841

# Acupuncture

**Kevin S Robins BAcC**
O ⊕ ✿ 🌐
Fees: £26–35; Second visit: £21–30
Plymouth PL4
01752 298834

**R D Eccles BAcC**
⊕ ⊕ ✿ 🌐
Fees: £26–35; Second visit: £21–30
Plymouth PL3,Kingsbridge TQ7,South
Brent TQ10
01803 732458

**Michael Chapman BAcC, AACP**
⊕ ⊕ ⊕ ✿ 🌐
Fees: £26–35; Second visit: £21–30
Sidmouth EX10
01395 578656

**Valerie Ann Davis BAcC**
⊕ O ⊕ ✿ 🌐
Fees: £26–35; Second visit: £21–30
Sidmouth EX10
01395 578050

**Roger Hill BAcC**
⊕ ⊕ ⓔ 🌐
Fees: £46–55; Second visit: £21–30
South Molton EX36
01769 572608

**Alan Brown BAcC**
O 🌐
Fees: <£25; Second visit: £21–30
Torquay TQ2
01803 329006

**Nicholas Clarke BAcC**
O ✿ 🌐
Fees: <£25; Second visit: <£20
Torquay TQ1
01803 297009

**Ruth Ann Gardener BAcC**
⊕ 🌐
Fees: £26–35; Second visit: £21–30
Torquay TQ1
01803 293346

**Lisa Bright BAcC**
⊕ ⊕ 🌐
Fees: £26–35; Second visit: £21–30
Totnes TQ9
01803 863872

**Stephen Hopwood BAcC,**
⊕ O ⊘ ✿ 🌐
Fees: £26–35; Second visit: £21–30
Totnes TQ9
01803 868282

**Marcus Mason BAcC**
⊕ ⊕ 🌐
Fees: £36–45; Second visit: £21–30
Totnes TQ9
07977 429321

**Michael Potter BAcC**
⊕ ⊕ ✿ 🌐
Fees: £26–35; Second visit: £21–30
Totnes TQ9
01803 863270

**Patricia Price BAcC**
O ⊕ 🌐 ✿ 🌐
Fees: £26–35; Second visit: £21–30
Totnes TQ9,Paignton TQ3
01803 865541

## GLOUCESTERSHIRE

**Edward Mander Lilac BAcC**
⊕ ⊕ ✿ 🌐
Fees: £36–45; Second visit: £21–30
Brockworth GL3
01242 261896

**Sylvia Apperly BAcC**
⊕ ⊕ ⊕ ⊘ 🌐
Fees: £26–35; Second visit: £21–30
Cheltenham GL52
07931 308562

**Daniel Blyth BAcC**
⊕ ⊕ ⊘ ✿ 🌐
Fees: £26–35; Second visit: £21–30
Cheltenham GL50
01242 241933

**Nicola Ellis AACP**
O ✿ 🌐
Fees: £26–35; Second visit: £31–40
Cheltenham GL53
01242 252252

**Caroline Hencher BAcC**
O ✿ 🌐
Fees: £36–45; Second visit: £21–30
Cheltenham GL52
01242 572406

**Mark Lester BAcC**
⊕ ⊕ ⊜ ❖ ⊜
**Fees:** £26–35; Second visit: £21–30
Cheltenham GL52
01242 238095

**Lucy Townsend AACP**
⊕ ❖ ⊜
**Fees:** £26–35
Cheltenham GL54
01451 831370

**Gwynne Tucker Brown AACP**
⊕ ❖ ⊜
**Fees:** £26–35; Second visit: £31–40
Cheltenham GL53
01242 228019

**Linda Upton BAcC**
⊕ ⊕ ⊜
**Fees:** £46–55; Second visit: £21–30
Cheltenham GL50
01242 584140

**Carol Thompson AACP**
O ⊘ ⊜
**Fees:** £36–45; Second visit: £31–40
Fairford GL7
01285 712123

**Jamie Gisby BAcC**
⊕ ⊕ ⊕ ⊜ ❖ ⊜
**Fees:** £36–45; Second visit: £21–30
Gloucester GL1
01452 505550

**Julian Kingscote BAcC**
⊕ ⊕ ⊕ ❖ ⊜
**Fees:** £36–45; Second visit: £21–30
Gloucester GL1
01452 505550

**Anthony Norton BAcC**
⊕ ⊕ ⊜ ⊜
**Fees:** £36–45; Second visit: £21–30
Gloucester GL19
01452 700306

**Colin Rogers BAcC**
⊕ ⊕ ❖ ⊜
**Fees:** £36–45; Second visit: £21–30
Gloucester GL1
01452 505550

**Vicki Brown BAcC**
⊕ ⊕ ⊘ ⊜
**Fees:** £36–45; Second visit: £21–30
Moreton-in-Marsh GL56
01608 652875

**Christina Edwards BAcC**
⊕ O ⊕ ⊘ ❖ ⊜
**Fees:** £36–45; Second visit: £21–30
Moreton-in-Marsh GL56
01608 650077

**David Smyth BAcC**
⊕ O ⊕ ❖ ⊜
**Fees:** £36–45; Second visit: £21–30
Ruardean GL17
01594 860169

**Andrew R Amer BAcC**
⊕ ⊕ ❖ ⊜
**Fees:** £26–35; Second visit: £21–30
Stroud GL5
01453 759444

**Susanne Boyd BAcC**
⊕ ⊜ ❖ ⊜
**Fees:** £26–35; Second visit: £21–30
Stroud GL5
01453 886868

**Movdeh Danesh BAcC**
O ❖
**Fees:** >£55; Second visit: >£50
Stroud GL5
01453 872334

**Sarah Parker BAcC**
⊕ ⊕ ❖ ⊜
**Fees:** £46–55; Second visit: £21–30
Stroud GL6
01453 836066

**Kim Wells BAcC**
⊕ ❖ ⊜
**Fees:** £26–35; Second visit: £21–30
Stroud GL5,London N8
01453 750796

**Meriel Darby BAcC**
⊕ ⊕ ⊜ ⊜
**Fees:** £26–35; Second visit: £21–30
Tewkesbury GL20
01380 725461

# Acupuncture

## SOMERSET

**Chris Binning BAcC**
✪ ⭕ 🆖 ✿ 🔄
Fees: £26–35; Second visit: £21–30
Weston-super-Mare BS22
01934 517913

**Yun Yan Zhou BAcC**
✪ 🔄 ⊘ 🔄
Fees: £26–35; Second visit: £21–30
Bath BA1
01225 483393

**Alex Jane Holloway BAcC**
✪ 🔄 ✿ 🔄
Fees: £36–45; Second visit: £21–30
Axbridge BS26
01934 750518

**Tamara Ashcroft-Nowicki BAcC**
✪ 🔄 ⊘ ✿ 🔄
Fees: £36–45; Second visit: £21–30
Bath
01225 466271

**Barbara Pickett BAcC**
⭕ ✪ 🔄 ✿ 🔄
Fees: £36–45; Second visit: £21–30
Bath BA2
01225 837171

**Damin Wan BAcC**
✪ Ⓒ ✿ 🔄
Fees: £26–35; Second visit: £31–40
Bath BA2
01225 337778

**Gisela Norman BAcC**
✪ 🔄 🆖 ✿ 🔄
Fees: £36–45; Second visit: £21–30
Bristol BS3
0117 983 8528

**Wendy Booth BAcC**
⭕ ✿ 🔄
Fees: £26–35; Second visit: £21–30
Cheddar BS27
01934 744481

**K Gardner AACP**
✪ ✪ 🔄 🆖 ✿ 🔄
Fees: £36–45; Second visit: £21–30
Cheddar BS27
01934 744574

**Hugh Tripp BAcC**
✪ 🔄 🔄
Fees: £36–45; Second visit: £21–30
Glastonbury BA6
01458 830080

**Topsey Mason AACP**
✪ ⭕ ⊘ ✿ 🔄
Fees: £36–45; Second visit: £31–40
Langport TA10
01963 220246

**Henry Bizon BAcC**
✪ 🔄 ✿ 🔄
Fees: £36–45; Second visit: £21–30
Taunton TA1
01823 271066

**Helen Hartnell AACP**
✪ 🔄 🆖 ⊘ 🔄
Fees: £36–45; Second visit: £21–30
Taunton TA2
01823 333355

**Allan Johnstone BAcC**
✪ ⭕ ✿ 🔄
Fees: £36–45; Second visit: £31–40
Taunton TA4
01984 656692

**Joseph Mo BAcC**
⭕ 🆖 ✿ 🔄
Fees: £26–35; Second visit: £21–30
Taunton TA2
01823 334143

**Robert Parnell BAcC**
✪ ⭕ 🔄 🆖 ✿ 🔄
Fees: £26–35; Second visit: £21–30
Wells BA5, Bristol BS3
01749 679014

**Richard Bertschinger BAcC**
✪ ✪ 🆖 ⊘ Ⓒ 🔄
Fees: £46–55; Second visit: £21–30
Yeovil BA21
01935 422488

**Lesley Jenkins BAcC**
✪ ⭕ 🔄 🆖 🔄
Fees: £46–55; Second visit: £21–30
Yeovil BA21
01935 422488

## WILTSHIRE

**Sue Bishop BAcC**
⊕ ⊕ ❊ ⊜
Fees: £46–55; Second visit: £21–30
Devizes SN10
01350 730042

**Jane Ford BAcC**
⊕ ⊜
Fees: £36–45; Second visit: £21–30
Devizes SN10
01380 730042

**Gaynor Maxwell-Scott BAcC**
⊕ ❊ ⊜
Fees: £36–45; Second visit: £21–30
Devizes SN10
01380 727101

**Hazel Andrews BAcC**
O ⊕ ❊ ⊜
Fees: £36–45; Second visit: £31–40
Swindon SN3
01793 827507

**Julia Bliss BAcC**
⊕ O ⊕ ❊ ⊜
Fees: £36–45; Second visit: £21–30
Swindon SN1
01793 512267

**Janice Booth BAcC**
⊕ O ⊕ ⓝ ❊ ⊜
Fees: £36–45; Second visit: £21–30
Swindon SN1
01793 465630

**Carole Dale BAcC**
O ❊ ⊜
Fees: £36–45; Second visit: £21–30
Swindon SN1
01793 642832

**Jeannie Willis BAcC**
⊕ ⊕ ❊ ⊜
Fees: £36–45; Second visit: £21–30
Swindon SN4
01793 855266

**Keith Murray BAcC**
⊕ ⊕ ❊ ⊜
Fees: £26–35; Second visit: £21–30
Bradford-on-Avon BA15
01225 868282

**Theresa Parr AACP**
O ⊕ ⓝ ⊘ ❊ ⊜
Fees: £26–35; Second visit: £21–30
Chippenham SN14
01249 463612

**Altair De Almeida BAcC**
⊕ ⊕ ⓝ ⊜
Fees: £36–45; Second visit: £21–30
Malvern WR14
01684 562528

**Paul Hougham BAcC**
⊕ ❊ ⊜
Fees: £46–55; Second visit: £31–40
Malvern WR14
01684 569704

**Salvador March BAcC**
⊕ ❊ ⊜
Fees: £46–55; Second visit: £21–30
Malvern WR14
01684 892023

**Jennie Sheringham BAcC**
⊕ ⊕ ❊ ⊜
Fees: £36–45; Second visit: £21–30
Malvern WR14
01684 565586

**Kenneth C Smith BAcC**
⊕ ⊘ ❊ ⊜
Fees: £26–35; Second visit: £21–30
Malvern WR14
01684 568744

**Guy Tomlinson BAcC**
⊕ ⊜
Fees: £36–45; Second visit: £21–30
Malvern WR14
01684 893238

**Katy Mitchell AACP**
⊕ ❊ ⊜
Fees: £36–45; Second visit: £21–30
Salisbury SP2
01722 336262

**Will Richardson BAcC, BMAS, AACP**
⊕ ⊕ ⓝ ⊜
Fees: £36–45; Second visit: £31–40
Salisbury SP2
01722 741314

# Acupuncture

**Russ Chapman BAcC**
⊕ ⊕ ⊛ ✿ ⊛
Fees: £36–45; Second visit: £21–30
Trowbridge BA14
01225 777456

**Pauline French BAcC**
⊕ ⊛ ✿ ⊛
Fees: £36–45; Second visit: £21–30
Warminster BA12, Salisbury SP2,
Salisbury SP3
01985 213927

# Homeopathy

## BRISTOL

**Lyn Clark RSHom**
⊕ ⚪ ⊛ ⊛ © ✿
Fees: £36–45; Second visit: £20–30
Bristol BS7
0117 944 5542

**Tony Conway RSHom**
⊕ ⚪ ⊛ ✿
Fees: £46–55; Second visit: £31–40
Bristol BS6
01458 440136

**Gosia Gray RSHom**
⊕ ⚪ ⊛ ⊛ © ✿
Fees: £46–55; Second visit: £20–30
Bristol BS6
0117 974 5084

**Leslie Harris RSHom**
⚪ ⊕ ⊛ ⊛ © ✿
Fees: £46–55; Second visit: £20–30
Bristol BS16
0117 902 8484

**Clare Long RSHom**
⊕ ⚪ ⊛ © ✿
Fees: £46–55; Second visit: £20–30
Bristol BS6
0117 942 9744

**A Maendl MFHom**
⚪ ⊕ ⊛ ⊛ ⊘ ✿
Fees: £36–45; Second visit: £20–30
Bristol BS9
0117 9626060

**Diane Murray RSHom**
⊕ ⊛ ⊛ ✿
Fees: >£55; Second visit: £31–40
Bristol BS8
0117 946 6035

**Daphne Nancholas RSHom**
⚪ ⊛ ©
Fees: £46–55; Second visit: £20–30
Bristol BS3
0117 966 0393

**Nicola Rowntree RSHom**
⊕ ⚪ ⊛ ✿
Fees: >£55; Second visit: £31–40
Bristol BS20,Bristol BS6,Bristol BS4
01275 818083

**David Spence MFHom**
⊛ ⊘
Bristol BS6
0117 973 1231

**Penelope Stirling RSHom**
⊕ ⚪ ⊛ ⊛ ✿
Fees: >£55; Second visit: £31–40
Bristol BS8
0117 927 3205

**Nigel Summerley RSHom**
⊕ ⊛ ⊛ ⊘ © ✿
Fees: £36–45; Second visit: £20–30
Bristol BS20
01275 818303

**Jane Whitehead RSHom**
⊕ ⚪ ⊛ ⊛ © ✿
Fees: £46–55; Second visit: £20–30
Bristol BS3
0117 963 6267

## CORNWALL

**Anne Clover FFHom,**
⊛ ⊘
Fees: £36–45; Second visit: £20–30
Falmouth TR11
01326 374996

**Bill Watson RSHom**
❂ O ⊕ ⊕ ⓦ Ⓔ ❧
**Fees:** >£55; Second visit: £20–30
Falmouth TR11
01326 241284

**Gill Dransfield RSHom**
O ⓦ Ⓔ
**Fees:** £36–45; Second visit: £20–30
Luxulyan PL30
01726 852367

**David Heap RSHom**
O ⓦ
**Fees:** £46–55; Second visit: £20–30
Newquay TR7
01637 873353

**Fiona D'Alwis RSHOm**
❂ O ⊕ ⓦ Ⓔ ❧
**Fees:** £36–45; Second visit: £20–30
Penzance TR18
01736 788547

**Mark Sullivan MFHom**
❂ ⊕ ⓦ Ⓔ ❧
**Fees:** >£55; Second visit: £20–30
Truro TR1
01872 273133

**Linda Wicks RSHom**
❂ O ⊕ ⓦ Ⓔ ❧
**Fees:** £36–45; Second visit: £20–30
Truro TR1, Redruth TR15
01872 240585

### DEVON

**Paul Nelson RSHom**
⊕ ⊕ ⓦ Ⓔ ❧
**Fees:** £36–45; Second visit: £20–30
Barnstaple EX32
01598 710010

**Carole Welch RSHom**
O ⓦ Ⓔ ❧
**Fees:** £36–45; Second visit: £20–30
Bideford EX39
01237 470847

**Barbara Povah RSHom**
O ⓦ Ⓔ
**Fees:** £25–35; Second visit: £20–30
Cullompton EX15
01823 680619

**Sandra Dean RSHom**
O ⓦ ❧
**Fees:** £36–45; Second visit: £20–30
Exeter EX2
01392 218968

**Pili Goss RSHom**
O ⓦ Ⓔ ❧
**Fees:** £36–45; Second visit: £20–30
Exeter EX4
01392 465342

**Lorna Hall RSHom**
❂ O ⊕ ⓦ Ⓔ ❧
**Fees:** £36–45; Second visit: £20–30
Exeter EX4
01392 425743

**Janine Jackson-Bruce RSHom**
O ⓦ ❧
**Fees:** £25–35; Second visit: <£20
Exeter EX1
01392 254354

**Marie Lloyd RSHom**
❂ O ⊕ ⓦ ⊘ Ⓔ
**Fees:** £36–45; Second visit: £20–30
Exeter EX2
01392 256348

**Antonia Maks RSHom**
O ⓦ Ⓔ ❧
**Fees:** £36–45; Second visit: £20–30
Exeter EX4
01392 490052

**Alison Morrish RSHom**
❂ ⊕ ⓦ ⊘ Ⓔ ❧
**Fees:** £46–55; Second visit: £31–40
Exeter EX1
01392 214074

**Margaret Ruth Eames MFHom**
O ⓦ ⊘ Ⓔ ❧
**Fees:** £25–35; Second visit: <£20
Ilfracombe EX34
01271 882427

**Dorothy West MFHom**
O ⓦ ⊘
**Fees:** £46–55; Second visit: £20–30
Ivybridge PL21
01752 892792

# Homeopathy

**Rod Holcombe MFHom**
⊕ ⊕ ⦿ ⊘ Ⓔ
**Fees:** £36–45; Second visit: £20–30
Kingsbridge TQ7
01548 853248

**Virginia Sykes RSHom**
⊕ ⊕ ⦿ Ⓔ ❀
**Fees:** £36–45; Second visit: £20–30
Newton Abbot TQ12
01626 334514

**Jayne Hill RSHom**
⊕ O ⊕ Ⓔ ❀
**Fees:** £36–45; Second visit: £20–30
Okehampton EX20,Exmouth
EX8,Newton Abbot TQ13
01837 54246

**Helen Swan RSHom**
⊕ ⊕ ⦿ Ⓔ ❀
**Fees:** £25–35; Second visit: £20–30
Paignton TQ4
01803 522889

**Serena Scrine RSHom**
⊕ ⊕ ⊘
Plymouth PL9
01752 401172

**Gordon Summers RSHom**
⊕ ⊕ ⊕ ⦿ Ⓔ ❀
**Fees:** £36–45; Second visit: £20–30
Plymouth PL3,Totnes TQ9,London N16
01803 732728

**Susanna Terry RSHom**
⊕ O ⊕ ⦿ Ⓔ
**Fees:** £46–55; Second visit: £20–30
Plymouth PL6
01837 840718

**Michael Hart MFHom**
⊕ O ⊕ ⦿ ⊘
**Fees:** £46–55; Second visit: £20–30
South Brent TQ10
01364 72440

**Nicholas Burton-Taylor RSHom**
⊕ O ⊕ ⦿ ⊘ Ⓔ ❀
**Fees:** £46–55; Second visit: £31–40
Tavistock PL19
01364 73721

**Andrew Terry RSHom**
⊕ O ⊕ ⦿ Ⓔ ❀
**Fees:** £46–55; Second visit: £20–30
Tavistock PL19
01837 840718

**Jane Hurley RSHom**
O
**Fees:** £46–55; Second visit: £31–40
Teignmouth TQ14
01626 770063

**Jeanne Harris RSHom**
⊕ ⊕ ⦿ Ⓔ
**Fees:** £36–45; Second visit: £20–30
Tiverton EX16, Barnstaple EX31
01884 256691

**Jennie Swan RSHom**
O Ⓔ ❀
**Fees:** £36–45; Second visit: £20–30
Torrington EX38
01805 623730

**Ursula Athene RSHom**
O ⊕ ⦿ Ⓔ ❀
**Fees:** £36–45; Second visit: £20–30
Totnes TQ9
01803 865955

**Christopher Gethin RSHom**
⊕ O ⊕ ⦿ Ⓔ
**Fees:** £46–55; Second visit: £31–40
Totnes TQ9,Newton Abbot TQ13
01364 652207

**Aileen Knapp RSHom**
O ⦿ Ⓔ
**Fees:** £25–35; Second visit: £20–30
Totnes TQ9
01803 866925

## GLOUCESTERSHIRE

**Karen Byers RSHom**
⊕ O ⊕ ⦿ ❀
**Fees:** £46–55; Second visit: £20–30
Cheltenham GL50
01242 238958

**Chloe Keef RSHom**
⊕ ⊕ ⦿ ❀
**Fees:** £46–55; Second visit: £20–30
Cheltenham GL50
01242 584140

**Patricia Moroney RSHom**
✛ O ⊕ ⓝ ⓔ ✿
Fees: £36–45; Second visit: £31–40
Cheltenham GL50,Stroud GL6,
Hightown L38
01452 812347

**Robert Nichols RSHom**
O ⓝ ⓔ ✿
Fees: £46–55; Second visit: £31–40
Gloucester GL50
01242 520704

**Gwenyth Mafham RSHom**
O ⊕ ⓝ ⓔ
Fees: £46–55; Second visit: £20–30
Moreton In Marsh GL56,Leamington
Spa CV31
01608 664537

**Kathlyn Drewett MFHom**
⊘
Newent GL18
01531 820689

**Peter Adams RSHom**
✛ ⊕ ⓝ ⓔ
Fees: >£55; Second visit: £20–30
Stroud GL5
01453 750796

**Hazel Rank-Broadley RSHom**
✛ O ⊕ ⓝ ✿
Fees: £46–55; Second visit: £20–30
Stroud GL5,Malmesbury SN16
01453 765985

**Polly Howell RSHom**
✛ O ⊕ ⓝ ⓔ
Fees: £36–45; Second visit: £20–30
Tetbury GL8, Bristol BS37
01666 503500

**Jill Peacey RSHom**
✛ ⊕ ⊕ ⓝ ⊘ ⓔ ✿
Fees: £36–45; Second visit: £20–30
Tetbury GL8
01666 503089

## SOMERSET

**Audrey Pearson MFHom**
O ⓝ ⓔ
Fees: £46–55; Second visit: <£20
Bath BA1
01225 858293

**Richard Napper RSHom**
✛ O ⊕ ⊕ ⓝ ⓔ ✿
Fees: £46–55; Second visit: £31–40
Bath BA1,Newport NP20,Cheddar
BS27
01225 460106

**Janet Snowdon RSHom**
✛ ⊕ ⓝ ⓔ
Fees: £46–55; Second visit: £31–40
Bath BA1
01225 337147

**Judith Mistral RSHom**
O ⓝ ⓔ
Fees: £46–55; Second visit: £20–30
Frome BA11
01373 463368

**Wendy Heath RSHom**
✛ O ⊕ ⓝ ⓔ ✿
Fees: £46–55; Second visit: £20–30
Clevedon BS21,Bristol BS6,Bristol BS2
01275 879706

**Gillian C How MFHom**
✛ ⊕ ⓝ
Fees: >£55; Second visit: £41–50
Clevedon BS21
01275 335533

**June Swainson RSHom**
O ⓔ ✿
Fees: £36–45; Second visit: £20–30
Clevedon BS21
01275 872162

**Karen Leadbeater RSHom**
O ⊕ ⊕ ⊘ ✿
Fees: £36–45; Second visit: £20–30
Bath BA1
01225 338687

**Mabel Smith RSHom**
O ⓔ ✿
Fees: £36–45; Second visit: £20–30
Bath BA2
01225 837363

# Homeopathy

**Ian Wiles MFHom**
🌀 ⊘
Bath BA2
01225 464187

**Alan Harvey RSHom**
🌀 O ⊕ ⊕ 🌀 🄴
Fees: >£55; Second visit: £31–40
Chard TA20, Honiton EX14, Ilminster
TA19
01460 63644

**Elizabeth Edleston RSHom**
🌀 O ⊕ 🌀 🄴
Fees: £36–45; Second visit: £20–30
Crewkerne TA18
01460 77990

**Gareth Morgan MFHom**
🌀 O ⊕ 🌀 ⊘
Fees: £46–55; Second visit: £31–40
Dulverton TA22, Taunton TA1
01398 323054

**Rita Tremain RSHom**
🌀 O ⊕ ⊕ 🌀 ⊘
Fees: £36–45; Second visit: £20–30
Dunster TA24, Minehead TA24
01643 821087

**Philip Jackson MFHom**
⊕ ⊘
Fees: £25–35; Second visit: <£20
Glastonbury BA6
01458 850594

**Roy Welford MFHom**
🌀 ⊕ ⊕ 🌀 ⊘
Fees: £46–55; Second visit: £20–30
Glastonbury BA6, Yeovil BA21, Bristol
BS6
01458 834100

**Judith Harold RSHom**
🌀 O ⊕ ⊕ 🌀 🄴
Fees: £25–35; Second visit: <£20
Horton TA19
01460 53013

**Dee Robertson RSHom**
O ⊕ 🌀 ⊘ 🄴 ✿
Fees: £46–55; Second visit: £20–30
Ilminster TA19
01460 52924

**Jeremy Swayne FFHom,**
⊕ 🌀 ⊘ 🄴
Fees: >£55; Second visit: £20–30
Shepton Mallet BA4
01749 860662

**Rowena Doble RSHom**
🌀 O ⊕ 🌀 🄴 ✿
Fees: £46–55; Second visit: £31–40
Somerton TA11
01458 850046

**Rebecca Hobbs MFHom**
⊘
Fees: >£55; Second visit: £31–40
Taunton TA4, Taunton TA1
01984 618237

**Nabeeh Marar RSHom**
🌀 ⊕ 🌀 ✿
Fees: £46–55; Second visit: £20–30
Taunton TA1
01823 272227

**Richard Savage MFHom**
🌀 O 🌀 ⊘
Fees: £46–55; Second visit: £20–30
Taunton TA1
01823 286251

**Phyllis Travell RSHom**
🌀 O ⊕ 🌀 ⊘ 🄴 ✿
Fees: £25–35; Second visit: <£20
Wellington TA21
01823 663836

**Anthony Bickley RSHom**
🌀 ⊕ 🌀
Fees: £46–55; Second visit: £31–40
Yeovil BA21
01935 422488

## WILTSHIRE

**Alison Fixsen RSHom**
🌀 O ⊕ 🌀 🄴 ✿
Fees: £36–45; Second visit: £20–30
Chippenham SN15
01380 850941

**Janet Gray MFHom**
O ⊘
Fees: >£55; Second visit: £20–30
Chippenham SN14
01225 891115

**Cherry Hillier RSHom**
O 🔵 € ✵
Fees: £36–45; Second visit: £20–30
Devizes SN10
01380 860316

**Michael Handford MFHom**
⊕ ⊘ ✵
Fees: >£55; Second visit: <£20
Marlborough SN8
01672 520366

**Vivian Hemery RSHom**
O 🔵 € ✵
Fees: £25–35; Second visit: £20–30
Marlborough SN8
01672 861676

**Pauline Waywell RSHom**
⊕ 🔵 € ✵
Fees: £36–45; Second visit: £20–30
Swindon SN1
01793 465629

**Andrew Ward FFHom, RSHom**
⊕ ⊕ ⊕ 🔵 ⊘ ✵
Fees: £46–55; Second visit: £31–40
Bradford-on-Avon BA15
01225 868282

**Jill Etheridge RSHom**
O ⊕ 🔵 € ✵
Fees: £36–45; Second visit: £20–30
Malvern WR14,Hereford HR2
01684 564266

**Annie Batchelor RSHom**
O 🔵 € ✵
Fees: £46–55; Second visit: £20–30
Salisbury SP1
01722 504747

**Marcus Christo RSHom**
⊕ 🔵 ✵
Fees: £36–45; Second visit: £20–30
Salisbury SP1,Warminster BA12
01722 411998

**John Michael English FFHom,**
O 🔵 €
Fees: >£55; Second visit: £20–30
Salisbury SP1
01722 410416

**Sheila Brewis RSHom**
⊕ 🔵 ⊘
Fees: £36–45; Second visit: £20–30
Trowbridge BA14
01373 834757

**Henrietta Wells RSHom**
🔵
Fees: £46–55; Second visit: £20–30
Warminster BA12
01985 850551

# Osteopathy

**BRISTOL**

**Ceridwen Bloor GOsC**
⊕ O 🔵
Fees: <£25; Second visit: £21–30
Bristol BS8
0117 929 3913

**Jeni Briggs GOsC**
⊕ 🔵
Fees: £26–35; Second visit: £31–40
Bristol BS3
0117 923 1138

**Juliana Cram GOsC**
⊕ ⊕ ⊕ 🔵 ⊘ ✵
Fees: £26–35; Second visit: £21–30
Bristol BS6
0117 973 0490

**C T Davis GOsC, BOA**
⊕ ⊕ 🔵
Fees: £26–35; Second visit: £21–30
Bristol BS6
0117 974 4313

# Osteopathy

**Ellen Hart GOsC**
⊕ O ⊕ ⊛ ✿
**Fees:** <£25; Second visit: £21–30
Bristol BS6
0117 924 9353

**Martin Matthews GOsC**
⊕ ⊛ ✿
**Fees:** <£25; Second visit: £21–30
Bristol BS6
0117 923 2802

**J H Thompson GOsC, BOA**
⊕ ⊛ ⊘
**Fees:** <£25; Second visit: £31–40
Bristol BS8
0117 927 2100

**Hugh Vickers GOsC, BOA**
⊕ ⊕ ⊛ ⓔ ✿
**Fees:** <£25; Second visit: £21–30
Bristol BS34
01454 610767

**Katherine Bench GOsC**
⊕ ⊕ ⊛ ⊘
**Fees:** £26–35; Second visit: £21–30
Bristol BS3
0117 966 9724

**Jocelyn Drew GOsC, BOA**
⊕ O ⊕ ⊛ ✿
**Fees:** £26–35; Second visit: £31–40
Bristol BS9
0117 938 5107

**A Harcourt GOsC, BOA**
⊕ ⊛
**Fees:** <£25; Second visit: £21–30
Bristol BS37
01454 326256

**Cheryl A Jones GOsC**
⊕ ⊕ ⊛
**Fees:** <£25; Second visit: £21–30
Bristol BS6
0117 974 1199

**David Richardson GOsC, BOA**
⊕ ⊛ ✿
**Fees:** £26–35; Second visit: £21–30
Bristol BS1
0117 922 7788

**Gabrielle Waldron GOsC**
⊕ ⊕ ⊛ ⊘ ✿
**Fees:** <£25; Second visit: £31–40
Bristol BS16
0117 949 1290

**Rebecca Winsor GOsC**
⊕ ⊕ ⊛ ⓔ
**Fees:** £26–35; Second visit: £21–30
Cotham BS6
0117 944 1793

**Giles Cleghorn GOsC**
⊕ ⊕ ⊛
**Fees:** £36–45; Second visit: £21–30
Redland BS6
0117 974 5084

**Nicholas Hounsfield GOsC, BOA**
⊕ ⊕ ⊛ ⊘ ✿
**Fees:** £26–35; Second visit: £21–30
Redland BS6
0117 974 5084

**Clare Ballard GOsC**
⊕ O ⊛
**Fees:** £26–35; Second visit: £21–30
St Andrews BS6
0117 942 1206

**Monika Wiesenthal GOsC, BOA**
O ⊛ ✿
**Fees:** £26–35; Second visit: £21–30
Stockwood BS14
01275 830241

**Mark Morgan GOsC**
⊕ ⊛ ✿
**Fees:** £26–35; Second visit: £21–30
Westbury-on-Trym BS10
0117 959 2000

## CORNWALL

**Nicola J Halse GOsC**
O ⊛
**Fees:** <£25; Second visit: £21–30
Bude EX23
01840 230032

**Deborah J Weatherhogg GOsC**
O ✿
**Fees:** <£25; Second visit: <£20
Bude EX23
01288 355692

**Rachael Hilliard GOsC**
⊕ ⦿ ✸
**Fees:** £26–35; Second visit: £21–30
Camborne TR14
01209 612197

**Matthew Brierley GOsC, BOA**
⊕ ⦿ ⊘ ✸
**Fees:** <£25; Second visit: <£20
Falmouth TR11
01326 312466

**Alistair M Tatton GOsC**
O ⦿
**Fees:** <£25; Second visit: <£20
Falmouth TR11
01326 319440

**Duncan Scobie GOsC, BOA**
⊕ ⦿ ✸
**Fees:** £26–35; Second visit: £21–30
Helston TR13
01326 563022

**David Wells GOsC, BOA**
⊕ ⊕
**Fees:** £26–35; Second visit: £21–30
Launceston PL15
01566 775005

**A E Banbury GOsC, BOA**
O ⊕ ⦿ ✸
**Fees:** <£25; Second visit: £21–30
Liskeard PL14
01579 342273

**Kathryn West GOsC**
⊕ ⦿ ✸
**Fees:** £26–35; Second visit: £21–30
Newquay TR7
01637 878645

**Jonathan Gore GOsC, BOA**
⊕ ⊕ ⦿ ✸
**Fees:** <£25; Second visit: £21–30
Redruth TR15
01209 712397

**Paul Keilbart GOsC**
O ⦿ ⓔ ✸
**Fees:** £26–35; Second visit: £21–30
St Austell PL25
01726 67788

**Nicholas Hilliard GOsC, BOA**
⊕ ⦿ ✸
**Fees:** £26–35; Second visit: £21–30
Truro TR26
01209 612197

**Jonathan Wills GOsC**
O ⦿ ✸
**Fees:** <£25; Second visit: £31–40
Truro TR1
01872 222701

**David A R Cormack GOsC, BOA**
⊕ ⦿
**Fees:** £26–35; Second visit: £21–30
Wadebridge PL27
01208 812048

## DEVON

**Alanna Bayley GOsC, BOA**
⊕ ⊕ ⦿ ✸
**Fees:** £36–45; Second visit: £21–30
Barnstaple EX31
01271 373346

**Lisa Flynn GOsC**
⊕ ⦿ ✸
**Fees:** <£25; Second visit: £21–30
Barnstaple EX32
01271 376456

**Coralie Foxwell GOsC, BOA**
⊕ ⊕ ⊕ ⦿
**Fees:** <£25; Second visit: <£20
Barnstaple EX31
01271 345546

**Nigel de Salengre GOsC**
⊕ ⊕ ⊕ ⦿
**Fees:** £36–45; Second visit: £21–30
Barnstaple EX31
01271 373346

**Peter Spencer GOsC,**
⊕ ⊕ ⊘
**Fees:** £36–45; Second visit: £21–30
Barnstaple EX31
01271 373346

**Robert Wheeler GOsC, BOA**
O ⦿ ✸
**Fees:** <£25; Second visit: £21–30
Braunton EX33
01271 814087

# Osteopathy

**B Ruth Swinney GOsC**
⊕ O ⊕ ⊛
**Fees:** <£25; Second visit: £31–40
Brixham TQ5
01803 850518

**Louis Bartlett GOsC, BOA**
⊕ ⊕ ⊛ ⓒ ⊛
**Fees:** £26–35; Second visit: £21–30
Crediton EX17
01363 774175

**Louise Ellison GOsC**
O ⊕ ⊛ ⊛
**Fees:** <£25; Second visit: <£20
Dartmouth TQ6
01803 835196

**Peter Hands GOsC, BOA**
⊕ ⊛ ⊘ ⊛
**Fees:** £26–35; Second visit: £21–30
Dawlish EX7
01626 863256

**Colin Crewdson GOsC, BOA**
⊕ ⊕ ⊛ ⓒ ⊛
**Fees:** £26–35; Second visit: £21–30
Exeter EX4
01392 221321

**Jane Dickson GOsC, BOA**
O ⊛
**Fees:** <£25; Second visit: <£20
Exeter EX4
01392 279761

**Warwick Downes GOsC, BOA**
⊕
**Fees:** <£25; Second visit: £31–40
Exeter EX4
01392 221321

**Paul Fillery GOsC, BOA**
⊕ ⊕ ⊛
**Fees:** £26–35; Second visit: £21–30
Exeter EX1
01392 410549

**Jennifer Hooper GOsC**
O ⊕ ⊕ ⊛ ⊛
**Fees:** <£25; Second visit: <£20
Exeter EX2
01392 427757

**Mary Riddle GOsC, BOA**
⊕ ⊛ ⊘ ⊛
**Fees:** £26–35; Second visit: £21–30
Exeter EX1
01392 273243

**Paul Thompson GOsC**
⊕ ⊛ ⊛
**Fees:** £26–35; Second visit: £21–30
Exeter EX4
01392 221321

**Colin Wayman GOsC, BOA**
O ⊛
**Fees:** <£25; Second visit: <£20
Exeter EX4
01392 279761

**Andrea Jackson GOsC, BOA**
⊕ O ⓒ ⊛
**Fees:** £26–35; Second visit: £21–30
Exmouth EX8
01395 270303

**Anthony C Smith GOsC, BOA**
⊕ ⊛
**Fees:** <£25; Second visit: £21–30
Exmouth EX8
01395 222666

**David Wasserman GOsC**
⊕ ⊕ ⊛ ⓒ
**Fees:** <£25; Second visit: £21–30
Holsworthy EX22
01409 254410

**Hannah Stewart GOsC, BOA**
⊕
**Fees:** <£25; Second visit: £21–30
Honiton EX14
01404 42023

**Michael Harris GOsC, BOA**
⊕ ⊛
**Fees:** £26–35; Second visit: £21–30
Ivybridge PL21
01752 896116

**Donald Graham A Moody GOsC**
⊕ ⊕ ⊛ ⊛
**Fees:** £26–35; Second visit: £21–30
Ivybridge PL21
01752 893253

**Sarah Bunting GOsC**
O ⓝ
Fees: £26–35; Second visit: £21–30
Modbury PL21, South Brent TQ10
01548 830849

**Peter J Baker GOsC, BOA,**
⊕ O ⓖ ⓝ Ⓔ ❁
Fees: <£25; Second visit: £21–30
Newton Abbot TQ12
01626 205400

**L Hopkins GOsC, BOA**
O ⓝ ❁
Fees: <£25; Second visit: £21–30
Newton Abbot TQ13
01364 652585

**Julia Young GOsC, BOA**
⊕ ⓝ
Fees: <£25; Second visit: <£20
Okehampton EX20
01837 55516

**Cherry Harris GOsC, BOA**
⊕
Fees: £36–45; Second visit: £21–30
Paignton TQ4
01803 527091

**Lynette Taylor GOsC**
O ⓝ ⊘ ❁
Fees: <£25; Second visit: <£20
Paignton TQ4
01803 556789

**Michael Bruce GOsC, BOA**
⊕ ⓝ ⊘ ❁
Fees: <£25; Second visit: £31–40
Plymouth PL7
01752 347663

**Alison Cameron GOsC, BOA**
⊕ ⓝ Ⓔ
Fees: <£25; Second visit: £21–30
Plymouth PL4
01752 223518

**Michael Hopkins GOsC, BOA,**
O ⊕ ⓝ ⊘
Fees: £26–35; Second visit: £21–30
Plymouth PL3
01752 229674

**James Oldham GOsC**
⊕ ⓖ ⓝ ⊘ ❁
Fees: <£25; Second visit: <£20
Plymouth PL5
07967 321450

**Charles Peers GOsC**
⊕ ⊕ ⓝ ⊘ ❁
Fees: <£25; Second visit: <£20
Plymouth PL1
01752 225567

**Sally Blyth GOsC, BOA**
O ⊕ ⓝ Ⓔ ❁
Fees: £26–35; Second visit: £21–30
Sidmouth EX10
01395 577473

**Donald Blyth GOsC, BOA**
O ⊕ ⓝ Ⓔ ❁
Fees: £26–35; Second visit: £21–30
Sidmouth EX10, Seaton EX12
01395 577473

**Barry Lonergan GOsC, BOA**
O ⓝ
Fees: <£25; Second visit: £31–40
Sidmouth EX10
01395 516845

**Penelope Price GOsC**
⊕ O ⓖ ⓝ ❁
Fees: £26–35; Second visit: £21–30
Sidmouth EX10
01395 578082

**Christian Chemin GOsC**
O ⓝ Ⓔ
Fees: £26–35; Second visit: £31–40
South Brent TQ10
01364 642790

**E A Ellison GOsC, BOA**
⊕ ⓖ ⓝ Ⓔ ❁
Fees: <£25; Second visit: <£20
South Brent TQ10
01364 73149

**Rebecca Popplewell GOsC, BOA**
O ⓖ ⓝ ❁
Fees: £26–35; Second visit: £21–30
South Molton EX36
01769 574830

# Osteopathy

**Amanda Coleshill GOsC, BOA**
⊕ ⊕ ⓝ ⊘ ✿
**Fees:** <£25; Second visit: £21–30
Tavistock PL19
01822 616103

**Philip Hartnoll GOsC**
○ ⊕ ⓝ ✿
**Fees:** £26–35; Second visit: £21–30
Tavistock PL19
01822 614814

**Alexander Evans GOsC**
⊕ ⊕ ⊕ ⓝ
**Fees:** <£25; Second visit: <£20
Teignmouth TQ14
01626 773222

**Sonia Mistely GOsC**
⊕ ⓝ Ⓔ
**Fees:** <£25; Second visit: £21–30
Teignmouth TQ14
01626 773339

**Harvey Fudge GOsC, BOA**
⊕ ⊕ ⊕ ⓝ ✿
**Fees:** <£25; Second visit: £21–30
Tiverton EX16
01884 258570

**Alan Brown GOsC**
○
**Fees:** £26–35; Second visit: £21–30
Torquay TQ2
01803 329006

**Victoria Latchem GOsC**
○ ⓝ ⊘ Ⓔ ✿
**Fees:** <£25; Second visit: £21–30
Totnes TQ9
01803 865356

**Jonathan Parker GOsC**
○ ⓝ ✿
**Fees:** <£25; Second visit: <£20
Totnes TQ9
01803 865841

## GLOUCESTERSHIRE

**Steven W Davies GOsC**
⊕ ⊕ ⓝ ✿
**Fees:** <£25; Second visit: £21–30
Cheltenham GL52
01242 574311

**Mark Lester GOsC**
⊕ ⓝ ✿
**Fees:** <£25; Second visit: £21–30
Cheltenham GL52
01242 238095

**Sarah Stevens GOsC**
⊕ ○ ⊕ ⓝ ⊘ Ⓔ
**Fees:** £36–45; Second visit: £21–30
Cheltenham GL52
01242 674607

**Clive Hayden GOsC, BOA**
⊕ ⊕ ⓝ ⊘
**Fees:** £46–55; Second visit: £21–30
Churchdown GL3
01452 714511

**Kathy Drake GOsC, BOA**
⊕ ○ ⊕ ⓝ ✿
**Fees:** £26–35; Second visit: £21–30
Cirencester GL7
01285 656393

**Rupert Peter Hanbury GOsC, BOA**
⊕ ⓝ ⊘ ✿
**Fees:** <£25; Second visit: £21–30
Cirencester GL7
01285 643958

**Martin Holding GOsC**
⊕ ⊕ ⓝ ✿
**Fees:** £36–45; Second visit: £21–30
Cirencester GL7, Windsor SL4
01285 659214

**James Martin GOsC, BOA**
⊕ ⊕ ⓝ ⊘ ✿
**Fees:** £26–35; Second visit: £31–40
Cirencester GL7, Swindon SN6
01285 643958

**Meg McDonald GOsC**
⊕ ⊕ ⓝ ✿
**Fees:** £36–45; Second visit: £21–30
Cirencester GL7
01285 643958

**Elizabeth Kendal GOsC**
⊕ ○ ⊕ ⓝ ⊘
**Fees:** £36–45; Second visit: £21–30
Gloucester GL1
01452 308799

**Clare Pitman GOsC**
Fees: £36–45; Second visit: £21–30
Gloucester GL3
01452 714511

**Caroline A Tash GOsC, BOA**
Fees: <£25; Second visit: £21–30
Gloucester GL2
01452 740818

**Rebecca Orchard GOsC**
Fees: £26–35; Second visit: £21–30
Hardwicke GL2
01452 722135

**Marianne Bennison GOsC**
Fees: £26–35; Second visit: £21–30
Lechlade GL7
01367 252264

**Mary O'Leary GOsC, BOA**
Fees: £26–35; Second visit: £31–40
Lechlade GL7
01367 252264

**Christopher Parsons GOsC, BO**
Fees: £46–55; Second visit: >£50
Mitcheldean GL17
01594 544566

**Hector Wells GOsC, BOA**
Fees: £26–35; Second visit: £31–40
Moreton-in-Marsh GL56
01608 652252

**Michael Rumney GOsC, BOA**
Fees: <£25; Second visit: £21–30
Stroud GL5
01453 750796

**Sarah Spencer Chapman GOsC, BOA**
Fees: £26–35; Second visit: £21–30
Stroud GL5
01453 758962

**Heather Stout GOsC, BOA**
Fees: £26–35; Second visit: <£20
Tetbury GL8
01666 502214

**Penny Kavallares GOsC, BOA**
Fees: £36–45; Second visit: £21–30
Tewkesbury GL20
01684 294368

**Michael Lloyd-Jones GOsC**
Fees: £36–45; Second visit: £21–30
Tewkesbury GL20
01684 294368

**Carmel Smythe GOsC**
Fees: <£25; Second visit: £31–40
Tewkesbury GL20
01684 294368

## SOMERSET

**Peter Cockhill GOsC, BOA**
Fees: <£25; Second visit: £21–30
Bath BA1
01225 460106

**Satyen P Gadher GOsC**
Fees: £26–35; Second visit: £21–30
Bath BA1
01225 427835

**Bevis Nathan GOsC, BOA**
Fees: £36–45; Second visit: £31–40
Bath BA1
01225 313153

**Alan O'Toole GOsC**
Fees: £26–35; Second visit: £21–30
Bath BA1
01225 426171

**Martin Sparkes GOsC, BOA**
Fees: £26–35; Second visit: £21–30
Bath BA1
01225 445888

# Osteopathy

**Terence Sutcliffe GOsC**
⊕ ⊕ ⊛ ⊛
**Fees:** £26–35; Second visit: £21–30
Bath BA1
01225 446089

**Belinda Eyers GOsC, BOA**
⊕ ⊛ ⊛
**Fees:** <£25; Second visit: £21–30
Chew Magna BS40
01275 333587

**Rebecca Osborne GOsC**
⊕ ⊛ ⊛
**Fees:** £26–35; Second visit: £21–30
Clevedon BS21,Westbury-on-Trym
BS10
01275 340360

**Andrew Sims GOsC**
⊕ ⊕ ⊕ ⊛ ⊛
**Fees:** £26–35; Second visit: £21–30
Clevedon BS21
01275 874832

**Alexander Prince GOsC**
⊕ ⊕ ⊛ ⊘ ⊛
**Fees:** £26–35; Second visit: £21–30
Portishead BS20
01275 818303

**Lucy Race GOsC, BOA**
⊕ ⊛ ⊘ ⊛
**Fees:** £26–35; Second visit: £21–30
Portishead BS20
01275 818303

**Alison Huxtable GOsC, BOA**
⊕ ⊕ ⊛ ⊛
**Fees:** £36–45; Second visit: £21–30
Weston-super-Mare BS22
01934 419933

**Ian Pitt GOsC**
O ⊛ ⊘ Ⓔ ⊛
**Fees:** £36–45; Second visit: £21–30
Weston-super-Mare BS23
01934 629116

**Peter Everett GOsC, BOA**
⊕ ⊕ ⊛ ⊘ ⊛
**Fees:** <£25; Second visit: £21–30
Winscombe BS25
01934 844764

**Janet White GOsC, BOA**
⊕ ⊛ Ⓔ
**Fees:** £26–35; Second visit: £21–30
Winscombe BS25
01934 843617

**Stephen Woods GOsC, BOA**
⊕ ⊕ ⊛ ⊛
**Fees:** <£25; Second visit: £21–30
Bridgwater TA6
01278 457730

**Andrew Knight GOsC, BOA**
⊕ ⊕ ⊛
**Fees:** £26–35; Second visit: £21–30
Castle Cary BA7
01963 351477

**Elizabeth Price GOsC, BOA**
⊕ ⊕ ⊛
**Fees:** £26–35; Second visit: £21–30
Crewkerne TA18,Bridport DT6
01460 78068

**Sally Welford GOsC, BOA**
⊕ ⊕ ⊕ ⊛ Ⓔ
**Fees:** <£25; Second visit: £31–40
Crewkerne TA18
01460 77990

**Stephen Plumb GOsC**
⊕ ⊘ Ⓔ ⊛
**Fees:** <£25; Second visit: £41–50
Frome BA11
01373 463548

**Alison Bevan GOsC, BOA**
⊕ ⊕ ⊛ ⊛
**Fees:** £26–35; Second visit: £21–30
Minehead TA24,Taunton TA2
01823 333535

**A Trevenen Pascoe GOsC, BOA**
⊕ ⊛ ⊘
**Fees:** <£25; Second visit: £21–30
Shepton Mallet BA4
01749 345259

**Robert Williams GOsC**
O ⊕ ⊛
**Fees:** £26–35; Second visit: £21–30
South Petherton TA13
01460 242490

**David Harrison GOsC, BOA**
⊕ O ⬤ ⊘
Fees: £26–35; Second visit: £21–30
Taunton TA1,Eastcote HA5,Cumbria
LA9
01823 275948

**Sara Kennard GOsC, BOA**
⊕ ⬤
Fees: <£25; Second visit: <£20
Taunton TA1
01823 332871

**Nicole Perret GOsC, BOA**
⊕ ⬤ ⊘
Fees: <£25; Second visit: £31–40
Taunton TA1
01823 444373

**Martha Price GOsC**
⊕ ⬤
Fees: <£25; Second visit: <£20
Taunton TA1
01823 332871

**Philip Walpole GOsC, BOA**
⊕ ⬤ ⬤ ✸
Fees: £26–35; Second visit: £21–30
Taunton TA1
01823 254456

**Richard Campion GOsC, BOA**
O ⬤
Fees: <£25; Second visit: £21–30
Wedmore BS28
01934 712489

**Detlef Campion GOsC, BOA**
O ⊘
Fees: <£25; Second visit: £21–30
Wedmore BS28
01934 712489

**Jennifer Hodgson GOsC**
⊕ ⬤ ⬤ Ⓔ ✸
Fees: <£25; Second visit: £21–30
Wells BA5
01749 679014

**Anthony Bickley GOsC**
⊕ ⬤ ⊘
Fees: £26–35; Second visit: £21–30
Yeovil BA21
01935 422488

**Rachel Cameron GOsC**
O ⬤ ⊘ Ⓔ ✸
Fees: £26–35; Second visit: £21–30
Yeovil BA20
01935 413840

**Elizabeth A Clayton GOsC, BOA**
⊕ ⬤ ⬤ ⊘ ✸
Fees: <£25; Second visit: £21–30
Yeovil BA21
01935 422488

**Lynda Kemp GOsC, BOA**
⬤ Ⓔ ✸
Fees: <£25; Second visit: £21–30
Yeovil BA20
01935 476855

**Kevin Partridge GOsC**
⊕ ⊕ ⬤ ⬤ ⊘ ✸
Fees: £26–35; Second visit: £21–30
Yeovil BA20,Shaftesbury SP7
01935 470804

## WILTSHIRE

**Charlotte Walker GOsC**
⊕ ⊕ ⬤ ⬤
Fees: £26–35; Second visit: £21–30
Devizes SN10
01380 728453

**Caspar W Hull GOsC, BOA**
⊕ ⬤ ⬤ ⊘ Ⓔ ✸
Fees: <£25; Second visit: £31–40
Melksham SN12
01225 704883

**Martin Preston GOsC, BOA**
⊕ ⬤ ⬤ Ⓔ ✸
Fees: £36–45; Second visit: £21–30
Pewsey SN9
01672 564646

**David Brunskill GOsC, BOA**
⊕ ⬤ ⊘
Fees: <£25; Second visit: £21–30
Swindon SN4
01793 848093

**Judith Hayes GOsC**
⊕ O ⬤ Ⓔ ✸
Fees: £26–35; Second visit: <£20
Swindon SN3
01793 432403

# Osteopathy

**Rebecca Hill GOsC, BOA**
✪ ⚪ ⊕ ⓝ ✿
Fees: £36–45; Second visit: £21–30
Swindon SN6,Gloucestershire GL7
01793 750504

**Jolyon Livingston GOsC, BOA**
✪ ⊕ ⓝ ⊘ ⓔ ✿
Fees: £36–45; Second visit: £21–30
Swindon SN6
01793 750504

**Pauline Mather GOsC**
✪ ⊕ ⓝ ⓔ ✿
Fees: <£25; Second visit: £21–30
Swindon SN1
01793 465629

**Joanne Butler GOsC**
✪ ⊕ ⓝ ✿
Fees: <£25; Second visit: £21–30
Bradford-on-Avon BA15
01225 868295

**Christian Sullivan GOsC**
✪ ⊕ ⓝ ⊘ ⓔ ✿
Fees: £26–35; Second visit: £21–30
Bradford-on-Avon BA15
01225 868282

**James Mackie GOsC, BOA**
✪ ⊕ ⓝ
Fees: £26–35; Second visit: £21–30
Fonthill Bishop SP3
01747 820021

**J Barnes GOsC, BOA**
✪ ⓝ ⊘ ⓔ ✿
Fees: £26–35; Second visit: £31–40
Salisbury SP1
01722 414214

**Simon Browning GOsC**
⚪ ⓝ ✿
Fees: £26–35; Second visit: £21–30
Salisbury SP1
01722 331317

**Rhian Watson GOsC**
✪ ⊕ ⊕ ⓝ ⊘ ✿
Fees: £26–35; Second visit: £21–30
Salisbury SP3
01747 820021

**Jonathan Penny GOsC**
✪ ⊕ ⊕ ⓝ ⓔ ✿
Fees: £26–35; Second visit: £21–30
Warminster BA12
01985 213927

# Chiropractic

### BRISTOL

**Jesper Jensen GCC, BCA**
✪ ⓝ ⊜
Fees: <£25; Second visit: £21–30
Bishopston BS7
0117 924 5842

**Christine Andrew GCC, BCA**
✪ ⓝ ✿
Fees: <£25; Second visit: £21–30
Bristol BS6
0117 973 0878

**Alison Archibald GCC, BCA**
✪ ⓝ ✿ ⊜
Fees: £36–45; Second visit: £21–30
Bristol BS8,Taunton TA2
0117 929 8384

**Elizabeth Armstrong GCC, MCA**
⚪ ✿
Fees: £26–35; Second visit: £21–30
Bristol BS6
0117 974 2508

**Louise Bashall GCC, BCA**
✪ ⓝ ✿
Fees: <£25; Second visit: £21–30
Bristol BS6
0117 973 0878

**Emma Brewer GCC, MCA**
✪ ⚪ ⊘ ⓔ ✿
Fees: £26–35; Second visit: £21–30
Bristol BS8
0117 970 6708

**Carol Clothier GCC, BCA**
Fees: £26–35; Second visit: £21–30
Bristol BS8
01453 755799

**Pamela Cronin GCC, BCA**
Fees: £36–45; Second visit: £21–30
Bristol BS35
01454 418259

**Diane Dear GCC, BAAC**
Fees: £26–35; Second visit: £21–30
Bristol BS9
0117 968 1294

**Claire Tanya Gordon GCC, BCA**
Fees: £36–45; Second visit: £21–30
Bristol BS8
01935 423138

**Hugh Hurst GCC, BCA**
Fees: £26–35; Second visit: £21–30
Bristol BS8
0117 974 4217

**Sasha Langman GCC, MCA**
Fees: £26–35; Second visit: £21–30
Bristol BS15
0117 914 5590

**Deborah A Le Roux GCC, BCA**
Fees: £26–35; Second visit: £21–30
Bristol BS48
01275 810296

**Eli Meldgaard GCC, BCA**
Fees: <£25; Second visit: £21–30
Bristol BS7
0117 924 5842

**James Scrimshaw GCC, BCA**
Fees: <£25; Second visit: £21–30
Bristol BS6
0117 942 0200

**Douglas Ingrams GCC, BCA**
Fees: £26–35; Second visit: £21–30
Clifton BS8,Bristol BS16
0117 974 4217

### CORNWALL

**Wayne Whittingham GCC**
Fees: £26–35; Second visit: <£20;
Second visit: £21–30
Hartley PL3
01752 770131

**Kathleen Tomes-Nicholson GCC, BCA**
Fees: £46–55; Second visit: £21–30
Bodmin PL31
01208 78777

**B Masters GCC, BCA**
Fees: £36–45; Second visit: £21–30
Launceston PL15,Launceston PL15
01566 773671

**Andrew Doody GCC**
Fees: £26–35; Second visit: £21–30
Liskeard PL14
01579 340654

**Richard Southam GCC**
Fees: £26–35; Second visit: £21–30
Liskeard PL14
01579 340654

**M Noone GCC, BCA**
Fees: £36–45; Second visit: £21–30
Newquay TR7
01637 878788

**Paul Stick GCC**
Fees: £36–45; Second visit: £21–30
Truro TR1
01872 262899

# Chiropractic

### J C Tillyard-Thomas GCC, MCA
⊕ ✿
**Fees:** £26–35; Second visit: £21–30
St Ives TR26
01736 797272

## DEVON

### Timothy Wallis GCC, BCA
⊕ ⓝ ✿ ⊜
**Fees:** <£25; Second visit: £21–30
Plymouth PL19
01822 616806

### Gavin Perry GCC, BAAC
⊕ ⓝ ⊘ ✿
**Fees:** £26–35; Second visit: £21–30
Plymouth PL25
01726 74347

### Tracy Dixon GCC, BCA
⊕ ⊕ ⓝ ✿ ⊙
**Fees:** £26–35; Second visit: £21–30
Barnstaple EX32
01271 345142

### Sharon L Read-Jones GCC, BCA
⊕ ⊕ ⊕ ⓝ ⊘ ✿
**Fees:** £26–35; Second visit: £21–30
Barnstaple EX32
01271 376776

### Julien Barker GCC, MCA
⊕ O ⓝ ⊘ ✿
**Fees:** £26–35; Second visit: £21–30
Dartmouth TQ6
07855 803260

### Giles T G Jackson GCC, BCA
O ⓝ ⊘ ⊜
**Fees:** £46–55; Second visit: £21–30
Exeter EX4
01392 467438

### Shona Loftus GCC, MCA
⊕ O ⊕ ⓝ ⊘ ✿
**Fees:** £26–35; Second visit: £21–30
Exeter EX4
01392 499115

### Stephen Masters GCC, BCA
⊕ ⊕ ⓝ ⊘ ✿ ⊜
**Fees:** £26–35; Second visit: £21–30
Exeter EX32
01271 345142

### Richard Stenning GCC, BCA
⊕ ⊕ ⓝ ⊘ ©
**Fees:** £26–35; Second visit: £21–30
Exeter EX13,Honiton EX14
01297 35844

### Mark Stone GCC, BCA
⊕ O ⊘ ✿ ⊜
**Fees:** £26–35; Second visit: <£20
Exeter EX31,Ilfracombe
EX31,Ilfracombe EX34
01271 327444

### Una Tracey GCC, MCA
⊕ O ⊕ ⓝ ⊘ © ✿
**Fees:** £26–35; Second visit: £21–30
Exeter EX4
01392 499115

### Andrea Strickland GCC, MCA
O ⓝ ✿
**Fees:** £26–35; Second visit: £21–30
Exmouth EX8
01395 265544

### Melanie Carpenter GCC, BCA
⊕ ⓝ ⊘ ✿ ⊜
**Fees:** <£25; Second visit: <£20
Newton Abbot TQ12
01626 202026

### Julia Verwey GCC, BCA
O ⊕ ⊘ ✿ ⊜
**Fees:** <£25; Second visit: <£20
Newton Abbot TQ12
01626 353334

### Frank Verwey GCC, BCA
⊕ O ⊕ ⊘ ✿ ⊜
**Fees:** <£25; Second visit: <£20
Newton Abbot TQ12
01626 353334

### Robyn Lopes GCC, MCA
⊕ ⊕ ⓝ © ✿
**Fees:** £26–35; Second visit: £21–30
Plymouth PL9
01752 407531

### J Hernandez Silva GCC, BCA
⊕ ⊕ ⓝ ✿ ⊜
**Fees:** £26–35; Second visit: £21–30
Plymouth PL3
01752 770131

# Chiropractic

**George R Walker GCC, BCA**
⊕ Ⓝ ❄ ⬡
**Fees:** £26–35; Second visit: £21–30
Plymouth PL3
01752 607008

**Frank Loftus GCC, MCA**
⊕ ⊕ Ⓝ ❄
**Fees:** £26–35; Second visit: £21–30
South Molton EX36
01769 572608

**Anthony Haslam GCC, BCA**
⊕ Ⓝ ❄ ⬡
**Fees:** Second visit: <£20
Torquay TQ1
01803 292131

**Christine Hourahane GCC, BCA, MCA**
⊕ Ⓝ ⊘
**Fees:** £26–35; Second visit: £21–30
Torquay TQ7
01548 561952

**Graeme Kurvers GCC, BCA**
⊕ Ⓝ
**Fees:** £26–35; Second visit: £21–30
Totnes TQ9
01803 866447

### GLOUCESTERSHIRE

**Teresa Pritchard GCC, MCA**
◯ Ⓝ ❄
**Fees:** £26–35; Second visit: £21–30
Berkeley GL13
01453 811881

**Gabrielle Swait GCC, MCA**
⊕ Ⓝ ⊘ ❄
**Fees:** £26–35; Second visit: £21–30
Gloucester GL52,Tewkesbury GL20
01242 676951

**Joanna Elvey GCC, MCA**
⊕ ⊕ Ⓝ ⊘ ⓔ
**Fees:** £36–45; Second visit: £21–30
Cheltenham GL52,Cheltenham GL51
01242 703901

**Robert Grace GCC, BCA**
⊕ ⊕ ⊘ ❄
**Fees:** <£25; Second visit: £21–30
Cheltenham GL52
01242 222111

**Rita Hemmings GCC, BCA**
⊕ Ⓝ ⓔ ⬡
**Fees:** £36–45; Second visit: £21–30
Cheltenham GL51
01242 513459

**Alison Jane Shaw GCC, BCA**
⊕ Ⓝ ❄
**Fees:** £36–45; Second visit: £21–30
Cheltenham GL50
01242 227440

**Christine Southerton GCC, MCA**
⊕ Ⓝ ❄
**Fees:** £36–45; Second visit: £21–30
Chipping Sodbury BS37
01454 320088

**Stuart Smellie GCC, BCA**
⊕ Ⓝ ⊘ ⬡
**Fees:** £26–35; Second visit: £21–30
Gloucester GL52
01242 252222

**Simon Spearing GCC, MCA**
⊕ ⊕ Ⓝ ⊘ ❄
**Fees:** £26–35; Second visit: £21–30
Cheltenham GL53
01242 263316

**Keith Walker GCC, BCA**
⊕ Ⓝ ⊘ ❄ ⬡
**Fees:** £26–35; Second visit: £21–30
Cheltenham GL50,Warwick CV37
01242 254000

**Dilys Bates GCC, MCA**
◯ Ⓝ ❄
**Fees:** £36–45; Second visit: £21–30
Gloucester GL2
01452 503910

**Irene Bayliss GCC, MCA**
⊕ ⊕ Ⓝ ⊘ ❄
**Fees:** £46–55; Second visit: £21–30
Gloucester GL7
01367 253304

**Charles Cutts GCC, BCA**
⊕ Ⓝ ⊘ ❄ ⬡
**Fees:** <£25; Second visit: £21–30
Gloucester GL1
01452 304386

# Chiropractic

**Alexander Morton GCC, MCA**
⊕ O ⦿ ❀
**Fees:** £26–35; Second visit: £21–30
Gloucester GL18
01531 822772

**Celia Herrmann GCC, MCA**
⊕ O ⊕
**Fees:** £36–45; Second visit: £41–50
Hucclecote GL3,Cheltenham GL50
01452 611854

**Tina Hamer GCC, MCA**
⊕ O ⊕ ⦿ ⊘ ❀
**Fees:** £36–45; Second visit: £21–30
Cheltenham GL53
01242 519019

**Sylvia Hemming GCC, MCA**
O ⊕ ⦿ ❀
**Fees:** £26–35; Second visit: £21–30
Moreton-in-marsh GL56
01608 650077

**Sue Johns GCC, MCA**
⊕ ⊕ ⦿ € ❀
**Fees:** £26–35; Second visit: £21–30
Stroud GL6
01453 836066

**Sunny Fitzpatrick GCC, BAAC, MCA**
⊕ ⦿ € ❀
**Fees:** £26–35; Second visit: £21–30
Gloucester GL54
01451 831654

**David Hubbard GCC, MCA**
⊕ ⊕ ⦿ ⊘
**Fees:** £46–55; Second visit: £21–30
Stroud GL5
01453 759444

**Paul D C Maunsell GCC, MCA**
⊕ O ⊕ ⦿ ❀
**Fees:** £26–35; Second visit: £21–30
Stroud GL5
01453 872229

**Helyn Morris GCC, MCA**
⊕ ⊕ ⦿ €
**Fees:** £26–35; Second visit: £21–30
Stroud GL6
01453 750796

**Lesley Rolfe GCC, MCA**
O ⦿ ❀
**Fees:** £36–45; Second visit: £21–30
Toddington GL54
01242 620429

## SOMERSET

**David Morley GCC, BCA**
⊕ ⦿ ⊘
**Fees:** <£25; Second visit: £21–30
Radstock BA3
01761 411412

**Simon Finemore GCC, BCA**
⊕ ⊕ ⦿ ⊘ ⊜
**Fees:** £36–45; Second visit: £21–30
Bath BA2
01225 484800

**Graham Matthews GCC, BAAC**
⊕
**Fees:** £36–45; Second visit: £21–30
Bath BA2
01225 421328

**G W A Courtis GCC, BCA**
⊕ ⦿ € ❀
**Fees:** £46–55; Second visit: £21–30
Bath BA1
01225 423333

**Peter Dixon GCC, BCA**
⊕ O ⊕ ⦿ ⊘ ❀
**Fees:** £36–45; Second visit: £21–30
Bath BA15
01225 862140

**Christopher Ford Dc GCC, BAAC**
⊕ ⊕ ⦿ € ❀
**Fees:** £36–45; Second visit: £21–30
Bath BA1
01225 421328

**D Marks GCC, BCA**
⊕ ⦿ ❀
**Fees:** £46–55; Second visit: £21–30
Bath BA1
01225 423333

**Anna Goodwin GCC, MCA**
⊕ ⊕ ⦿ ⊘ € ❀
**Fees:** £26–35; Second visit: £21–30
Bath BA15
01225 869208

**Alison Rigby GCC, BCA**
**Fees:** £36–45; Second visit: £21–30
Bath BA9
01963 32986

**David Aberdeen GCC, BCA**
**Fees:** £36–45; Second visit: £21–30
Bristol BS9
0117 962 3135

**June Gregory GCC, MCA**
**Fees:** £26–35; Second visit: £21–30
Bicknoller TA4
01984 656179

**Ruth Turner GCC, BCA**
**Fees:** <£25; Second visit: £21–30
Bristol BS7
0117 924 5842

**Nick Shipton GCC, MCA**
**Fees:** £26–35; Second visit: £21–30
Evercreech BA4,Castle Cary BA7,Frome
BA11
01749 830952

**Ray Jones GCC, BCA**
**Fees:** £26–35; Second visit: £21–30
Frome BA11
01373 463098

**Ann Tynan GCC, MCA**
**Fees:** £26–35; Second visit: £21–30
Glastonbury BA6
01458 833779

**Mary Wilkinson GCC, MCA**
**Fees:** £36–45; Second visit: £21–30
Minehead TA24,Exeter EX4,Taunton
TA1
01643 841660

**T C Jay GCC, BCA**
**Fees:** £26–35; Second visit: £21–30
Taunton TA1
07823 333973

**Sarah Kendal GCC, MCA**
**Fees:** <£25; Second visit: £21–30
Watchet TA23
01984 640270

**Sally White GCC, MCA**
**Fees:** £26–35; Second visit: £21–30
Watchet TA23
01984 640625

**A Young GCC, BCA**
**Fees:** <£25; Second visit: £21–30
Yeovil BA21
01935 423138

**Martin Young GCC, BCA**
**Fees:** £46–55; Second visit: £21–30
Yeovil BA21
01935 423138

## WILTSHIRE

**Robert Jolly GCC, BCA**
**Fees:** £36–45; Second visit: £21–30
Swindon SN4
01793 845300

**Jan Blankenstein GCC, BCA**
**Fees:** £36–45; Second visit: £21–30
Swindon SN3
01793 820599

**Mark Blokland GCC, BCA**
**Fees:** £36–45; Second visit: £21–30
Swindon SN4
01793 845300

**Graeme Cooper GCC, MCA**
**Fees:** £36–45; Second visit: £21–30
Swindon SN11
01249 812015

**Patricia Allinson GCC, MCA**
**Fees:** £26–35; Second visit: £21–30
Little Bedwyn SN8
01672 870391

# Chiropractic

### Juliana Blanch GCC, MCA
⊕ ⓝⓗ ⊘ ⓔ ❀
**Fees:** £26–35; Second visit: £21–30
Malmesbury SN16
01666 575125

### Jennifer Casemore GCC
⊕ ⓝⓗ ⊘ ⓔ ⓖ
**Fees:** £46–55; Second visit: £21–30
Salisbury SP1
01722 328606

### Caroline Davidson-Brewer GCC, MC
O ⊘
**Fees:** £36–45; Second visit: £21–30
Salisbury SP1
01722 328458

### Niamh Futcher GCC, MCA
⊕ O ⊕ ⓝⓗ ⊘ ❀
**Fees:** £26–35; Second visit: £21–30
Salisbury SP2,Marlborough SN8
01722 338620

### Nigel Hunt GCC, BAAC
⊕ O ⓝⓗ ⊘ ❀
**Fees:** £36–45; Second visit: £21–30
Salisbury SP1
01722 328606

### Brian Livingston GCC, MCA
⊕ O ⓔ ❀
**Fees:** £26–35; Second visit: £21–30
Salisbury SP2
01722 336106

### Ewen Merry GCC, BCA
⊕ ⓝⓗ ❀ ⓖ
**Fees:** £26–35; Second visit: £21–30
Worcester WR2
01905 428956

### Neill Saunders GCC, BAAC
ⓝⓗ ❀
**Fees:** £26–35; Second visit: £21–30
Swindon SN7
01367 244313

### M C Copland-Griffiths GCC, BCA
⊕ ⊕ ⓝⓗ ⊘ ❀ ⓖ
**Fees:** £36–45; Second visit: £21–30
Trowbridge BA14
01225 752199

### Joy-Elisabet Gill GCC, MCA
⊕ ⊕ ⊕ ⊘ ❀
**Fees:** £26–35; Second visit: £21–30
Trowbridge BA14,Westbury BA13
01225 764324

### Stuart Prior GCC, BCA
⊕ O ⊕ ⓝⓗ ❀
**Fees:** £36–45; Second visit: £21–30
Trowbridge BA14
01380 871 555

### Chris Richardson GCC, BCA
⊕ O ⊕ ⊘ ❀
**Fees:** £36–45; Second visit: £21–30
Warminster BA12
01985 217158

### David West GCC, MCA
⊕ ⓝⓗ ❀
**Fees:** £26–35; Second visit: £21–30
Wootton Bassett SN4
07977 271099

# Western Herbal Medicine

## BRISTOL

### B Baker MNIMH
⊕ O ⊕ ⊕ ⓝⓗ ❀
**Fees:** £26–35; Second visit: £21–30
Bristol BS16
0117 931 4367

### Jutta Blumenthal AMH
⊕ O ⊕ ⓝⓗ ❀
**Fees:** £26–35; Second visit: £21–30
Bristol BS4
0117 933 2799

**A Freeman MNIMH**
O ❀
Fees: £26–35; Second visit: £21–30
Bristol BS6
0117 924 6681

**J Green MNIMH**
O ⓝ Ⓔ ❀
Fees: £26–35; Second visit: £21–30
Bristol BS7
0117 924 8133

**D J Keogh MNIMH**
✛ ⊕ ⓝ ❀
Fees: £26–35; Second visit: <£20
Bristol BS6
0117 974 1199

**M Lyons MNIMH,**
Fees: £46–55; Second visit: £21–30
Bristol BS9
07968 364591

**D Petzsch MNIMH**
✛ O ⊕
Fees: £26–35; Second visit: £21–30
Bristol BS8
0117 946 6035

**S Redfern MNIMH**
✛ O ⊕ ⓝ ❀
Fees: £26–35; Second visit: £21–30
Bristol BS7
0117 944 4448

## CORNWALL

**Marilyn Scott IRCH**
✛ ⊕ ⓝ ❀
Fees: £26–35; Second visit: <£20
Hayle TR27, Falmouth TR11
01736 850941

**J A Hemming MNIMH**
✛ O ⊕ ⓝ Ⓔ
Fees: £26–35; Second visit: <£20
Penzance TR18
01736 360522

**M Holzamer MNIMH**
✛ ⊕
Fees: £26–35; Second visit: £21–30
Redruth TR15
01872 261516

## DEVON

**K Krzyzak MNIMH**
✛ ⊕ ❀
Fees: £26–35; Second visit: £21–30
Barnstaple EX32
01271 345733

**A Stobart MNIMH**
O ⓝ
Fees: £26–35; Second visit: <£20
Crediton EX17
01363 777531

**A Clay MNIMH,**
✛ ⓝ ⊘
Fees: £36–45; Second visit: £21–30
Exeter EX1
01392 253222

**S Y Mills MNIMH**
✛ ⊕ ⓝ ❀
Fees: £26–35; Second visit: <£20
Exeter EX4
01392 213899

**C Roguski MNIMH**
O ⓝ ❀
Fees: £36–45; Second visit: £21–30
Exeter EX3
01392 873747

**K A Willis MNIMH**
O ❀
Fees: £36–45; Second visit: £21–30
Exmouth EX8
01395 223307

**A Seal MNIMH**
✛ ⊕ ⓝ
Fees: £26–35; Second visit: <£20
Kingsbridge TQ7
01548 511347

**S Bristow MNIMH**
✛ O ⊕ ⓝ ❀
Fees: £36–45; Second visit: <£20
North Tawton EX20
01837 82210

**N Brydon MNIMH**
✛
Fees: £46–55; Second visit: £21–30
Ottery St Mary EX11
01404 815925

# Western Herbal Medicine

**Hilary Loder IRCH**
✚ ○ ⊕ ⓝ ✿
Fees: £26–35
South Molton EX36
01769 520319

## GLOUCESTERSHIRE

**A Hyland MNIMH**
✚ ⊕ ⓝ ⊘ ✿
Fees: £26–35; Second visit: <£20
Cheltenham GL50,Oxford OX1
01242 522136

**A Livesey MNIMH**
✚ ○ ⊕ ⓝ ⊘ Ⓔ ✿
Fees: £26–35; Second visit: <£20
Cheltenham GL53,Hailsham
BN27,Cheltenham GL50
01242 236675

**P J Rea MNIMH**
✚ ⓝ Ⓔ ✿
Fees: £26–35; Second visit: <£20
Forest of Dean GL17,Hailsham
BN27,Exeter EX4
01594 542517

**R Heyluer MNIMH**
✚ ⊕ ⓝ ⊘ ✿
Fees: <£25; Second visit: <£20
Gloucester GL12
07866 116725

**Annie Hood MNIMH**
○ ⓝ Ⓔ ✿
Fees: £26–35; Second visit: <£20
Tewkesbury GL20,Hailsham BN27
01684 292443

## SOMERSET

**S Hawkey MNIMH**
⊕ ⓝ ⊘ Ⓔ ✿
Fees: £36–45; Second visit: £21–30
Bath BA1
01225 427999

**M L Macmillan MNIMH**
✚ ⊕ ⓝ ✿
Fees: £26–35; Second visit: £21–30
Bath BA1
01225 427999

**N McNair MNIMH**
✚ ⊕ ⓝ Ⓔ ✿
Fees: £36–45; Second visit: £21–30
Bath BA1
01225 427999

**Andrew Johnson AMH**
✚ ⊕ ⊕ ✿
Fees: £46–55; Second visit: £21–30
Bath BA6
01458 833382

**Anita G Ferguson IRCH**
○ ⓝ ✿
Fees: £36–45; Second visit: £21–30
Bristol BS41
01275 393869

**Ned Reiter MNIMH**
✚ ○ ⊕ ⊕ ⓝ ⊘ ✿
Fees: £26–35; Second visit: <£20
Glastonbury BA6
01458 833663

**L Crockett MNIMH**
✚ ○ ⊕ ⓝ ✿
Fees: £26–35; Second visit: £21–30
Shepton Mallet BA4
01749 344395

**J M Sinclair MNIMH**
✚ ⊕ ✿
Fees: £26–35; Second visit: <£20
Taunton TA1
01823 681349

**Laura Stannard MNIMH**
✚ ⊕ ⓝ ✿
Fees: £26–35; Second visit: £21–30
Taunton TA1
01823 667104

**H Templeton MNIMH**
✚ ⊕ ⊕ ⊘
Fees: £26–35; Second visit: <£20
Taunton TA1
01398 331558

**R Blackwell MNIMH**
○
Fees: £46–55; Second visit: <£20
Wedmore BS28
01934 712848

# Western Herbal Medicine

## WILTSHIRE

**Alicia Sawaya AMH**
⊕  ⊕  🆖
Fees: £26–35; Second visit: £21–30
Swindon SN8
01672 871278

# Chinese Herbal Medicine

## BRISTOL

**Kwosinh Banh RCHM**
⊕  ⊕  ❀
Fees: <£25; Second visit: <£20
Bristol BS6
0117 942 7467

**Xiao Tong Fang RCHM**
⊕  🆖  ❀
Fees: <£25
Bristol BS23
01934 420202

**Helen Fielding RCHM**
⊕  O  ⊕  🆖
Fees: £26–35; Second visit: £21–30
Bristol BS8
0117 946 6035

**Quiyu Huang RCHM**
⊕  ⊕  ❀
Fees: <£25; Second visit: <£20
Bristol BS6
0117 9427467

## CORNWALL

**Kate Wilson RCHM**
⊕  O  🆖
Fees: £26–35; Second visit: £21–30
Truro TR19
01736 810394

## DEVON

**Simon King RCHM**
⊕  ⊕
Fees: £26–35; Second visit: <£20
Exeter EX4
01392 217422

**Kim Lay Im RCHM**
⊕  🆖  ⊘  ❀
Fees: £26–35; Second visit: £21–30
Plymouth PL4
01752 227841

**Nick Clarke RCHM**
O  ⊘  ❀
Fees: <£25; Second visit: <£20
Torquay TQ1
01803 297009

**Michael Potter RCHM**
⊕  ⊕  🆖  ❀
Fees: £26–35; Second visit: £21–30
Totnes TQ9
01803 863270

## GLOUCESTERSHIRE

**Daniel Blyth RCHM**
⊕  ⊕  ⊘  ❀
Fees: £26–35; Second visit: £21–30
Cheltenham GL50
0124 241933

**Linda Upton RCHM**
⊕  ⊕
Fees: £36–45; Second visit: £21–30
Cheltenham GL50
01242 584140

## SOMERSET

**Matthew Jackson RCHM**
⊕  O  ⊘  ❀
Fees: £26–35; Second visit: <£20
Bath BA6
01458 850594

# Chinese Herbal Medicine

**Robert Parnell RCHM**

✚ ◯ 🔵 ✦
**Fees:** £26–35; Second visit: £21–30
Bath BA5
01749 679014

**Damin Wan RCHM**

✚ 🔵 ✦
**Fees:** £36–45; Second visit: £31–40
Bath BA2
01225 337778

**Alison Courtney RCHM**

✚ ◯ 🔵 🔵 ⊘
**Fees:** £26–35; Second visit: £21–30
Taunton TA23
01984 634908

# Trent

Derbyshire
Leicestershire & Rutland
Lincolnshire
Nottinghamshire
South Yorkshire

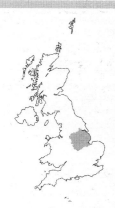

## Acupuncture

### DERBYSHIRE

**Susan Leah Nelson BAcC**
⊕ ⊕ ✿ ⊛
**Fees:** £36–45; Second visit: £21–30
Ashbourne DE6
01335 346096

**Joan Stewart AACP**
⊘ ⊛
**Fees:** £36–45; Second visit: £31–40
Bakewell DE45
01629 812834

**Trish Bailey AACP**
O ⊘ ⊛
**Fees:** £36–45; Second visit: £21–30
Belper DE56
01773 525038

**Grahame Gargini BAcC**
⊕ ⊕ ✿ ⊛
**Fees:** £26–35; Second visit: £21–30
Burton-on-Trent DE14
01283 516444

**Victor Ong BAcC**
⊕ O ⊕ ✿ ⊛
**Fees:** £46–55; Second visit: £31–40
Burton-on-Trent DE13,Cannock WS11
01543 472454

**Robin Croley BAcC**
⊕ ⊕ ✿ ⊛
**Fees:** £26–35; Second visit: £21–30
Chesterfield S41,Chesterfield S45
01246 273462

**Roderick Edlin BAcC**
⊕ ⊕ ✿ ⊛
**Fees:** £26–35; Second visit: £21–30
Derby DE22
01332 299133

**Caroline Hathaway BAcC**
⊕ O ⊕ ✿ ⊛
**Fees:** £26–35; Second visit: £21–30
Derby DE74,Loughborough LE11
01509 672708

**Joby Jackson BAcC**
⊕ ⊕ ✿ ⊛
**Fees:** £46–55; Second visit: £21–30
Derby DE22
01332 299133

**Ky Phong Lam BAcC**
⊕ ⊛
**Fees:** £26–35; Second visit: £21–30
Derby DE24
01332 384136

# Acupuncture

**Xiujie Luan BAcC**
⊕ O ⊕ ⚫ ✿ ⚫
Fees: <£25; Second visit: <£20
Derby DE22
01332 203279

**Anne Pottinger BAcC**
⊕ ⊕ ✿ ⚫
Fees: £36–45; Second visit: £21–30
Derby DE3
01332 521270

**Amir Qurban BAcC**
⊕ ⚫ © ✿ ⚫
Fees: <£25; Second visit: <£20
Derby DE23,Derby DE24
01332 763163

**Peter Robinson BAcC**
⊕ ⊕ ⚫
Fees: £26–35; Second visit: £21–30
Glossop SK13
01457 860860

## LEICESTERSHIRE & RUTLAND

**Michael Cooke BAcC**
O ✿ ⚫
Fees: £26–35; Second visit: £21–30
Hinckley LE10
01455 233995

**Gill Kelsey BAcC**
O ⊕ ⊕ ✿ ⚫
Fees: £36–45; Second visit: £21–30
Hinckley LE10
01455 449309

**Richard Farrer BAcC, AACP**
O ⊘ ⚫
Fees: £36–45; Second visit: £31–40
Leicester LE2
0116 271 2520

**Susmita Patel BAcC**
⊕ ⊕ ⚫ ✿ ⚫
Fees: £26–35; Second visit: £21–30
Leicester LE2
0116 270 8149

**Zheng Duan Reeve-Chen BAcC**
⊕ ✿ ⚫
Fees: £36–45; Second visit: £21–30
Leicester LE2
0116 221 8989

**Josephine Smith BAcC**
O ⊕ © ✿ ⚫
Fees: £36–45; Second visit: £21–30
Leicester LE3
0116 224 1326

**Emma Diamond BAcC**
O © ✿ ⚫
Fees: <£25; Second visit: £21–30
Leicester LE4
0116 299 6715

**Jo Tait AACP**
O ⊘ ⚫
Fees: £36–45; Second visit: £31–40
Leicester LE9
01455 285949

**Cathryn Colville AACP**
O ⊘ ⚫
Fees: £26–35; Second visit: £31–40
Loughborough LE11
01509 215614

**Nigel Pomfrett BAcC**
O ⊕ ✿ ⚫
Fees: £36–45; Second visit: £21–30
Loughborough LE11
01509 261131

**Vasanthy Watt BAcC**
⊕ ✿ ⚫
Fees: £46–55; Second visit: £21–30
Loughborough LE12
01509 413111

**Anne Etherton BAcC**
⊕ O ✿ ⚫
Fees: £36–45; Second visit: £21–30
Loughborough LE12,Nottingham NG9
01509 672457

**Angela Piggott BAcC**
⊕ ⚫ ✿ ⚫
Fees: £36–45; Second visit: £21–30
Lutterworth LE17
01455 559975

**Stella-Marie Welton BAcC**
⊕ ⊕ ✿ ⚫
Fees: £46–55; Second visit: £21–30
Market Harborough LE16
01858 410820

**Alec Welton BAcC**
✪ ⊕ ✿ ⊜
**Fees:** £46–55; Second visit: £21–30
Market Harborough LE16
01858 410820

**J T Woodings BMAS,**
O ⊘ ⊜
**Fees:** £26–35; Second visit: £31–40
Oakham LE15
01572 822556

## LINCOLNSHIRE

**Fiona Hedworth BAcC**
O
**Fees:** £26–35; Second visit: £21–30
Grantham NG31
01476 561987

**Deepa Panigrahi BAcC**
✪ O ⊕ ✿ ⊜
**Fees:** £26–35; Second visit: £21–30
Grimsby DN41,Grimsby DN31
01472 882578

**Sean Alexander Barkes BAcC**
✪ ⊘ ⊜
**Fees:** £26–35; Second visit: £21–30
Lincoln LN6
01522 809371

**Jane Seabrook BMAS, AACP**
✪ ⊜ ⊘ ✿ ⊜
**Fees:** £26–35; Second visit: £31–40
Lincoln LN2
01522 529000

**M Nielsen AACP**
✪ ⊕ ⊘ ⊜
**Fees:** £26–35; Second visit: £21–30
Louth LN11
01507 602323

**Louise Lipman BAcC**
✪ ⊕ ✿ ⊜
**Fees:** £36–45; Second visit: £21–30
Stamford PE9
01780 480889

## NOTTINGHAMSHIRE

**Erika Jones BAcC**
✪ ⊕ ⊜ ✿ ⊜
**Fees:** £36–45; Second visit: £21–30
Mansfield NG18
01623 626842

**Jennifer Oldham BAcC**
✪ ⊕ ⊜
**Fees:** £26–35; Second visit: £21–30
Mansfield NG18
01623 658224

**E M Aldred BAcC**
✪ ⊕ ⊜
**Fees:** £36–45; Second visit: £21–30
Nottingham NG3
0115 947 2131

**Val Clayson BAcC**
✪ O ⊕ ✿ ⊜
**Fees:** £46–55; Second visit: £21–30
Nottingham NG3
0115 962 4445

**Martin Dean BAcC**
O ✿
**Fees:** £36–45; Second visit: £21–30
Nottingham NG9
0115 9251184

**Nicholas Haines BAcC**
✪ ⊕ ✿ ⊜
**Fees:** £36–45; Second visit: £21–30
Nottingham NG5
0115 960 8855

**Kate Howard BAcC**
✪ O ⊕ ✿ ⊜
**Fees:** £36–45; Second visit: £21–30
Nottingham NG10
0115 973 2087

**Alison Mowbray BAcC**
✪ O ⊕ ✿ ⊜
**Fees:** £26–35; Second visit: £21–30
Southwell NG25
01636 815550

**Hannah Townsend BAcC**
✪ ✿ ⊜
**Fees:** £46–55; Second visit: £21–30
Southwell NG25
01636 816156

# Acupuncture

**Anna Davies AACP**
⊕ ⓝ ✿ ⚙
Fees: £26–35; Second visit: £31–40
Sutton-in-Ashfield NG17
01623 442722

## SOUTH YORKSHIRE

**Terri Patsalides BAcC**
O ✿ ⚙
Fees: <£25; Second visit: £21–30
Doncaster DN4
01302 328896

**Douglas Sutherland BAcC**
⊕ ⊕ ✿ ⚙
Fees: £36–45; Second visit: £21–30
Doncaster DN4,Leeds LS8
01302 311322

**George Chia BAcC, AACP**
⊕ ✿ ⚙
Fees: £26–35; Second visit: £21–30
Sheffield S10
0114 276 1997

**Patricia Delfosse BAcC**
⊕ O ⊕ ✿ ⚙
Fees: £36–45; Second visit: £21–30
Sheffield S11
0114 267 0540

**Karia Jose N Denobrega AACP, BAcC**
O ✿ ⚙
Fees: £26–35; Second visit: £31–40
Sheffield S11
0114 236 1066

**Dan Jiang BAcC**
O ⓝ ✿ ⚙
Fees: £26–35; Second visit: <£20;
Second visit: £21–30
Sheffield S10
0114 266 2051

**Nawaiz Nazir BAcC**
⊕ ⊕ ⊘ ⚙
Fees: £26–35; Second visit: £21–30
Sheffield S7
0114 258 9408

**Clare Oakley AACP**
O ⚙
Fees: £26–35; Second visit: £31–40
Sheffield S10
0114 268 1447

**Xing Zena Wang BAcC**
⊕ O ⊕ ⓝ ✿ ⚙
Fees: £26–35; Second visit: £21–30
Sheffield S11, Doncaster DN2,
Sheffield S7
0114 235 3701

**Julie Lynne Wisbey BAcC**
O ✿ ⚙
Fees: £36–45; Second visit: £21–30
Sheffield S11
07815 173982

**Liqin Zhao BAcC**
⊕ ✿ ⚙
Fees: £26–35; Second visit: £21–30
Sheffield S2
0114 255 6789

**Maria J N de Nobrega BAcC, AACP**
O ⓝ ⊘ ✿ ⚙
Fees: <£25
Sheffield S11
0114 2361066

# Homeopathy

## DERBYSHIRE

**Dawn Keyse RSHom**
⊕ ⊕ ⓝ € ✿
Fees: £25–35; Second visit: £31–40
Bakewell DE45
01298 872595

**Tony Grinney RSHom**
⊕ ⊕ ⓝ ⊘ € ✿
Fees: £46–55; Second visit: £20–30
Belper DE56,Liverpool L17
01773 820220

**Lorraine Hart RSHom**
⊕ 🅜 ✹
Fees: £36–45; Second visit: £20–30
Belper DE56
01773 828032

**Shannon Gerrard RSHom**
⊕ O ⊕ 🅜 ⊘ Ⓔ ✹
Fees: £36–45; Second visit: £20–30
Buxton SK17
01298 78614

**Jo Hale RSHom**
⊕ ⊕ 🅜 Ⓔ ✹
Fees: £46–55; Second visit: £20–30
Derby DE22
01332 299133

**Jane Cosgrove RSHom**
⊕ ⊕ 🅜 ⊘ Ⓔ ✹
Fees: £36–45; Second visit: £20–30
Dronfield S18
01246 411067

**Jackie Stanton RSHom**
⊕ O ⊕ 🅜 Ⓔ ✹
Fees: £36–45; Second visit: £20–30
Glossop SK13
01457 861940

**Adam Martanda RSHom**
⊕ 🅜 Ⓔ ✹
Fees: £46–55; Second visit: £31–40
Matlock DE4
01629 824098

## LEICESTERSHIRE & RUTLAND

**Andrew Meyer RSHom**
⊕ ⊕ ⊕ 🅜
Fees: £36–45; Second visit: £20–30
Leicester LE9
01332 760976

**Amita Raja MFHOm**
⊘
Fees: >£55; Second visit: >£50
Leicester LE9
0116 286 2386

## LINCOLNSHIRE

**Annie Hall RSHom**
⊕ O ⊕ 🅜 Ⓔ ✹
Fees: £46–55; Second visit: £20–30
Louth LN11,Lincoln LN1
01507 600185

**Beryl Taylor RSHom**
⊕ O ⊕
Fees: £36–45; Second visit: £20–30
Scunthorpe DN15
01724 734477

## NOTTINGHAMSHIRE

**Dorothy Mellors RSHom**
O 🅜 Ⓔ ✹
Fees: £36–45; Second visit: £20–30
Mansfield NG18
01773 872008

**Victoria Karney MFHom**
O ⊕ ⊕ 🅜
Fees: >£55; Second visit: £31–40
Nottingham NG15
0115 963 3676

**Louisa Lera RSHom**
⊕ ⊕ 🅜 ✹
Fees: £46–55; Second visit: £20–30
Nottingham NG5
0115 9608855

**Fiona F Robertson RSHom**
⊕ ⊕ 🅜 ⊘ Ⓔ ✹
Fees: £36–45; Second visit: £20–30
Nottingham NG7
0115 978 1006

**Elke Rohn RSHom**
⊕ O 🅜 Ⓔ ✹
Fees: £36–45; Second visit: £20–30
Worksop S81,Rotherham
S66,Rotherham S65
01909 591246

## SOUTH YORKSHIRE

**Susan Bedford RSHom**
O ⊕ 🅜 ⊘
Fees: £46–55; Second visit: £20–30
Doncaster DN1
01302 329311

# Homeopathy

**David Fitton MFHom**
⊘
Mexborough S64
01709 585171

**John Butler RSHom**
⊕ ⊕ ⊕ ⦿ ⦿ ⓔ ❀
Fees: £46–55; Second visit: £20–30
Sheffield S10, High Peak SK22
0114 276 9500

**Liza Chera RSHom**
⊕ ⦿ ⊕ ⦿ ⓔ
Fees: £46–55; Second visit: £20–30
Sheffield S10
01298 22606

**Susanne Hartley RSHom**
⊕ ⦿ ⊕ ⦿ ⓔ
Fees: £46–55; Second visit: £20–30
Sheffield S8, Sheffield S10
0114 250 7767

**Lynda Kenyon RSHom**
⊕ ⦿ ⊕ ⦿ ⓔ ❀
Fees: £46–55; Second visit: £20–30
Sheffield S7
0114 243 9147

**Clare Relton RSHom**
⊕ ⊕ ⊕ ⦿ ⊘ ❀
Fees: £46–55; Second visit: £20–30
Sheffield S10
0114 2769500

**Pat Strong MFHom**
⊕ ⊕ ⦿ ⓔ ❀
Fees: £46–55; Second visit: £31–40
Sheffield S10, Retford DN22
0114 276 9500

**Elaine Weatherley-Jones RSHom**
⊕ ⦿ ⊘ ⓔ
Fees: £36–45; Second visit: £31–40
Sheffield S10
0114 278 4600

**Annie Williams RSHom**
⊕ ⊕ ⦿ ⓔ
Fees: £46–55; Second visit: £20–30
Sheffield S10
0114 276 9500

# Osteopathy

**DERBYSHIRE**

**Elizabeth Taylor GOsC**
⊕ ⦿
Fees: £26–35; Second visit: £21–30
Ashbourne DE6
01335 300440

**Ian Rumboldt GOsC**
⊕ ⊕ ⊘ ❀
Belper DE56
01773 820220

**Warren G Hutson GOsC, BOA**
⊕ ⦿ ⊘ ❀
Fees: <£25; Second visit: £31–40
Buxton SK17
01298 23551

**Graham Scarr GOsC**
⊕ ⦿ ⊕ ⊘ ⦿
Buxton SK17
01298 78008

**Alan Smith GOsC, BOA**
⊕ ⦿ ⊕ ⊘ ❀
Castle Donnington DE74
01332 853777

**Simeon Hempsall GOsC, BOA**
⊕ ⦿ ⊘ ❀
Fees: £26–35; Second visit: £21–30
Chesterfield S41
01246 550538

**Clive Rickard GOsC**
⊕ ⊘ ❀
Fees: <£25; Second visit: <£20
Chesterfield S40, Rotherham S60
01246 277711

**Sanni Stratton GOsC**

○ ⊘ ✿

Fees: £26–35; Second visit: £21–30
Chesterfield S41
01246 550538

**Gerry Hale GOsC, BOA**

⊕ ⊕ ⊘ ✿

Derby DE3,Burton-on-Trent DE14
01332 521270

**Robert Shaw GOsC**

⊕ ⊘ ✿

Derby DE1
01332 371184

**Paul Ashburner GOsC, BOA**

⊕ ⊗ ✿

Fees: <£25; Second visit: £21–30
Derby DE21
01332 663342

**Ann Dickinson GOsC**

○ ⊘ ✿

Derby DE7
01332 792808

**Charles Dunning GOsC, BOA**

⊕ ✿ ⊜

Derby DE3
01332 521270

**Anne Hawkins GOsC**

⊕ ⊕ © ✿

Fees: £26–35; Second visit: £21–30
Derby DE23
01332 383951

**Joy Potts GOsC, BOA**

○ ⊗ ✿

Fees: <£25; Second visit: £21–30
Derby DE22
01332 556293

**Vanessa Ellis GOsC**

⊕ ⊕ ⊘ ✿

Fees: <£25; Second visit: £21–30
Dronfield S18
01246 411067

**Melvyn Johnson GOsC**

⊕ ○ ⊕ ⊘ ✿

Ilkeston DE7
0115 930 6582

**Rachel Mallaband GOsC**

⊕ ⊗ ✿

Fees: £26–35; Second visit: £21–30
Ilkeston DE7
0115 930 8255

**Adam W Lancashire GOsC**

⊕ ⊕ ⊕ ⊘ ✿

Fees: £36–45; Second visit: £41–50
Ripley DE5
01773 512249

**Leslie Cox GOsC**

○ ⊘ ✿ ⊜

Swadlincote DE12
01530 271680

**Julie Vaughan GOsC**

⊕ ⊘ ⊜

Hinckley LE10
01455 233484

**John Lovett GOsC, BOA**

⊕ ⊘

Leicester LE18
0116 257 1234

**Mark Leason GOsC, BOA**

⊕ ⊗ ✿

Fees: <£25; Second visit: £31–40
Leicester LE3
0116 282 6142

**Alison Leason GOsC, BOA**

⊕ ⊕ ⊘ ✿

Leicester LE3
0116 282 6142

**Marie O'Connell GOsC, BOA**

⊕ ⊕ ⊘ ✿

Leicester LE3
0116 282 6142

**Neil Smith GOsC, BOA**

⊕ ⊕ ⊘ ✿

Leicester LE2
0116 270 5348

**Graham Spowage GOsC, BOA**

⊕ ⊕ ⊗ ⊘ © ✿

Fees: £26–35; Second visit: £21–30
Leicester LE2
0116 270 5348

# Osteopathy

**James Butler GOsC, BOA**
🔵 ⊘ ❄
Loughborough LE11
01509 262880

**Jan Lowe GOsC, BOA**
🔵 ⓝ ⊘ ❄
Fees: <£25; Second visit: £21–30
Market Harborough LE16
01858 410071

**Charles Hassett GOsC, BOA**
🔵 ⊘ ❄
Melton Mowbray LE13
01664 480568

**Mitchell Lovett GOsC**
🔵 ⊕ ⓑ ⊘
Melton Mowbray LE13
0116 257 1234

## LINCOLNSHIRE

**Walter James Mason GOsC**
🔵 ⓝ ❄
Fees: <£25; Second visit: £21–30
Boston PE22
01754 820447

**Jo Sunner GOsC**
⊕ ⓝ ⊘ © ❄
Fees: £26–35; Second visit: £21–30
Bourne PE10
01778 391714

**Victor M Henighan GOsC, BOA**
🔵 ⓝ ⊘ ❄
Fees: £26–35; Second visit: £21–30
Gainsborough DN21
01427 678754

**Mark Duffree GOsC, BOA**
🔵 ⊘ ❄
Fees: £36–45
Grantham NG31
01476 590845

**Shelley Garnham GOsC**
ⓝ ⊘ ❄
Fees: £26–35; Second visit: £21–30
Grantham NG31
01476 563062

**Peter Burgess GOsC**
🔵 ⊕ ⓝ ⊘ ❄
Fees: £26–35; Second visit: £21–30
Grimsby DN31
01472 250800

**Hugh de la Hoyde GOsC, BOA**
🔵 ⓝ ❄
Fees: £26–35; Second visit: £21–30
Grimsby DN33
01472 877969

**Patrick Searle-Barnes GOsC, BOA**
🔵 ⊕ ⓝ ⊘ © ❄
Fees: £26–35; Second visit: <£20
Lincoln LN1
01522 537103

**Stephen Tyreman GOsC, BOA**
🔵 ⓝ ⊘ ❄
Fees: £26–35; Second visit: <£20
Lincoln LN1
01522 537103

**Stella Arden GOsC, BOA**
🔵 ⓞ ⓑ ⓝ ❄
Fees: <£25; Second visit: £31–40
Louth LN11
01507 608166

**David Etchell GOsC**
🔵 ⓞ ⓑ ⓝ ⊘ ❄
Fees: <£25; Second visit: <£20
Market Rasen LN7
01472 859517

**Saroja Etchell GOsC**
ⓞ ⓑ ⊘ ❄
Fees: <£25; Second visit: <£20
Nettleton, Market Rasen LN7
01472 859517

**P T Steeper GOsC, BOA**
🔵 ⓑ ⓝ ❄
Fees: <£25; Second visit: £21–30
Scunthorpe DN15
01724 854132

**Jonathan Townsend GOsC**
🔵 ⓝ ❄
Fees: <£25; Second visit: £21–30
Sleaford NG34
01529 414894

**Sarah Summerland GOsC**
⊕ ⊕ 🔵 🔵
Fees: <£25; Second visit: £21–30
Spalding PE11
01775 725530

**Anthea J Bentley GOsC**
⊕ ⊕ 🔵
Fees: £36–45; Second visit: £21–30
Stamford PE9
01780 480889

**Helen Branson GOsC, BOA**
⊕ 🔵 🔵
Fees: <£25; Second visit: £21–30
Stamford PE9
01780 763670

**Susan Nicholson GOsC, BOA**
⊕ O 🔵 🔵
Fees: £26–35; Second visit: £21–30
Stamford PE9
01780 759127

**Perry Westbrook GOsC**
⊕ 🔵 🔵
Fees: £36–45; Second visit: £21–30
Stamford PE9
01780 480889

## NOTTINGHAMSHIRE

**Ruth Campbell GOsC**
O 🔵
Fees: £26–35; Second visit: £21–30
Beeston NG9
0115 972 4079

**John Allfree GOsC, BOA,**
⊕ 🔵 ⊘ 🔵
Fees: <£25; Second visit: £21–30
Mansfield NG18
01623 641611

**James Booth GOsC**
⊕ ⊕ 🔵 ⊘ 🔵
Fees: £26–35; Second visit: £21–30
Nottingham NG2
0115 914 3311

**Graham G Broughton GOsC**
O ⊕ 🔵 🔵
Fees: <£25; Second visit: £21–30
Nottingham NG5
0115 960 5068

**Vaughan Cooper GOsC, BOA**
O 🔵
Fees: £36–45; Second visit: £21–30
Nottingham NG10
0115 946 1699

**Thomas W Edwards GOsC, BOA**
⊕ ⊕ 🔵
Fees: <£25; Second visit: £31–40
Nottingham NG2
0115 969 6085

**Rebecca Emerton GOsC, BOA**
⊕ 🔵 🔵
Fees: £26–35; Second visit: <£20
Nottingham NG13
01773 530268

**Imogen Hemingway GOsC**
⊕ ⊕ 🔵 ⊘ Ⓔ 🔵
Fees: £26–35; Second visit: £21–30
Nottingham NG16
01773 530268

**Paul Randall GOsC**
⊕ ⊕ 🔵 🔵
Fees: £26–35; Second visit: £21–30
Retford DN22
01777 706000

## SOUTH YORKSHIRE

**Julia Cawthorne GOsC**
⊕ ⊕ 🔵 🔵
Fees: £26–35; Second visit: £21–30
Barnsley S71
01226 200855

**Tracey Wood GOsC**
⊕ 🔵 ⊘ 🔵
Fees: £26–35; Second visit: £21–30
Doncaster DN1
01302 768638

**Kenneth Hall GOsC, BOA**
⊕ 🔵 🔵
Fees: £26–35; Second visit: £21–30
Doncaster DN2
01302 768706

**Daniel Sharpe GOsC**
⊕ 🔵 ⊘ 🔵
Fees: £36–45; Second visit: £21–30
Rotherham S60
01709 366661

# Osteopathy

**Kevin Beckwith GOsC**
Fees: £26–35; Second visit: £21–30
Sheffield S13
0114 269 4909

**Paul Donnelly GOsC, BOA**
Fees: £26–35; Second visit: £21–30
Sheffield S11
0114 267 1901

**William Eakins GOsC, BOA**
Fees: <£25; Second visit: £21–30
Sheffield S21
0114 248 0524

**Laurence-Marie Fourdrignier GOsC**
Fees: £26–35; Second visit: £21–30
Sheffield S13
0114 269 4909

**Lisa Halse GOsC, BOA**
Fees: £26–35; Second visit: £21–30
Sheffield S7
0114 250 9900

**Christopher Johnson GOsC**
Fees: £26–35; Second visit: £21–30
Sheffield S10
0114 276 9500

**Paul Krzok GOsC**
Fees: £26–35; Second visit: £21–30
Sheffield S1
0114 279 9766

**Susan Pawsey GOsC, BOA**
Fees: <£25; Second visit: £21–30
Sheffield S10
0114 230 3201

**Kim Thompson GOsC, BOA**
Fees: <£25; Second visit: £21–30
Sheffield S32
07980 755937

# Chiropractic

**DERBYSHIRE**

**G Carruthers GCC, BCA**
Fees: £36–45; Second visit: £21–30
Chesterfield S41
01246 200311

**Richard Nelson GCC, BCA**
Fees: £36–45; Second visit: £21–30
Derby DE1
01332 224820

**Sophie Hardy GCC, BCA**
Fees: £26–35; Second visit: £21–30
Derby DE3
01332 511119

**K R Jeffery GCC, BCA**
Fees: £26–35; Second visit: £21–30
Derby DE22
01332 346760

**Ian Reed GCC, BCA**
Fees: £36–45; Second visit: £21–30
Derby DE1
01332 224820

**Shaun Knighton GCC, BCA**
Fees: £26–35; Second visit: <£20
Heanor DE75
01773 762346

**Lee Goodwin GCC, BCA**
✦ ✦ ✦ ● ©
Fees: £26–35; Second visit: <£20
Shirebrook NG20
01623 743078

**Claire Brown GCC, MCA**
✦ ✦ ✦
Fees: <£25; Second visit: <£20
Sandiacre NG10
0115 939 0504

## LEICESTERSHIRE & RUTLAND

**Timothy Hutchful GCC, BCA**
✦ ● ✦ ●
Fees: £26–35; Second visit: £21–30
Leicester LE2
0116 254 2380

**Liam Mulvany GCC, MCA**
✦ O ✦ ●
Fees: £36–45; Second visit: £21–30
Leicester LE5,Nottingham NG5
0116 251 1647

**Neil Painter GCC, BCA**
✦ ●
Fees: £26–35; Second visit: £21–30
Leicester LE2
0116 271 2255

**Colin Rose GCC, BCA**
✦ ● ⊘ © ✦ ●
Fees: £26–35; Second visit: £21–30
Leicester LE2
0116 254 2380

**Thomas S Jeppesen GCC, BCA**
✦ ✦ ●
Fees: £36–45; Second visit: £21–30
Leicester LE2
0116 270 7948

**Tracy Norris GCC, BCA**
✦ ● ⊘
Fees: £26–35; Second visit: £21–30
Loughborough LE11
01509 219800

**Maria Faulks GCC, BCA**
✦ ● ✦
Fees: £26–35; Second visit: £21–30
Market Harborough LE16
01858 410820

**Rhiannon Jones GCC, MCA**
✦ O ●
Fees: £36–45; Second visit: £21–30
Oakham LE15
01572 737868

**Alan Watt GCC, MCA**
✦ O ✦ ✦
Fees: £26–35; Second visit: £21–30
Quorn LE12
01509 413111

## LINCOLNSHIRE

**Jamal Ashley GCC, BCA**
✦ ● ⊘ ✦ ●
Fees: £26–35; Second visit: £21–30
Brigg DN20
01652 650032

**Paul Woods GCC, MCA**
O © ✦
Fees: £26–35; Second visit: £21–30
Cleethorpes DN35
01472 601099

**Julia Kidson GCC, BCA**
✦ ● ✦ ●
Fees: £46–55; Second visit: £21–30
Brigg DN20
01652 650032

**Darren Barnes-Heath GCC, BCA**
✦ ● ⊘ ✦
Fees: £36–45; Second visit: £21–30
Lincoln LN1
01522 538450

**Douglas Clark GCC, BCA**
✦ ● ⊘ ✦
Fees: £36–45; Second visit: £21–30
Lincoln LN1
01522 538450

**Anita Compton GCC, BCA**
✦ ● ⊘ ✦
Fees: £36–45; Second visit: <£20
Lincoln LN2
01522 530645

**Mandy Hensman GCC, BCA**
✦ ● ⊘ ✦
Fees: £36–45; Second visit: £21–30
Lincoln LN1
01522 538450

# Chiropractic

**Mark Broe GCC, BCA**
⊕ ⊕ 🕲 🕸
**Fees:** £26–35; Second visit: <£20
Louth LN11
01507 610007

**Francis Usher GCC, BCA**
O 🕲
**Fees:** £36–45; Second visit: £21–30
Scunthorpe DN17
01724 844453

## NOTTINGHAMSHIRE

**John Goman GCC, MCA**
⊕ O ⊕ 🕲 🕸
**Fees:** £36–45; Second visit: £21–30
Carrington NG5
0115 960 8855

**Derek Allen GCC, BCA**
⊕ 🕲 ⊘ 🕸 🕲
**Fees:** £26–35; Second visit: £21–30
Mansfield NG18,Barnsley S75
01623 421401

**Colin Crossley GCC, BCA**
⊕ ⊕ 🕲 ⊘ Ⓔ 🕸
**Fees:** £26–35; Second visit: £21–30
Mansfield NG18
01623 635333

**Norman Tomlin GCC, MCA**
O ⊕ Ⓔ 🕸
**Fees:** £26–35; Second visit: £21–30
Mansfield NG18,Loughborough
LE11,Loughborough LE11
01623 640758

**Daphne Tomlin GCC, MCA**
O 🕸
**Fees:** £26–35; Second visit: £41–50
Mansfield NG18
01623 640758

**Elaine Aldred GCC, BCA**
⊕ ⊕ ⊕ 🕲 ⊘ 🕲
**Fees:** £36–45; Second visit: £21–30
Nottingham NG3
0115 947 2131

**John Anthony GCC, BAAC**
⊕ O 🕲 🕸
**Fees:** <£25; Second visit: <£20
Nottingham NG16
0115 854 8459

**Emma Crafts GCC, MCA**
🕲
**Fees:** £26–35; Second visit: £21–30
Nottingham NG13
01949 20646

**Chris Dowson GCC, MCA**
⊕ O 🕲 Ⓔ 🕸
**Fees:** £26–35; Second visit: £21–30
Nottingham NG5
0115 841 1544

**Jonna F Pedersen GCC, BCA**
⊕ 🕲
**Fees:** £26–35; Second visit: £21–30
Nottingham NG5
0115 985 7785

**Rashmi Seth GCC, MCA**
⊕ O ⊕ ⊕ 🕲 ⊘ 🕸
**Fees:** £26–35; Second visit: £21–30
Nottingham NG5
0115 967 9198

**Annie Wright GCC, BAAC**
⊕ O ⊕ 🕲 🕸
**Fees:** <£25; Second visit: £21–30
Nottingham NG9
0115 943 0247

**Sigrid P De Vries GCC, BCA**
⊕ ⊕ 🕲 ⊘ 🕸
**Fees:** £36–45; Second visit: <£20
Retford DN22
01777 860377

**Simon King GCC, BCA**
⊕ 🕲 🕸
**Fees:** £36–45; Second visit: £21–30
Retford DN22
01777 710720

**Bryon Sanders GCC, BCA**
O ⊘
**Fees:** £36–45; Second visit: <£20
Ruddington NG11
0115 974 3312

# Chiropractic

**Julie McKay GCC, BAAC**
Fees: £26–35; Second visit: £21–30
West Bridgford NG2
0115 982 5353

## SOUTH YORKSHIRE

**Peter Welsh GCC, BCA**
Fees: £36–45; Second visit: £21–30
Clifton S65, Sheffield S17
01709 720200

**Peter Oxenvad GCC, BCA**
Fees: <£25; Second visit: £21–30
Doncaster DN1
01302 739063

**A W D Robinson GCC, BCA**
Fees: £36–45; Second visit: £21–30
Doncaster DN1
01302 739063

**Andrew Carr GCC, BCA**
Fees: £36–45; Second visit: £21–30
Sheffield S10, Sheffield S10,
Sheffield S35
0114 266 6076

**Isobel Stevenson GCC, MCA**
Fees: £36–45; Second visit: £31–40
Sheffield S10
0114 276 9500

**Gitte Steffensen GCC, BCA**
Fees: £26–35; Second visit: £21–30
Sheffield S8
0114 274 5656

**Dorthe Mikkelsen GCC, BCA**
Fees: <£25; Second visit: £21–30
Sheffield S8
0114 274 5656

**Ulrik Sandstrom GCC, BCA**
Fees: £36–45; Second visit: £21–30
Sheffield S8
0114 274 5656

# Western Herbal Medicine

## DERBYSHIRE

**J Paulson MNIMH**
Belper DE56, Hope Valley S33,
Hope Valley S33
01773 820220

**C Dobie MNIMH**
Fees: £36–45; Second visit: <£20
Buxton SK17, Hailsham BN27
01298 84661

**A M C Charles-Clenne MNIMH**
Derby DE1
01332 208400

**Xin Lu MNIMH**
Fees: <£25; Second visit: <£20
Derby DE22, China 1300
01332 203279

## LEICESTERSHIRE & RUTLAND

**T J Walters MNIMH**
Houghton on the Hill LE7
0116 243 2527

**Sylvia Bates AMH**
Leicester LE4
0116 267 3171

# Western Herbal Medicine

## J D Hyde MNIMH
⊕ 🔵 ⓔ ✿
**Fees:** £46–55; Second visit: £31–40
Leicester LE2,Exeter EX4
0116 254 3178

## Irene Sleath AMH
○ 🔵 ✿
Leicester LE9
01455 274239

## M A Ure MNIMH
○ ⓔ ✿
**Fees:** £26–35; Second visit: <£20
Leicester LE3,Hailsham BN27
0116 255 1412

## Jinchun Guo MNIMH
⊕ 🔵 ⊘ ✿
Loughborough LE11
01509 234678

## L Harris MNIMH
⊕ 🔵 ✿
**Fees:** <£25; Second visit: <£20
Oakham LE15
01572 771231

## LINCOLNSHIRE

### A C Hyde MNIMH
⊕ ⊕ ⓔ
**Fees:** £46–55; Second visit: £31–40
Grantham NG31
01476 400100

### A Stableford MNIMH
⊕ 🔵 ⓔ ✿
**Fees:** £46–55; Second visit: <£20
Lincoln LN1
01522 543207

### T L Norris MNIMH
⊕ ○ ⓔ ✿
**Fees:** £26–35; Second visit: <£20
Scunthorpe DN16
01724 867385

## NOTTINGHAMSHIRE

### John Allfree MNIMH,
⊕ ⊕ 🔵 ⊘ ✿
**Fees:** £46–55; Second visit: £21–30
Mansfield NG18
01623 641611

## E M Aldred MNIMH
⊕ ⊕
**Fees:** £36–45; Second visit: £21–30
Nottingham NG3
0115 947 2131

## K Antonis MNIMH
⊕ ⊕ ⓔ ✿
**Fees:** £26–35; Second visit: <£20
Nottingham NG1,Nottingham NG9
0115 943 1204

## M Murphy MNIMH
⊕ ○ ✿
**Fees:** £46–55; Second visit: £21–30
Nottingham NG5
01623 402428

## Karen Pickup MNIMH
Nottingham NG8
0115 928 2928

## A Smith MNIMH
⊕ ⊕ 🔵 ⊘ ✿
**Fees:** £26–35; Second visit: <£20
Nottingham NG9
0115 917 3120

## SOUTH YORKSHIRE

### J E Alton MNIMH
⊕ ⊕ 🔵 ⓔ ✿
**Fees:** £26–35; Second visit: <£20
Sheffield S11
0114 268 2468

### C Bendle MNIMH
⊕ ⊕ ⊕ 🔵 ⓔ ✿
**Fees:** £26–35; Second visit: <£20
Sheffield S10,Hailsham
07941 414497

### S Bottomley MNIMH
⊕ ⊕ 🔵
**Fees:** £26–35; Second visit: <£20
Sheffield S7
0114 258 6480

### R James MNIMH
⊕ ⊕ 🔵 ✿
**Fees:** £26–35; Second visit: <£20
Sheffield S11
0114 268 2468

## Western Herbal Medicine

**Jeanette Kozimer IRCH**
❸ ⓫ ⓦ ❉
**Fees:** £46–55; Second visit: £31–40
Sheffield S11
0114 266 2321

**J Meakin MNIMH**
❸ O ⓫ ⓦ ❉
**Fees:** £26–35; Second visit: £21–30
Sheffield S42
01246 567202

**E Pitt MNIMH**
❸ O ⓫ ❉
**Fees:** £26–35; Second visit: <£20
Sheffield S11
07767 238486

**Delphine Sayre MNIMH**
O ⓦ
**Fees:** <£25; Second visit: <£20
Sheffield S8
0114 255 8338

## Chinese Herbal Medicine

**Richard Farrer RCHM**
O ⓦ ❉
**Fees:** £36–45; Second visit: £31–40
Leicester LE2
0116 271 2520

**Vasanthy Watt RCHM**
❸ ❉
**Fees:** £46–55; Second visit: £21–30
Leicester LE12
01509 413111

**Jiuchun Guo RCHM**
❸ ⊕ ⓦ ❉
**Fees:** <£25; Second visit: <£20
Loughborough LE11
01509 234678

**Andrew Kemp RCHM**
❸ ⓫ ❉
**Fees:** £36–45; Second visit: £21–30
Nottingham NG5
07957 456252

**Kang Situ RCHM**
O ⊘ ❉
**Fees:** <£25; Second visit: <£20
Nottingham NG7
0115 985 9096

**Xing Zena Wang RCHM**
❸ O ⓫ ⓦ ❉
**Fees:** £36–45; Second visit: £21–30
Sheffield S11, Doncaster DN2,
Sheffield S7
0114 235 3701

## Ayurvedic Medicine

**Sonal Bhavsar AMAUK**
❸ O ⓦ ❉
**Fees:** £26–35; Second visit: <£20
Leicester LE4
0116 233 8288

**Kanu Patel AMAUK**
❸ ❉
**Fees:** <£25
Leicester LE4
0116 266 3939

# Ayurvedic Medicine

**Amritlal Vadolia AMAUK**
O ⊕ ⊛ ✿
**Fees:** <£25; Second visit: <£20
Leicester LE3
0116 289 2021

**Nishu Sharma AMAUK**
O ⊛ ⊘
**Fees:** £36–45; Second visit: £21–30
Mansfield NG18
07870 430815

# West Midlands

Hereford & Worcester
Shropshire
Staffordshire
Warwickshire
West Midlands

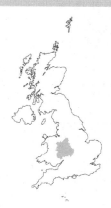

## Acupuncture

### HEREFORD & WORCESTER

**Jennifer Perry BAcC**
O Ⓔ ✿ ☻
Fees: £26–35; Second visit: £21–30
Bromsgrove B61
01527 876618

**Anne Stone AACP**
O ✿ ☻
Fees: £36–45; Second visit: £31–40
Droitwich WR9
01905 774432

**Jacqueline Turner BAcC**
⊕ O ⊕ ⊕ ☻
Fees: £36–45; Second visit: £21–30
Droitwich WR9,
Birmingham B14, Worcester WR7
01905 794894

**David Burness BAcC**
⊕ ☻ ✿ ☻
Fees: £36–45; Second visit: £21–30
Evesham WR11
01789 751414

**Andrea Hipwell BAcC**
O ✿ ☻
Fees: £36–45; Second visit: £21–30
Hereford HR1, Worcester WR7
01432 850016

**Diana Pullen BAcC**
⊕ ⊕ ✿ ☻
Fees: £36–45; Second visit: £21–30
Hereford HR2
01432 279653

**Gabrielle Rann BAcC**
O ⊕ Ⓔ ✿ ☻
Fees: £36–45; Second visit: £31–40
Hereford HR2
01432 870980

**Vanessa Hamilton BAcC**
⊕ ⊕ ⊕ ✿ ☻
Fees: £26–35; Second visit: £21–30
Hereford HR4
01432 273234

**Wendy Palette BAcC**
⊕ ⊕ Ⓔ ✿ ☻
Fees: £36–45; Second visit: £21–30
Kidderminster DY10
01562 777142

# Acupuncture

**Rhona Watson AACP**
⊕ ⊛ ∅ ⊕
**Fees:** £26–35; Second visit: £21–30
Kidderminster DY11
01562 67129

**Ben Stevens BAcC**
⊕ ⊕ ✿ ⊛
**Fees:** £36–45; Second visit: £21–30
Ledbury HR8
01531 634220

**Caroline Newton AACP**
○ ⊛ ∅ ⊕
**Fees:** £26–35; Second visit: £31–40
Leominster HR6
01568 709005

**James Hayllar BAcC**
⊕ ⊛ ✿ ⊛
**Fees:** £26–35; Second visit: £21–30
Pershore WR10
01386 556553

**Wendy Kaye Hooper BAcC**
⊕ ○ ⊕ ⊕ ⊛ ∅ ✿ ⊛
**Fees:** <£25; Second visit: £21–30
Redditch B97
01527 544642

**Lynn Owen BAcC**
⊕ ✿ ⊛
**Fees:** £26–35; Second visit: £21–30
Redditch B98
01527 596664

**Janie Shepherd BAcC**
○ ⊛
**Fees:** £36–45; Second visit: £21–30
Ross-on-Wye HR9
01989 565536

**Sue Marston BAcC**
⊕ ✿ ⊛
**Fees:** £36–45; Second visit: £21–30
Stourport-on-Severn DY13
01562 742628

**Zhenghong Qi BAcC**
⊕ ⊕ ⊛ ✿ ⊛
**Fees:** £26–35; Second visit: £21–30
Worcester WR1
01905 25252

**Katrina Weight BAcC**
⊕ ○ ✿ ⊛
**Fees:** <£25; Second visit: £21–30
Worcester WR5
01905 352060

## SHROPSHIRE

**Heather Keeling AACP**
○ ∅ ⊛
**Fees:** £36–45; Second visit: £31–40
Bridgnorth WV16
07966 550251

**Bronwen Lloyd-Hughes BAcC**
⊕ ○ ⊕
Bridgnorth WV16
01746 764421

**Hugh Ruxton BAcC**
⊕ ⊕ ✿ ⊛
**Fees:** £26–35; Second visit: £21–30
Bridgnorth WV16
01746 761050

**Jill Parker AACP**
⊕ ○ ∅ ⊛
**Fees:** £26–35; Second visit: £31–40
Bridgnorth WV16, Wolverhampton
WV6,Bridgnorth WV16
01746 762187

**Tess Reynolds BAcC**
○ ✿ ⊛
**Fees:** £36–45; Second visit: £21–30
Ellesmere SY12
01691 622006

**Clare Unitt BAcC**
⊕ ○ ⊕ ✿ ⊛
**Fees:** £26–35; Second visit: £21–30
Ludlow SY8
01584 879756

**Panos Barlas AACP**
○ ∅ ⊛
**Fees:** £46–55; Second visit: £31–40
Market Drayton TF9
01630 673944

**Julie Barwise AACP**
○ ∅ ⊛
**Fees:** £26–35; Second visit: £31–40
Shrewsbury SY3
01743 282506

**Helen Geddes AACP**
✪ O ⊘ ⊕
**Fees:** £26–35; Second visit: £21–30
Shrewsbury SY3
01743 270280

**Gillian Lockwood BAcC**
✪ O ⊕ ✿ ⊕
**Fees:** £36–45; Second visit: £21–30
Shrewsbury SY3
01743 248878

**Frankie Reid BMAS**
O ⊘ ⊕
**Fees:** £36–45; Second visit: £31–40
Shrewsbury SY3,Shrewsbury SY3
01743 282500

**Megan MacDonald BAcC**
O ⊘ ✿ ⊕
**Fees:** £26–35; Second visit: £21–30
Shrewsbury SY4
01939 220483

**Philip Cartwright BMAS**
✪ ⊕ 🅝 ⊘ ⊕
**Fees:** £26–35; Second visit: £21–30
Telford TF1
01952 641222

**Richard Fallows AACP**
✪ 🅝 ⊕
**Fees:** £36–45; Second visit: £21–30
Telford TF1
01952 260983

**Diane Hallett BAcC**
✪ ⊕ ⊕ Ⓔ ✿ ⊕
**Fees:** £36–45; Second visit: £21–30
Telford TF2,Shrewsbury SY2,Bishops
Castle SY9
01952 620138

**Lynn Spence BAcC**
✪ O ⊕ ✿ ⊕
**Fees:** £26–35; Second visit: £21–30
Telford TF7
01952 581251

**Liz Castle BAcC**
✪ ⊕ ⊕ ✿ ⊕
**Fees:** £26–35; Second visit: £21–30
Whitchurch SY13
01948 880170

## STAFFORDSHIRE

**Anne Bourne BAcC**
✪ ⊕ 🅝 ✿ ⊕
**Fees:** £36–45; Second visit: £21–30
Leak ST13
01260 274085

**Ian Markham BAcC**
✪ ⊕ ✿ ⊕
**Fees:** £46–55; Second visit: £21–30
Leek ST13,Derby DE1,
Stoke-on-Trent ST4
01298 84661

**Helen Pearce AACP**
✪ ⊕
**Fees:** £36–45; Second visit: £31–40
Newcastle-under-Lyme ST5
01782 717047

**Clare Dobie BAcC**
✪ ⊕ ✿ ⊕
**Fees:** £46–55; Second visit: £21–30
Stafford ST17
01298 84661

**Stephen Henson BAcC**
O ⊘ ✿ ⊕
**Fees:** £26–35; Second visit: £21–30
Stoke-on-Trent ST12
01782 372668

**Sara Blackhurst AACP**
✪ ✿ ⊕
**Fees:** £26–35; Second visit: £21–30
Stoke-on-Trent ST7
0161 247 5315

**Ho Ching Chow BAcC**
O ⊕ ✿ ⊕
**Fees:** £26–35; Second visit: £21–30
Stoke-on-Trent ST7
01270 872544

**Susan Evans BAcC**
✪ ⊕ ✿ ⊕
**Fees:** £36–45; Second visit: £21–30
Stone ST15
01785 616010

**Ebrahim Dabestani BMAS**
✪ ⊘ ✿ ⊕
**Fees:** £26–35; Second visit: £21–30
Tamworth B77
01827 251251

# Acupuncture

## Nicole Blest AACP
⊕ 🔘 ⊘ ✿ 💯
**Fees:** £36–45; Second visit: £21–30
Uttoxeter ST14
01889 563645

## Valerie A Swingler BAcC
⊕ ✿ 💯
**Fees:** £26–35; Second visit: £21–30
Uttoxeter ST14
01283 221563

---

**WARWICKSHIRE**

## Sally Lissaman BAcC
⊕ O ⊕ € ✿ 💯
**Fees:** £36–45; Second visit: £21–30
Bubbenhall CV8
07961 533799

## Vivienne Brown BAcC
O 💯
**Fees:** £46–55; Second visit: £21–30
Leamington Spa CV31
01926 422388

## Paul Cooney BAcC
⊕ ⊕ ✿ 💯
**Fees:** £26–35; Second visit: £21–30
Leamington Spa CV31
01926 833368

## Anne-Marie Cullen BAcC
⊕ 🔘 ✿ 💯
**Fees:** £36–45; Second visit: £21–30
Leamington Spa CV31
01926 336964

## Kerry Anne Grady BAcC
O ✿ 💯
**Fees:** £36–45; Second visit: £21–30
Leamington Spa CV31
01926 316450

## Jacqueline D'Arcy BAcC
⊕ ✿ 💯
**Fees:** £36–45; Second visit: £21–30
Leamington Spa CV32
01926 408285

## Martin Grasby BAcC
⊕ ⊕ ✿ 💯
**Fees:** £36–45; Second visit: £21–30
Leamington Spa CV32
01926 450990

## Natalie Guillamon BAcC
⊕ ⊕ ✿ 💯
**Fees:** £36–45; Second visit: £21–30
Leamington Spa CV32
01926 316500

## Martine Gallie BAcC
⊕ ⊕ ✿ 💯
**Fees:** £36–45; Second visit: £21–30
Leamington Spa CV32,Kenilworth CV8
01926 450990

## Deborah Collins BAcC
O ⊕ ✿ 💯
**Fees:** >£55; Second visit: £21–30
Leamington Spa CV32,Warwick CV34
01926 885600

## Gillian Doughty AACP
⊘ 💯
**Fees:** £26–35; Second visit: £21–30
Leamington Spa CV32,Warwick CV34
01926 436321

## Gerry Bishop BAcC
⊕ ⊕ ✿ 💯
**Fees:** £46–55; Second visit: £21–30
Leamington Spa CV33
01926 450990

## Lois Francis BAcC
⊕ O ⊕ ✿ 💯
**Fees:** £36–45; Second visit: £21–30
Nuneaton CV11
024 7634 3100

## Tim Metford BAcC
⊕ O ⊕ ✿ 💯
**Fees:** £36–45; Second visit: £21–30
Nuneaton CV11
024 7634 3100

## Janet Kaldesic AACP
O ✿ 💯
**Fees:** £46–55; Second visit: £41–50
Nuneaton CV13
01455 213953

## Jill Drew BAcC, AACP
⊕ ⊕ ⊕ 🔘 ✿ 💯
**Fees:** £36–45; Second visit: £31–40
Rugby CV21
01788 568410

**Paula McPhail BAcC**
**Fees:** £36–45; Second visit: £21–30
Rugby CV21
01788 568896

**Audrey Canale-Parola BAcC**
**Fees:** £36–45; Second visit: £21–30
Rugby CV22
01788 817961

**Jose Lacey BAcC**
**Fees:** £26–35; Second visit: £21–30
Rugby CV22
01788 813777

**Jenny Cowgill BAcC**
**Fees:** £46–55; Second visit: £21–30
Stratford-upon-Avon CV37
01789 299228

**Rosemary John AACP**
**Fees:** £26–35; Second visit: £31–40
Studley B80
01527 852534

**Erika Fitzgibbon BAcC**
**Fees:** £46–55; Second visit: £21–30
Warwick CV34
01926 400558

**David R Millard BAcC**
**Fees:** £36–45; Second visit: £21–30
Warwick CV34
0800 956 1465

**Jan Still BAcC**
**Fees:** £46–55; Second visit: £21–30
Warwick CV34
01926 406558

**Celia Tudor-Evans BAcC**
**Fees:** £26–35; Second visit: £21–30
Warwick CV34
01926 493638

**Janette Harper BAcC**
**Fees:** £26–35; Second visit: £21–30
Warwick CV35
01926 842205

## WEST MIDLANDS

**Tuong van Long BAcC**
**Fees:** £26–35; Second visit: £21–30
Birmingham B7
0121 328 9642

**Katy Kerr BAcC**
**Fees:** £36–45; Second visit: £21–30
Birmingham B11
0121 449 1454

**Michael Baird BMAS**
**Fees:** £26–35; Second visit: £21–30
Birmingham B13
0121 449 0971

**Michael Scully BAcC**
**Fees:** £36–45; Second visit: £21–30
Birmingham B13
0121 444 9515

**Merlin Young BAcC**
**Fees:** £36–45; Second visit: £21–30
Birmingham B13,Oldbury B68
0121 421 3480

**Margaret Ehrenberg BAcC**
**Fees:** £26–35; Second visit: £21–30
Birmingham B14
0121 441 2757

**Nick Lampert BAcC**
**Fees:** £26–35; Second visit: £21–30
Birmingham B14
0121 441 2757

**Linda Winstanley BAcC**
**Fees:** £36–45; Second visit: £21–30
Birmingham B14
0121 444 5650

# Acupuncture

**Charmian Wylde BAcC**
Fees: £26–35; Second visit: £21–30
Birmingham B14
0121 441 2757

**Daphne Barker BAcC**
Fees: £26–35; Second visit: £21–30
Birmingham B15
0121 456 1946

**Ai-Ling Zhou BAcC**
Fees: £26–35; Second visit: £21–30
Birmingham B23
0121 350 2018

**Ramesh Parmar BAcC**
Fees: £36–45; Second visit: £21–30
Birmingham B28
0121 733 1357

**Kim Wager BAcC**
Fees: £36–45; Second visit: £21–30
Birmingham B29
07775 570185

**Janine Davis BAcC**
Fees: £26–35; Second visit: £21–30
Birmingham B45
0121 445 3118

**Nan Fellows BAcC**
Fees: <£25; Second visit: £21–30
Birmingham B45
0121 445 3118

**Chris Morgana Leeson BAcC**
Fees: £36–45; Second visit: £21–30
Birmingham B46
01675 464369

**Margaret McNeill BAcC**
Fees: £36–45; Second visit: £21–30
Birmingham B46, Tamworth B79
01675 465726

**Brian Clensy BAcC**
Fees: £26–35; Second visit: £21–30
Coventry CV1
024 7655 5114

**Carol Fawkes BAcC**
Fees: £26–35; Second visit: £21–30
Coventry CV3
024 7650 5997

**Rose Severs BAcC**
Fees: £36–45; Second visit: £21–30
Coventry CV3
024 7630 1918

**Roger Beresford BAcC**
Fees: £26–35
Coventry CV5
024 7671 5535

**Sheila Leddington Wright AACP**
Fees: £26–35; Second visit: £21–30
Coventry CV5
024 76673741

**Bikram Singh Deol BAcC**
Fees: >£55; Second visit: £21–30
Coventry CV5
024 7667 0147

**Jo Rochford BAcC**
Fees: £36–45; Second visit: £21–30
Coventry CV7
01676 533064

**C A Byrne BAcC**
Fees: £26–35; Second visit: £21–30
Solihull B45
0121 706 5959

**Fabienne Alsing BAcC**
Fees: £46–55; Second visit: £21–30
Solihull B90
01564 702186

**Ron Franks BAcC**
○ ✿ ⊕
Fees: £36–45; Second visit: £21–30
Solihull B90
0121 693 4455

**Anne Garland BAcC**
⊕ ○ ⊕ ✿ ⊕
Fees: £36–45; Second visit: £21–30
Solihull B91
0121 705 1979

**Anne Hands AACP**
⊕ ⊕ ✿ ⊕
Fees: £26–35; Second visit: £21–30
Solihull B91
0121 704 2068

**Julian Morgan BAcC**
○ ⊕ ✿ ⊕
Fees: >£55; Second visit: £21–30
Solihull B91
0121 704 4909

**Ian Pardoe BMAS**
⊕ ○ ⊕ ⊘ ✿ ⊕
Fees: £26–35; Second visit: £21–30
Solihull B91
0121 711 3117

**Edward Garland BAcC**
⊕ ⊕ ⊕ ✿ ⊕
Fees: £36–45; Second visit: £21–30
Solihull B93
01564 772246

**Jane Morgan BAcC**
○ ✿ ⊕
Fees: >£55; Second visit: £21–30
Solihull B95
01564 795342

**Robert Clark BAcC**
○ ⓔ ✿ ⊕
Fees: £26–35; Second visit: £21–30
Stourbridge DY7
01384 877375

**Jane Bleasdale BAcC**
⊕ ⊕ ✿ ⊕
Fees: £36–45; Second visit: £21–30
Stourbridge DY8
01384 375271

**Tony Concannon BAcC**
⊕ ⊕ ⊕ ⊘ ✿ ⊕
Fees: £46–55; Second visit: £21–30
Stourbridge DY8
01384 379141

**Clare Ingram BAcC**
○ ⊕ ✿ ⊕
Fees: £26–35
Stourbridge DY9
01562 777773

**Helen Wall BAcC**
○ ⊕ ✿ ⊕
Fees: £36–45; Second visit: £21–30
Sutton Coldfield B76
0121 351 1381

**Paul Clusker BAcC**
⊕ ⊕ ⊕ ✿ ⊕
Fees: £36–45; Second visit: £21–30
Walsall WS2, Sutton Coldfield B73
01922 620047

**Pete A Evans AACP**
⊕ ⊕ ⊕ ✿ ⊕
Fees: £26–35; Second visit: £21–30
Wolverhampton WV5
01902 894613

**Sheila Plant BAcC**
○ ⊕
Fees: £26–35; Second visit: £21–30
Wolverhampton WV6
01902 424720

**Julia Rose BAcC**
⊕ ⊕ ✿ ⊕
Fees: £36–45; Second visit: £21–30
Wolverhampton WV7
01902 374555

**Letty Wevers AACP**
⊕ ○ ⊕ ✿ ⊕
Fees: £36–45; Second visit: £31–40
Wolverhampton WV7
01902 374555

# Homeopathy

## HEREFORD & WORCESTER

**Jeremy Sherr RSHom**
⊕ ⬤ Ⓔ ✿
Fees: >£55; Second visit: £31–40
Great Malvern WR14
01684 563192

**Anne Finch RSHom**
⊕ ⊕ ⬤ Ⓔ ✿
Fees: £36–45; Second visit: £20–30
Ledbury HR8, Newent GL18,
Gloucester GL1
01531 634220

**Suzanne Noble RSHom**
⊕ ⊕ ⬤ Ⓔ
Fees: £36–45; Second visit: £20–30
Leominster HR6, Hereford HR1
01568 750462

**Barbara Winton RSHom**
⊕ ⬤ ⊕ ⬤ Ⓔ ✿
Fees: £36–45; Second visit: £20–30
Leominster HR6, Hereford HR2
01544 388814

**Stella Berg RSHom**
⊕ ⬤ ⊕ ⬤ Ⓔ
Fees: £36–45; Second visit: £31–40
Ross On Wye HR9
01989 561060

**Paul Downey MFHom**
⊕ ⬤ ∅
Fees: £36–45; Second visit: £20–30
Ross-on-Wye HR9
01989 763535

## SHROPSHIRE

**Fiona Robertson RSHom**
⊕ ⬤ ⬤ Ⓔ ✿
Fees: £36–45; Second visit: £20–30
Bishops Castle SY9
01588 638416

**Len Marlow RSHom**
⊕ ⊕ ⬤ Ⓔ ✿
Fees: £36–45; Second visit: £20–30
Bridgnorth WV16
01746 768886

**Yanisa De Winter RSHom**
⊕ ⬤ ⊕ ⬤ Ⓔ
Fees: £36–45; Second visit: £20–30
Radbrook Green SY3
01743 873197

**Rosalind McGregor MFHom**
⬤
Fees: £25–35; Second visit: £20–30
Shrewsbury SY7
01588 660392

## STAFFORDSHIRE

**Jill Povey RSHom**
⊕ ⊕ ⬤ Ⓔ ✿
Fees: £36–45; Second visit: £20–30
Leek ST13
01538 385346

**Anthony Flowers RSHom**
⊕ ⬤ ⊕ ⬤ ✿
Fees: £46–55; Second visit: £20–30
Lichfield WS14
01892 863472

**Margaret Bevington RSHom**
⊕ ⊕ Ⓔ ✿
Fees: £46–55; Second visit: £20–30
Newcastle-under-Lyme ST5
01782 615184

**Lesley Foulkes RSHom**
⊕ ⊕ ⬤ ✿
Fees: £36–45; Second visit: £20–30
Newcastle-under-Lyme ST5
01782 615184

**Elspeth Larkin RSHom**
⊕ ⊕ ⬤ Ⓔ ✿
Fees: £46–55; Second visit: £20–30
Newcastle-under-Lyme ST5
01782 615184

**Janice Marshall RSHom**
⬤ ✿
Fees: <£25; Second visit: £20–30
Newcastle-under-Lyme ST5, Alsager
01782 380034

# Homeopathy

## WARWICKSHIRE

**Claire Pickin MFHom**
⊕ ⊕ ⦿
Fees: >£55; Second visit: £31–40
Leamington Spa CV32
01926 651496

**Penelope Holcroft MFHom**
⊕ ⦿ ⊘
Fees: >£55; Second visit: £20–30
Rugby CV22
01788 813777

**Sara G Byfyeld RSHom**
⊕ O ⊕ ⊕ ⦿ © ✿
Fees: £46–55; Second visit: £20–30
Southam CV47
01926 813974

**Sheryl Conran-Brown RSHom**
⊕ ⊕ ⦿
Fees: >£55; Second visit: £31–40
Southam CV47
01926 810491

## WEST MIDLANDS

**Robynn C Ormond MFHom**
O ⊕ ⊘
Fees: >£55; Second visit: £31–40
Birmingham B29
0121 472 1965

**Mary Millicent Rayner MFHom**
⦿
Fees: £46–55; Second visit: £41–50
Birmingham B38
0121 458 6595

**Sheila Oxspring RSHom**
⊕ O ⊕ ⊕ ⦿ ⊘ © ✿
Fees: £36–45; Second visit: £20–30
Bromsgrove B60
01527 837783

**Gaynor Sandell RSHom**
⊕ ⊕ ⦿ © ✿
Fees: £36–45; Second visit: £20–30
Bromsgrove B60
01527 873894

**Maggie Curley MFHom**
⊕ ⊕ ⊕ ⦿ ⊘
Fees: >£55; Second visit: £31–40
Coventry CV1
024 7622 2505

**Melvyn Smith RSHom**
⊕ ⦿ ✿
Fees: £46–55; Second visit: £20–30
Smethwick B66
01684 562371

**Mollie Hunton FFHom,**
O ⦿
Fees: >£55; Second visit: £20–30
Stourbridge DY8
01384 373111

**David Smith MFHom**
⊕ O ⦿ ✿
Fees: £36–45; Second visit: £41–50
Sutton Coldfield B73,Solihull
B91,Birmingham B15
0121 355 2155

# Osteopathy

## HEREFORD AND WORCESTERSHIRE

**Richard Hughes GOsC**
⊕ ⦿ © ✿
Fees: £26–35; Second visit: £21–30
Bewdley DY12
07961 352058

**Michelle Davies GOsC**
O ⊕ ⦿ © ✿
Fees: £26–35; Second visit: £21–30
Bromyard HR7
07966 493994

**J E Edwards GOsC**
⦿ ⊘ ✿
Fees: <£25; Second visit: £21–30
Droitwich WR9
01905 772458

# Osteopathy

**Rachel Quickenden GOsC**
✚ 🜨 🆖 💥
**Fees:** <£25; Second visit: <£20
Evesham WR11
01386 421821

**Russell Sutton GOsC**
✚ 🜨 🆖 ⊘ 💥
**Fees:** <£25; Second visit: £31–40
Evesham WR11
01386 421821

**Bernadette Trevillion GOsC, BOA**
✚ 🆖 ⊘ 💥
**Fees:** <£25; Second visit: £21–30
Evesham WR11
01386 830314

**Robert W Blackburn GOsC, BOA**
✚ 🜨 🆖 ⊘ 💥
**Fees:** £26–35; Second visit: £21–30
Hereford HR1
01432 273234

**Nicholas Handoll GOsC, BOA**
✚ 🜨 🆖 💥
**Fees:** >£55; Second visit: £31–40
Hereford HR2
01432 356655

**Sarah Hope GOsC**
O 🆖 💥
**Fees:** <£25; Second visit: £31–40
Hereford HR2
01981 580371

**Pushpa Rathod GOsC**
✚ 🜨 🆖 💥
**Fees:** £26–35; Second visit: £21–30
Hereford HR2,Ludlow SY8
01432 279653

**David C Grand GOsC, BOA**
✚ 🜨 🆖
**Fees:** <£25; Second visit: £21–30
Kidderminster DY10
01562 822115

**N V Kavanagh GOsC, BOA**
✚ 🆖 ⊘
**Fees:** <£25; Second visit: £21–30
Kidderminster DY10
01562 822115

**Jodi Davies GOsC**
✚ 🆖 💥
**Fees:** £26–35; Second visit: £21–30
Ledbury HR8
01531 635080

**Beverly Gyde GOsC**
✚ 🆖 💥
**Fees:** £26–35; Second visit: £21–30
Ledbury HR8
01531 635080

**Sally Lansdale GOsC**
✚ 🆖
**Fees:** <£25; Second visit: £21–30
Leominster HR6
01568 610610

**Simon Lichtenstein GOsC**
✚ 🆖 💥
**Fees:** <£25; Second visit: £21–30
Leominster HR6
01568 610610

**Ashley Robinson GOsC, BOA**
O
**Fees:** £36–45; Second visit: £21–30
Leominster HR6
01568 709194

**Andrea Pegler GOsC, BOA**
✚ O 🆖
**Fees:** <£25; Second visit: £21–30
Worcester WR1
01905 26450

**Vivienne Marks GOsC, BOA**
✚ O 🆖 Ⓔ 💥
**Fees:** <£25; Second visit: £21–30
Worcester WR1
01905 26450

**Andrea Meyer GOsC, BOA**
✚ Ⓔ
**Fees:** £26–35; Second visit: £21–30
Worcester WR1
01905 26450

**Agnes King GOsC**
✚ ⊘ Ⓔ 💥
Worcester WR14
01684 568744

**Terry Moule GOsC, BOA**
⊕ ⊘ Ⓔ ❀ 🏵
Worcester WR14
01684 568800

**Kenneth Smith GOsC**
⊕ ⊘ Ⓔ ❀
Worcester WR14
01684 568744

**Harriet Yeoman GOsC**
⊕ ⊕ ⊕ ⊘
Worcester WR14
01684 575379

**Amy Vowles GOsC**
⊕ ⊕ ⊘ ❀
Worcester WR2
01905 424877

**Guy Ledger GOsC, BOA**
⊕ O ⊘ ❀
Worcester WR7
01386 793945

**Peter Jones GOsC, BOA**
⊕ O 🅽
Fees: £26–35; Second visit: £21–30
Worcester WR8
01684 594654

**Joanna Young GOsC**
⊕ ⊘ ❀
Worcester WR9
01905 345409

## SHROPSHIRE

**Elspeth Keeling-Howard GOsC**
⊕ O ⊘ ❀
Fees: £26–35; Second visit: £21–30
Church Stretton SY6
01694 724866

**Lynne Aitken GOsC**
O ⊘ ❀
Fees: £26–35; Second visit: £21–30
Craven Arms SY7
01588 660204

**Tilly Teresa Calvert GOsC**
⊕ O ⊕ 🅽 ⊘
Fees: £26–35; Second visit: £21–30
Ludlow SY8
01584 879756

**Janine Lees GOsC, BOA**
⊕ ⊕ ⊘ ❀
Fees: £26–35; Second visit: £21–30
Market Drayton TF9
01630 656546

**Fiona Adlard GOsC**
O ⊘
Fees: £26–35; Second visit: £21–30
Shrewsbury SY3
01743 248543

**Susan Allen GOsC**
⊕ O
Fees: £26–35; Second visit: £21–30
Shrewsbury SY2
01743 365746

**Richard Allen GOsC, BOA**
⊕ ⊘
Fees: £26–35; Second visit: £21–30
Shrewsbury SY2
01743 365746

**Alison Allott GOsC**
O ⊘
Fees: <£25; Second visit: <£20
Shrewsbury SY3
01743 243273

**Denis McTurk GOsC**
⊕ O ⊘
Fees: £36–45; Second visit: £21–30
Shrewsbury SY18
01686 412456

**Russell White GOsC**
⊕ ⊕ ⊘ ❀
Fees: £26–35; Second visit: £21–30
Shrewsbury SY1
01743 357076

## STAFFORDSHIRE

**Roy Hughes GOsC, BOA**
⊕ ❀
Fees: £26–35; Second visit: £21–30
Burntwood WS7
01543 684980

**Peter Noon GOsC, BOA**
O 🅽 ❀
Fees: <£25; Second visit: <£20
Cannock WS12
01543 424075

# Osteopathy

**David Cooper GOsC**
🅾 🎵 💲
**Fees:** <£25; Second visit: £21–30
Newcastle-under-Lyme ST5
01782 633483

**Sharon Bradbury GOsC**
⊕ 🎵 💲
**Fees:** £26–35; Second visit: £21–30
Newcastle-under-Lyme ST5
01782 610500

**Mark Corson GOsC, BOA**
⊕ ⊕ 🎵 💲
**Fees:** <£25; Second visit: £21–30
Stafford ST16
01785 226848

**David Heath GOsC**
⊕ ⊕ 🎵 ©
**Fees:** £26–35; Second visit: £21–30
Stoke-on-Trent ST4
01782 658555

**Kendall Chew GOsC, BOA**
⊕ 🎵 © 💲
**Fees:** £26–35; Second visit: £21–30
Stoke-on-Trent ST7
01270 875020

**Martin Davies GOsC, BOA**
⊕ ⊕ 🎵 © 💲
**Fees:** £26–35; Second visit: £21–30
Stoke-on-Trent ST7
01270 883242

**Ian Whyte GOsC, BOA**
⊕ ⊕ ⊘ ⊜
**Fees:** £26–35; Second visit: £21–30
Stone ST15
01785 816481

**C Jane Easty GOsC, BOA**
⊕ ⊕ 🎵 ⊘
**Fees:** £36–45; Second visit: £41–50
Tamworth B79
01827 65568

**Jennifer Candlish GOsC, BOA**
⊕ 🅾 🎵 💲
**Fees:** £26–35; Second visit: £21–30
Uttoxeter ST14
01889 564883

## WARWICKSHIRE

**Sarah Pank GOsC, BOA**
⊕ ⊕ ⊕ 🎵 💲
**Fees:** <£25; Second visit: £31–40
Altrincham WA15
0161 929 8101

**John Williams GOsC**
🅾 💲
**Fees:** £26–35; Second visit: £21–30
Atherstone CV10
01827 712436

**Brian Collins GOsC**
⊕ 🅾 🎵
**Fees:** £26–35; Second visit: £21–30
Nuneaton CV11
024 7638 7449

**William Garland GOsC, BOA**
⊕ ⊕ 🎵
**Fees:** <£25; Second visit: £21–30
Rugby CV21
01788 560646

**Stephen Harris GOsC**
⊕ ⊕ 🎵 💲
**Fees:** £36–45; Second visit: £31–40
Rugby CV21,London W1T
01788 579595

**Adam Sheridan GOsC, BOA**
⊕ 🎵 © 💲
**Fees:** <£25; Second visit: £21–30
Rugby CV21
01788 560646

**Rebecca Houghton GOsC**
🅾 🎵 💲
**Fees:** <£25; Second visit: £31–40
Stratford-upon-Avon CV37
01789 731144

**Laurence Kirk GOsC**
⊕ ⊕ 🎵 💲
**Fees:** £26–35; Second visit: £21–30
Stratford-upon-Avon CV37
01789 267888

**James Kitchen GOsC, BOA**
⊕ ⊕ ⊕ 🎵 💲
**Fees:** £36–45; Second visit: £31–40
Stratford-upon-Avon CV37
01789 414289

# Osteopathy

**Alison Donley GOsC**
Fees: £26–35; Second visit: £21–30
Warwick CV34
01926 411497

## WEST MIDLANDS

**John R Coleman GOsC, BOA**
Fees: £26–35; Second visit: £21–30
Birmingham B36
0121 783 2914

**Peter Dutton GOsC, BOA**
Fees: <£25; Second visit: £21–30
Birmingham B31
0121 478 2802

**David Evans GOsC, BOA**
Fees: £26–35; Second visit: £21–30
Birmingham B30
0121 443 5500

**Thomas Harper GOsC, BOA**
Fees: £26–35; Second visit: £21–30
Birmingham B3,Nuneaton CV11
0121 236 2169

**Edwin G M Helder GOsC, BOA**
Fees: £26–35; Second visit: £21–30
Birmingham B31
0121 478 2802

**Justine Knowles GOsC**
Fees: £26–35; Second visit: £21–30
Birmingham B29
0121 472 4673

**Andrew Leask GOsC**
Fees: £26–35; Second visit: £21–30
Birmingham B2
0121 632 5332

**Stephen Ling GOsC, BOA**
Fees: £26–35; Second visit: £21–30
Birmingham B23
0121 350 2018

**Mamta Narayan GOsC, BOA**
Fees: £26–35; Second visit: £21–30
Birmingham B43
0121 357 9078

**Bharpoor Sohal GOsC, BOA**
Fees: £26–35; Second visit: £21–30
Birmingham B2
0121 632 5332

**Gordon Irving GOsC, BOA**
Fees: <£25; Second visit: £21–30
Bromsgrove B60
01527 872291

**Jackie Salter GOsC, BOA**
Fees: £26 35; Second visit: £21–30
Brierley Hill DY5
01384 483081

**Jim Cahill GOsC**
Fees: £36–45; Second visit: £21–30
Coventry CV4
024 7647 4466

**Joanne Sheridan GOsC, BOA**
Fees: <£25; Second visit: £21–30
Coventry CV1
024 7655 5114

**Deborah Bayley GOsC**
Fees: £26–35; Second visit: £21–30
Coventry CV36
0808 144 0909

**Carol Fawkes GOsC**
Fees: <£25; Second visit: >£50
Coventry CV3
024 7650 5997

**Richard Friend GOsC**
Fees: £26–35; Second visit: £21–30
Coventry CV1
024 7655 5114

# Osteopathy

**K H Lord GOsC, BOA**
🅞 🅝🅗
Fees: <£25; Second visit: £31–40
Coventry CV5
024 7667 3940

**Jane-Marian O'Connor GOsC, BOA**
🅞 🅝🅗 🅐 🅢
Fees: £36–45; Second visit: £21–30
Coventry CV32
01926 335932

**Everard Peters GOsC**
🅞 🅐 🅢
Fees: £26–35; Second visit: £21–30
Coventry CV31
01926 338168

**Suzanne Stanley-Smith GOsC, BOA**
🅔 🅞 🅖 🅝🅗 🅐 🅢
Fees: <£25; Second visit: £21–30
Coventry CV32
01926 424146

**Joseph Stapleton GOsC**
🅔 🅞 🅖 🅝🅗 🅢
Fees: £26–35; Second visit: £21–30
Coventry CV5
024 7669 1100

**Richard S Walker GOsC, BOA,**
🅔 🅞 🅝🅗 🅐 🅔
Fees: <£25; Second visit: £31–40
Coventry CV5
024 7667 7444

**Fiona Passey GOsC, BOA**
🅔 🅖 🅝🅗 🅐 🅢
Fees: £26–35; Second visit: £21–30
Halesowen B63
0121 585 8555

**Clare De Souza GOsC, BOA**
🅔 🅖 🅝🅗
Fees: £26–35; Second visit: £21–30
Solihull B93
01564 772246

**Tom Munden GOsC, BOA**
🅔 🅖 🅝🅗 🅢
Fees: £36–45; Second visit: £21–30
Solihull B93
01564 772246

**Jay Patel GOsC, BOA**
🅔 🅞 🅝🅗 🅢
Fees: £26–35; Second visit: £21–30
Solihull B91
0121 705 8353

**Paul Robinson GOsC**
🅔 🅖 🅝🅗 🅐 🅢
Fees: £26–35; Second visit: £21–30
Solihull B90
01564 702186

**Peter Rees GOsC**
🅔 🅞 🅖 🅝🅗 🅢
Fees: £26–35; Second visit: £21–30
Stourbridge DY8
01384 375271

**Barbara Stopczynska GOsC, BOA**
🅔 🅞 🅖 🅝🅗 🅢
Fees: £26–35; Second visit: £21–30
Sutton Coldfield B74
0121 352 1983

**David Jones GOsC**
🅔 🅞 🅖 🅝🅗
Fees: £26–35; Second visit: £21–30
Walsall WS1
01922 622521

**Jennifer Budd GOsC**
🅔 🅖 🅝🅗 🅐 🅢
Fees: £36–45; Second visit: £21–30
Wolverhampton WV1
01902 426486

**Geoff Hale GOsC, BOA**
🅔 🅖 🅝🅗
Fees: £26–35; Second visit: £21–30
Wolverhampton WV6
01902 429353

# Chiropractic

## HEREFORD & WORCESTER

**YenYang Co GCC, BCA**
⊕ ○ ⬤ Ⓔ ⬤
**Fees:** £36–45; Second visit: £21–30
Broadway WR12
01386 852463

**Judy Magnay GCC, MCA**
○ ⬤ ⬤
**Fees:** £26–35; Second visit: £21–30
Checkley HR1
01432 850443

**Helen Nunn GCC, BCA**
⊕ ⬤
**Fees:** £26–35; Second visit: £21–30
Hereford HR1
01432 352928

**Bruce Fraser GCC, MCA**
⊕ ○ ⊕ ⬤ ⬤
**Fees:** £26–35; Second visit: £21–30
Hereford HR1,Hereford HR2,
Gloucester GL3
01989 740325

**Jenni Turvey GCC, MCA**
⊕ ○ ⬤
**Fees:** £36–45; Second visit: £21–30
Ross-on-wye HR9
01989 762220

**Emma Gillett GCC, MCA**
⊕ ⊕ ⊕ ⬤ ⊘
**Fees:** £36–45; Second visit: £21–30
West Malvern WR14
01684 891463

**Patricia Ridler GCC, MCA**
⊕ ⬤
**Fees:** £36–45; Second visit: £21–30
Worcester WR10
01386 554209

**Alex Morton GCC, MCA**
⊕ ○ ⬤
**Fees:** £26–35; Second visit: £21–30
Worcester WR14
01684 566646

## SHROPSHIRE

**Martyn Spencer GCC, BAAC**
⊕
**Fees:** <£25; Second visit: <£20
Bucknell SY7
01547 530891

**Nigel P Fullerton GCC, BCA**
⊕ ⬤ ⬤
**Fees:** £26–35; Second visit: £21–30
Ludlow SY8
01584 874200

**Helen Lightfoot GCC, MCA**
○ ⊕ ⬤ ⊘ ⬤
**Fees:** £26–35; Second visit: £21–30
Market Drayton TF9
01630 647508

**Charles Kusiar Snr GCC, BCA**
○ ⬤ ⬤
**Fees:** £36–45; Second visit: <£20
Shrewsbury SY2
01743 343926

**B Matthews MNIMH**
⊕ ⊕ ⬤ ⬤
**Fees:** <£25; Second visit: <£20
Shrewsbury SY23
01974 282605

**Thomas D Gwilliam GCC, BCA**
⊕ ⬤ Ⓔ ⬤ ⬤
**Fees:** £26–35; Second visit: £21–30
Telford TF1
01952 242596

**Bridget McElwain GCC, BCA**
⊕ ⊕ ⬤ ⬤ ⬤
**Fees:** £26–35; Second visit: £21–30
Telford TF1
01952 242596

**Samantha Ostle GCC, MCA**
○ ⬤ ⊘ ⬤
**Fees:** £26–35; Second visit: £21–30
Telford TF6
01952 677002

**Simon David Pierce GCC, BCA**
⊕ ⬤ ⬤ ⬤
**Fees:** £26–35; Second visit: £21–30
Wellington TF1
01952 242596

# Chiropractic

## STAFFORDSHIRE

**Victoria Stanley GCC, BCA**
⊕ ⚫ ⊘ ❄
Fees: £26–35; Second visit: <£20
Stoke on Trent ST4
01782 627133

**Christina Rudd GCC, MCA**
O ⊘ ❄
Fees: £36–45; Second visit: £21–30
Burntwood WS7
01543 683495

**Pia Antrobus GCC, BCA**
⊕ ⊕ ⚫ ⊘ Ⓔ ❄ ⚫
Fees: £26–35; Second visit: £21–30
Lichfield WS14
01543 256844

**Jane Hvas GCC, BCA**
⊕ ⚫ ⊘ ⚫
Fees: £26–35; Second visit: £21–30
Stoke on Trent ST17
01782 614040

**Fiona Barney GCC, BAAC**
⊕ ⊕ ⚫ ⊘ ❄
Fees: £26–35; Second visit: <£20
Tamworth
01827 69762

**Amanda Green GCC, BCA**
⊕ ⚫ ⊘ Ⓔ ❄
Fees: £36–45; Second visit: £21–30
Tamworth B79
01827 310910

**Karen Jacobsen GCC, BCA**
⊕ ⚫ ⊘ ⚫
Fees: £26–35; Second visit: £21–30
Walton-on-the-hill ST17
01785 614040

## WARWICKSHIRE

**Rachel Newey GCC, MCA**
O ⚫ ❄
Fees: £36–45; Second visit: £31–40
Kenilworth CV8
01926 854094

**Carl Seal GCC, BAAC, MCA**
⊕ ⊕ ⚫ ❄
Fees: £26–35; Second visit: £21–30
Kenilworth CV8
01926 857545

**Michael Chester GCC, BAAC, MCA**
O ❄
Fees: £26–35; Second visit: £21–30
Rugby CV21
01788 536452

**Joy Lynch GCC, MCA**
⊕ ⚫ ❄
Fees: £26–35; Second visit: £21–30
Rugby CV21
01788 551913

**Gary Frogley GCC, MCA**
O ⚫ ❄
Fees: <£25; Second visit: £21–30
Rugby CV22
01773 8567380

**Deirdre Edwards GCC, MCA**
⊕ ⊕ ⚫ ⊘ ❄
Fees: £36–45; Second visit: £21–30
Stratford-upon-avon CV37
01789 294313

**Patricia McIntosh GCC, MCA**
O ⚫ Ⓔ ❄
Fees: £26–35; Second visit: £31–40
Warwick CV34
01926 491756

**Bronwen Hurley GCC, MCA**
⊕ O ⊕ ⚫ ❄
Fees: <£25; Second visit: £21–30
Warwick CV35
01926 640380

## WEST MILDLANDS

**Kevin Grant GCC, MCA**
⊕ ⊕ ⚫ ❄
Fees: £26–35; Second visit: £21–30
Birmingham B13,Bristol BS37
0121 449 9515

**Jo Hanstead GCC, MCA**
⊕ ⊕ ⊕ ⚫ Ⓔ ❄
Fees: £26–35; Second visit: £21–30
Birmingham B14
0121 443 1580

# Chiropractic

**Barbara Husband GCC, MCA**
⊕ ⊕ ⊕ ❀
**Fees:** £26–35; Second visit: £21–30
Birmingham B13
0121 449 9515

**James Rousseau GCC, BCA**
⊕ ⊕ ❀ ⊕
**Fees:** £26–35; Second visit: £21–30
Birmingham B12
0121 449 7766

**Mark Sammons GCC, MCA**
⊕ O ⊕ ⊕ ❀
**Fees:** £36–45; Second visit: £21–30
Birmingham B27
0121 706 4279

**Charles Sawyer GCC**
⊕ ⊕ ❀ ⊕
**Fees:** >£55; Second visit: £21–30
Birmingham B91
0121 705 1876

**Leslie Smith GCC, MCA**
⊕ ⊕ ⊕ ⊘
**Fees:** £26–35; Second visit: £21–30
Birmingham B14
0121 443 3478

**Lynn Wilkes GCC, MCA**
⊕ O ⊕ ⊕ Ⓔ ❀
**Fees:** £36–45; Second visit: £21–30
Birmingham B13
0121 449 9815

**John Duncombe GCC, MCA**
⊕ ⊕ ⊕ ❀
**Fees:** £26–35; Second visit: £21–30
Birmingham B13
0121 449 9515

**Lawrence Dawson GCC, BCA**
⊕ ⊕ ⊘ ❀ ⊕
**Fees:** £46–55; Second visit: £21–30
Birmingham B72
0121 321 1755

**Wendy Lymer GCC, MCA**
O ⊘ ❀
**Fees:** £26–35; Second visit: £21–30
Bromsgrove B60
01527 831972

**Tim Beardsley GCC, BCA**
⊕ ⊕ ⊘ Ⓔ ❀
**Fees:** £36–45; Second visit: £21–30
Bromsgrove B60
01527 831467

**Robert Hatfield GCC, BCA**
⊕ ⊘ ❀ ⊕ ⊕
**Fees:** £46–55; Second visit: £21–30
Coventry CV2
024 7645 2357

**Susan Faulkner GCC, MCA**
⊕ O ⊕ ⊕ ⊕ ❀
**Fees:** £26–35; Second visit: £21–30
Coventry CV4
024 7647 3727

**Helen James GCC, MCA**
⊕ O ⊕ ⊕ ❀
**Fees:** £26–35; Second visit: £21–30
Coventry CV47
01295 770369

**Kathryn Falconer GCC**
⊕ ⊕ ❀
**Fees:** £26–35; Second visit: <£20
Dudley DY9
01562 887388

**David Evans GCC, BCA**
⊕ ⊕ ⊘ ❀ ⊕
**Fees:** £26–35; Second visit: £21–30
Shirley B90
0121 744 6627

**Rashna Tucker GCC, BCA**
⊕ ⊕ ⊘ ❀ ⊕
**Fees:** £26–35; Second visit: £21–30
Shirley B90
0121 744 6627

**C Scott-Dawkins GCC, BCA**
⊕ ⊕ ⊕ ⊘
**Fees:** £46–55; Second visit: £21–30
Solihull B90
0121 744 6627

**Annette O'Neill GCC**
⊕ ⊕ ❀ ⊕
**Fees:** >£55; Second visit: £21–30
Solihull B91
0121 705 1876

# Chiropractic

**Jane Simblet GCC, BAAC, MCA**
➕ ⭕ 🔵 🔴 ✳️
**Fees:** £36–45; Second visit: £21–30
Solihull B91
0121 243 7749

**Oliver Crawford GCC, BCA**
➕ 🔴 ✳️
**Fees:** £26–35; Second visit: <£20
Stourbridge DY9
01562 887388

**John Lange GCC, BCA**
➕ 🔴 ⊘ ✳️ 🔘
**Fees:** £46–55; Second visit: £21–30
Sutton Coldfield B72,Solihull B90
0121 321 1755

**Ann Loveday GCC, MCA**
➕ 🔵 ⊘ ✳️
**Fees:** £26–35; Second visit: £21–30
Sutton Coldfield B73
0121 355 1554

**Paul Malone GCC, BCA**
➕ 🔵 🔴 ⊘ ✳️ 🔘
**Fees:** £26–35; Second visit: £21–30
Walsall WS1
01922 634959

**David Malone GCC, BAAC**
➕ ✳️
**Fees:** £46–55; Second visit: £21–30
Walsall WS1
01922 634959

**Henryk G Kulyha GCC, BCA**
➕ 🔴 ⊘ ✳️ 🔘
**Fees:** £26–35; Second visit: £21–30
Wolverhampton WV1
01902 772446

**John Oliver GCC, BCA**
🔴 ✳️
**Fees:** £26–35; Second visit: £21–30
Wolverhampton WV16
01746 769073

# Western Herbal Medicine

## HEREFORD & WORCESTER

**Helen Jones IRCH**
⭕ 🔵 ✳️
**Fees:** <£25; Second visit: <£20
Hay-on-Wye HR3
01497 820265

**C O Barnes MNIMH**
⭕ ✳️
**Fees:** <£25; Second visit: <£20
Hereford HR1
01432 274584

**R McOnegal MNIMH**
⭕ 🔴
**Fees:** £26–35; Second visit: £21–30
Hereford HR1
01432 820148

**Philip Weeks AMH**
➕ ✳️
**Fees:** £36–45; Second visit: £21–30
Hereford HR1
01432 360233

## SHROPSHIRE

**L Idoux MNIMH**
⭕
**Fees:** £26–35; Second visit: <£20
Oswestry SY11
01743 352533

**G Shakespeare MNIMH**
➕ 🔵 🔴 ⊘ ✳️
**Fees:** £26–35; Second visit: <£20
Telford TF7
07932 798574

**Nicky Jevon AMH**
⭕ ✳️
**Fees:** £36–45
Shropshire SY10
01691 671119

## STAFFORDSHIRE

**K P Lewis MNIMH**
⭕ ✳️
**Fees:** £36–45; Second visit: £21–30
Featherstone WV10
01902 863466

**C Dobie MNIMH**

✚ 〇 ⊕ 🔵 🔅
Fees: £36–45; Second visit: <£20
Leek ST13
01298 84661

**Clive Rooker AMH**

✚ 〇 ⊕ ⌀ 🔅
Fees: £36–45; Second visit: <£20
Lichfield WS14
01543 481497

**C Menzies-Trull MNIMH**

〇 🔅
Fees: £26–35; Second visit: <£20
Newcastle under Lyme ST5
01782 713977

**E E Lear MNIMH**

〇 🔅
Stone ST15
01785 813366

## WARWICKSHIRE

**A J Kaye MNIMH**

〇 ⊕ ⌀ € 🔅
Fees: £36–45; Second visit: £21–30
Fillongley CV7
01676 542142

**T Checklin MNIMH**

✚ 〇 ⊕ 🔵 ⌀
Fees: £36–45; Second visit: £31–40
Leamington Spa CV32
01926 316500

**J A Jones MNIMH**

✚ ⊕
Leamington Spa CV32
01926 316500

## WEST MIDLANDS

**Alan Payne AMH**

✚ ⊕ 🔵
Fees: £26–35; Second visit: <£20
Birmingham B79
01827 68374

**N Lopez MNIMH**

✚ 〇 ⊕ 🔅
Fees: £26–35; Second visit: <£20
Birmingham B12
0121 249 0338

**N Peterson MNIMH**

〇 🔵 € 🔅
Fees: £36–45; Second visit: £21–30
Birmingham B13
0121 449 4213

**Susanna Russon AMH**

✚ ⊕ 🔵 🔅
Fees: £36–45; Second visit: £21–30
Birmingham B38
0121 459 3535

**J Wright MNIMH**

✚ 🔅
Fees: £26–35; Second visit: <£20
Birmingham B9
0121 687 4448

**M J Burns MNIMH**

〇
Fees: >£55; Second visit: £41–50
Coventry CV3
024 7644 5441

**Abigail Francis AMH**

✚ 〇 ⊕ 🔵 🔅
Fees: £26–35; Second visit: <£20
Coventry CV8,Nottingham
NG16,Leamington Spa CV31
01926 857237

**A Chiotis MNIMH**

✚ 〇 🔅
Wolverhampton WV14
01902 404347

**G Hale MNIMH**

✚ ⊕ ⌀
Fees: £26–35; Second visit: <£20
Wolverhampton WV6
01902 429353

# Chinese Herbal Medicine

**Margaret Ehrenberg RCHM**
✪ ⊕ ✿
**Fees:** £26–35; Second visit: <£20
Birmingham B14
0121 441 2757

**Nick Lampert RCHM**
✪ ⊕ ✿
**Fees:** £26–35; Second visit: <£20
Birmingham B14
0121 441 2757

**Jacqueline Turner RCHM**
✪ O ⊕ ⊕
**Fees:** £26–35; Second visit: <£20
Birmingham B14, Droitwich
WR9, Worcester WR7
0121 443 1580

**Qing Yun Yao RCHM**
✪ ⊕ ⊕ ✿
**Fees:** £26–35; Second visit: £21–30
Birmingham B29, Redditch B97
0121 414 0287

# Scotland

Aberdeenshire
Angus
Argyll & Bute
Ayrshire
Dumfries & Galloway
East Lothian
Edinburgh
Fife
Glasgow
Highland

Inverclyde
Midlothian
Moray
North Lanarkshire
Orkney Islands
Perth & Kinross
Renfrewshire
Scottish Borders
South Lanarkshire
Stirling

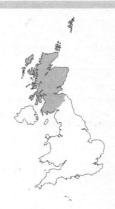

## Acupuncture

### ABERDEENSHIRE

**Kathleen Powderly BAcC**
O ⊘ ✿ ☻
Fees: £26–35; Second visit: £21–30
Aberdeen AB15
01224 326264

**Robert Wilson BAcC**
⊕ ⊕ ☻
Fees: £26–35; Second visit: £21–30
Aberdeen AB10
01224 572727

**Sheila Harper BAcC**
⊕ O ⊕ ✿ ☻
Fees: £26–35; Second visit: £21–30
Aberdeen AB22
01224 707157

**Claire Oldroyd AACP**
O ⊘ ✿ ☻
Fees: £46–55; Second visit: £31–40
Aberdeen AB21
01651 862399

**Elizabeth Ann Ross AACP**
O ☻
Fees: £36–45; Second visit: £41–50
Ellon AB41,Inverurie AB51
01651 851812

**Ishbel Spence BAcC**
O ⓔ ✿ ☻
Fees: £26–35; Second visit: £21–30
Peterhead AB42,Ellon AB41,Aberdeen
AB22
01779 472006

### ANGUS

**Kevin G McGhee BAcC**
⊕ ⊕ ⊘ ✿ ☻
Fees: £26–35; Second visit: £21–30
Broughty Ferry DD5
01382 737808

**Neil Falconer BAcC**
⊕ ✿ ☻
Fees: <£25
Dundee DD5
01382 774200

### ARGYLL & BUTE

**Marjorie Ann Sneddon AACP**
O ⊘ ☻
Fees: £36–45; Second visit: £31–40
Helensburgh G84
01436 679258

# Acupuncture

## AYRSHIRE

**Kathleen A Taylor AACP**
O ⊘ ☺
Fees: £26–35; Second visit: £21–30
Ayr KA7
01292 263295

**Tracey Telfer AACP**
⊕ O ⊕ ☺
Fees: £26–35; Second visit: £31–40
Galston KA4
01563 829040

**Jan de Vries BAcC**
⊕ ⊘ ✿ ☺
Fees: <£25; Second visit: <£20
Troon KA10,Glasgow G2,
Edinburgh EH1
01292 311414

## DUMFRIES & GALLOWAY

**Anne Leitch BAcC**
⊕ ⊕ ⊛ ⊘ ☺
Fees: £46–55; Second visit: £21–30
Dumfries DG1
01387 259944

**Lynda Sharp BAcC**
⊕ ⊕ ⊛ ✿ ☺
Fees: £26–35; Second visit: £21–30
Dumfries DG1
01387 267617

**Fred Smithers BAcC**
⊕ ⊕ ⊛ ☺
Fees: £46–55; Second visit: £21–30
Dumfries DG1
01387 259944

## EAST LOTHIAN

**Rona Smith AACP**
O ✿ ☺
Fees: £36–45; Second visit: £31–40
Tranent EH34
01875 340722

## EDINBURGH

**Andrea Battermann AACP**
⊕ ⊕ ☺
Fees: £36–45; Second visit: £21–30
Edinburgh EH8
0131 661 6052

**Jonathan Clogstoun-Willmott BAcC**
⊕ ⊕ ☺
Fees: £36–45; Second visit: £21–30
Edinburgh EH3
0131 225 1875

**Julia Edmonds BAcC**
⊕ O ✿ ☺
Fees: £36–45; Second visit: £21–30
Edinburgh EH8
0131 652 9995

**Quintus Farrell BAcC**
⊕ O ⊕ ✿ ☺
Fees: £26–35; Second visit: £21–30
Edinburgh EH1
0131 225 8092

**Jian Feng BAcC**
⊕ ☺
Fees: £26–35; Second visit: £21–30
Edinburgh EH3
0131 538 3303

**Rachael Forrest BAcC**
⊕ ⊕ ⊕ ✿ ☺
Fees: £26–35; Second visit: £21–30
Edinburgh EH3,Edinburgh EH3
0131 558 3303

**Sue Kingston BAcC**
O ✿ ☺
Fees: £36–45; Second visit: £21–30
Edinburgh EH4
0131 312 8494

**Sarah Price BAcC**
⊕ ⊕ ☺
Fees: £26–35; Second visit: £21–30
Edinburgh EH1
0131 225 8092

**Ming Chen Robertson BAcC**
⊕ ⊕ ✿ ☺
Fees: £36–45; Second visit: £31–40
Edinburgh EH6
0131 554 7888

**Jim Welsh BAcC**
O ✿ ⬤
Fees: £26–35; Second visit: £21–30
Edinburgh EH10
0131 466 7005

**Fiona Wolfenden BAcC**
⬤ ⬤ ✿ ⬤
Fees: £26–35; Second visit: £21–30
Edinburgh EH3,Edinburgh EH10
0131 3152130

## FIFE

**Catalina L Bowes BAcC**
⬤ ⬤ ✿ ⬤
Fees: £36–45; Second visit: £21–30
Dunfermline KY12
01383 314200

**A C Fawzi AACP**
⬤ ⬤ ⬤ ⬤
Fees: £36–45; Second visit: £31–40
Glenrothes KY7
01592 748832

**Jane Martin BAcC**
⬤ ⬤ ✿ ⬤
Fees: £26–35; Second visit: £21–30
Kirkcaldy KY1,St Andrews KY16
01592 264722

## GLASGOW

**Debbie Barbour AACP**
⬤ O ⬤ ⬤
Fees: £36–45; Second visit: £31–40
Glasgow G46,Glasgow G64
0141 585 7831

**Judith Bryden BAcC**
⬤ ⬤ ✿ ⬤
Fees: £26–35; Second visit: £21–30
Glasgow G64
0141 762 4162

**Myra Bunis BAcC, AACP**
⬤ ⬤ ⬤
Fees: £36–45; Second visit: £31–40
Glasgow G44
0141 633 3338

**David Campbell BMAS**
O ⊕ ⊘ ⬤
Fees: £36–45; Second visit: £21–30
Glasgow G77
0141 639 1853

**Ruth Chappell BAcC**
⬤ ⬤ ⬤ ✿ ⬤
Fees: £26–35; Second visit: £21–30
Glasgow G3
0141 332 4924

**Wei-Xiong Chen BAcC**
⬤ ✿ ⬤
Fees: £26–35; Second visit: £21–30
Glasgow G4
0141 357 1313

**Rhona Fraser BAcC**
⬤ ⬤ Ⓔ ✿ ⬤
Fees: £26–35; Second visit: £21–30
Glasgow G4
0141 552 4420

**Alan Hunter BAcC**
⬤ ⬤ ✿
Fees: £36–45; Second visit: £21–30
Glasgow G12,Glasgow G42
0141 339 5859

**Linda Miller BAcC**
⬤ O ⬤ ✿ ⬤
Fees: £46–55; Second visit: £21–30
Glasgow G63
01360 850215

**Caroline Rankin AACP**
⬤ O ✿ ⬤
Fees: £26–35; Second visit: £21–30
Glasgow G65
01236 823715

**Tom Williams BAcC**
O ✿ ⬤
Fees: £26–35; Second visit: £21–30
Glasgow G46
0141 638 8801

## HIGHLAND

**P J Boxx BAcC, BMAS,**
⬤ O Ⓔ ✿ ⬤
Carrbridge PH23
01479 841545

# Acupuncture

**Juliette Lowe BAcC**
⊕ O ⊕ ✿ 📖
**Fees:** £26–35; Second visit: £21–30
Inverness IV17,Alness IV17
01463 713614

## MIDLOTHIAN

**Gail Heatley  AACP**
⊕ ⊕ ✿ 📖 ⊘ 📖
**Fees:** £26–35; Second visit: £21–30
Loanhead EH20
07977 702456

## MORAY

**Annie Griffiths AACP**
O 📖 ✿ 📖
**Fees:** £26–35; Second visit: £31–40
Forres IV36
01309 676050

**Judy Light BAcC**
⊕ O ⊕ ⊕ ✿ 📖
**Fees:** £26–35; Second visit: £21–30
Forres IV36,Fochabers IV32
01309 671190

## PERTH & KINROSS

**Lou Radford BAcC**
O ⊕ ✿ 📖
**Fees:** £36–45; Second visit: £21–30
Aberfeldy PH15
01887 830242

**Patricia Magnus AACP**
O ⊘ 📖
**Fees:** £26–35; Second visit: £21–30
Auchterarder PH3
01764 660311

**Deborah Thomson BAcC,**
📖 ⊘ 📖
**Fees:** >£55; Second visit: £21–30
Crieff PH6
01764 679006

**Lynne A Gallagher AACP**
O 📖 ⊘ ✿ 📖
**Fees:** £36–45; Second visit: £31–40
Perth PH2
01738 442681

## RENFREWSHIRE

**Karen Campbell BAcC**
⊕ ⊕ ✿ 📖
**Fees:** £26–35
Johnstone PA5
01505 355502

**Neil D Scott-Kiddie BAcC**
⊕ O ⊕ ⊕ 📖 ✿ 📖
**Fees:** £26–35; Second visit: £21–30
Paisley PA1,Perth PH2
0141 889 8416

**Margaret O Williams AACP**
O ⊕ 📖 ⊘ ✿ 📖
**Fees:** £26–35; Second visit: £21–30
Paisley PA72
01680 300343

## SCOTTISH BORDERS

**Nicola Jones AACP**
O ⊘ ✿ 📖
**Fees:** £36–45; Second visit: £31–40
Hawick TD9
01450 870008

**Susan Meredith BAcC**
⊕ O ✿ 📖
**Fees:** £36–45; Second visit: £21–30
Hawick TD9
01450 370243

**Sally Vint AACP**
⊕ 📖 ⊘ 📖
**Fees:** £46–55; Second visit: £41–50
Hawick TD9
01450 860225

## STIRLING

**Mairi Menzies AACP**
⊕ 📖 ✿ 📖
**Fees:** £36–45; Second visit: £41–50
Callander FK17
01877 331351

## ABERDEENSHIRE

**Elaine Cairney RSHom**
⊕ ⊕ ⊛ ⓔ ✿
**Fees:** >£55; Second visit: £41–50
Aberdeen AB25,Forfar DD8
01224 636378

**Neil Spence FFHom, RSHom**
⊕ O ⊕ ⊛ ⊘ ⓔ ✿
**Fees:** >£55; Second visit: £41–50
Aberdeen AB25
01224 636378

**Anne Douglas MFHom**
⊕ ⊕ ⊛ ⊘
**Fees:** >£55; Second visit: £31–40
Aberdeen AB12
01224 876000

**Garton MFHom**
⊛ ⊘
Aberdeen AB15
01224 641560

**Murdoch J Shirreffs MFHom**
O ⊛ ⊘ ✿
**Fees:** >£55; Second visit: £31–40
Aberdeen AB10
01224 321998

**June Third-Carter MFHom**
⊕ ⊘ ✿
**Fees:** £25–35; Second visit: <£20
Fraserburgh AB43
01346 532998

## ANGUS

**Susan McAllion MFHom**
⊛ ⊘
Dundee DD2
01382 423141

**Liz Ellis MFHom**
⊕ O ⊕ ⊛ ⊘
**Fees:** >£55; Second visit: £20–30
Montrose DD10
01674 675213

## AYRSHIRE

**Maureen Scott MBE MFHom**
⊕ ⊛ ⊘ ⓔ ✿
**Fees:** £46–55; Second visit: £20–30
Ayr KA10
01292 288882

## DUMFRIES & GALLOWAY

**John K K Neil MFHom**
⊛ ⊘ ⓔ
Castle Douglas DG7
01644 420234

**Marion Gardner RSHom**
O ⊛ ✿
**Fees:** £36–45; Second visit: £20–30
Dalbeattie DG5
01556 620388

**Teresa Maxwell RSHom**
⊕ O ⊕ ⊛ ⓔ ✿
**Fees:** £36–45; Second visit: <£20
Dumfries DG1
01387 267617

**Christine Hudson RSHom**
O ⊛ ⓔ
**Fees:** £36–45; Second visit: £31–40
Lockerbie DG11
01576 710251

## EDINBURGH

**Helen Campbell FFHom, RSHom**
O ⊛ ⓔ ✿
**Fees:** £36–45; Second visit: £20–30
Edinburgh EH48
01501 730935

**Jennie Castell RSHom**
O ⊛ ⊘ ⓔ
**Fees:** £46–55; Second visit: £20–30
Edinburgh EH10,Selkirk TD7
0131 447 5364

**Jonathan Clogstoun-Willmott RSHom**
⊕ ⊕ ⊛ ⓔ
**Fees:** >£55; Second visit: £20–30
Edinburgh EH3
0131 225 1875

# Homeopathy

**Heinke Groth Woodbridge RSHom**
⊕ ⊕ ⊛ Ⓔ ❀
**Fees:** >£55; Second visit: £20–30
Edinburgh EH9
0131 229 9933

**Pat Hannaford MFHom**
⊕ ⊛ Ⓔ
**Fees:** >£55; Second visit: £20–30
Edinburgh EH9
0131 225 6617

**Rachel Harrison MFHom**
O ⊛ ⊘
**Fees:** £36–45; Second visit: £20–30
Edinburgh EH6,Edinburgh EH15
0131 554 1274

**Jane Patricia McGee RSHom**
⊕ O
**Fees:** £36–45; Second visit: £20–30
Edinburgh EH16,Dalkeith
EH22,Anstruther KY10
0131 667 2662

**Paula Millwood RSHom**
⊕ ⊕ Ⓔ
**Fees:** £46–55; Second visit: £31–40
Edinburgh EH3,Cupar KY15
0131 558 3303

**P S Mukherji MFHom**
O ⊛ ⊘ Ⓔ ❀
**Fees:** £46–55; Second visit: £20–30
Edinburgh EH10
0131 445 5668

**Kathi Parker RSHom**
⊕ ⊕ ⊛ Ⓔ ❀
**Fees:** £46–55; Second visit: £31–40
Edinburgh EH1,Whitley Bay NE26
0131 557 8286

**Rebecca Preston RSHom**
⊕ ⊕ ⊛ Ⓔ ❀
**Fees:** >£55; Second visit: £31–40
Edinburgh EH6
0131 554 7888

**Eva Tombs-Heirman RSHom**
⊕ ⊕ ⊕ ⊛ ⊘ Ⓔ ❀
**Fees:** >£55; Second visit: £20–30
Edinburgh EH10
0131 228 3234

## GLASGOW

**Mabel Aghadiuno MFHom**
⊛ ⊘
Glasgow G12
0141 637 3316

**Gabriel E Blass RSHom**
⊕ ⊕ ⊕ ⊛ ❀
**Fees:** £46–55; Second visit: £31–40
Glasgow G77,Glasgow G44,Glasgow
G1 5
0141 639 3644

**Valerie A Conway MFHom**
⊕ ⊕ ⊛ ❀
**Fees:** >£55; Second visit: £31–40
Glasgow G4
0141 339 0894

**Robert Jamieson MFHom**
⊕ ⊛ ⊘ Ⓔ
Glasgow G40
0141 531 6610

**Steven Kayne FFHom**
⊛ ⊘ Ⓔ ❀
**Fees:** £25–35; Second visit: <£20
Glasgow G76
0141 644 4344

**Gill Keith RSHom**
⊕ ⊛ Ⓔ ❀
**Fees:** >£55; Second visit: £31–40
Glasgow G3
0141 946 9330

**William Lang MFHom**
⊕ ⊛
**Fees:** £25–35; Second visit: <£20
Glasgow G41
0141 6320203

**R W Leckridge FFHom,**
⊛ ⊘
Glasgow G12
0141 211 1600

**Russell Malcolm FFHom,**
⊕ O ⊕ ⊛ ⊘ Ⓔ ❀
**Fees:** £46–55; Second visit: £41–50
Glasgow G3
0141 331 0393

**Alan Gordon Mathieson FFHom**
O ⊕ ⓦ ⊘ ⓔ ✿
Fees: >£55; Second visit: £31–40
Glasgow G12
0141 2111616

**K M Ohri MFHom**
⊕ ⓦ ⊘ ✿
Fees: >£55; Second visit: £31–40
Glasgow G72
0141 641 3729

**Leonard A Rosengard MFHom**
O ⊕ ⓦ ⊘ ⓔ ✿
Fees: £36–45; Second visit: <£20
Glasgow G73
0141 647 2800

**Thomas Whitmarsh FFHom,**
ⓦ ⊘ ✿
Fees: >£55; Second visit: £41–50
Glasgow G12
0141 211 1623

## HIGHLAND

**Vivien Maule RSHom**
⊕ O ⊕ ⓦ ⊘ ✿
Fees: >£55; Second visit: £31–40
Inverness IV3
01463 713614

## INVERCLYDE

**Anne M Pettigrew MFHom**
O ⊕ ⓦ ⊘ ⓔ
Fees: >£55; Second visit: £20–30
Greenock PA16
01475 888155

**Iain Stewart McLellan MFHom**
⊕ ⓦ ⊘
Fees: £36–45; Second visit: £20–30
Kilmacolm PA13
01505 872155

## NORTH LANARKSHIRE

**John Carlin RSHom**
⊕ O ⊕ ⊕ ⓦ ✿
Fees: £25–35; Second visit: £20–30
Airdrie ML6
01236 754935

## ORKNEY ISLANDS

**Patricia Mayborne RSHom**
⊕ O ⊕ ⓦ ⓔ ✿
Fees: £36–45; Second visit: £20–30
Stromness KW16
01856 851587

## PERTH & KINROSS

**Jude Wills-Hunt RSHom**
⊕ O ⓦ ⓔ
Fees: £46–55; Second visit: £20–30
Newtownmore PH20
01540 673358

## SOUTH LANARKSHIRE

**Anne Robb MFHom**
⊕ ⓦ
Fees: >£55; Second visit: £31–40
Lanark ML11
01555 662812

## STIRLING

**Liz Bradley MFHom**
⊕ ⊕ ⊕ ⓦ ⊘ ✿
Fees: >£55; Second visit: <£20
Stirling FK7
01786 451669

# Osteopathy

## ABERDEENSHIRE

**Peter Wilson PhD GOsC**
⊕ ⊕ ⊕ ⊛
Fees: £26–35; Second visit: £21–30
Aberdeen AB15
01224 622572

**Colin Ross GOsC**
⊕ ⊛
Fees: <£25; Second visit: £21–30
Aberdeen AB15
01224 310500

**Catherine Tiphanie GOsC**
⊕ ⊕ ⊛ ⊘
Fees: £26–35; Second visit: £21–30
Aberdeen AB10
01224 572727

**Robert Wilson GOsC**
⊕ ⊕ ⊛ ⊘
Fees: £26–35; Second visit: £21–30
Aberdeen AB10
01224 572727

**Fiona M Davison GOsC**
⊕ ⊕ ⊛ Ⓔ ✿
Fees: £26–35; Second visit: £21–30
Aberdeen AB25
01224 635999

**Gillian M Mitchell GOsC, BOA**
⊕ ⊛ ✿
Fees: <£25; Second visit: £31–40
Aberdeen AB25
01224 643803

**Maggie Brooks GOsC, BOA**
⊕ ⊕ ⊛ ✿
Fees: £26–35; Second visit: £21–30
Aberdeen AB23
01224 822956

## ANGUS

**Kevin McGhee GOsC, BOA**
⊕ ⊕ ⊛ ✿
Fees: £26–35; Second visit: £21–30
Dundee DD5
01382 737808

## ARGYLL & BUTE

**K Brimelow GOsC**
⊕ ⊛
Fees: <£25; Second visit: £21–30
Oban PA34
01631 565226

## AYRSHIRE

**Robert Johnston GOsC**
⊕ ⊕ ⊛ ⊘ Ⓔ ✿
Fees: <£25; Second visit: <£20
Ayr KA7
01292 441368

**Isla Brown GOsC**
⊕ Ⓞ ⊛ ✿
Fees: <£25; Second visit: £21–30
Kilmarnock KA4
01563 822244

**Faith Gardner GOsC,**
⊕ ⊘
Fees: <£25; Second visit: £21–30
Kilmarnock KA7
01292 611808

**Yvonne Potts GOsC, BOA**
Ⓞ ⊛ ✿
Fees: <£25; Second visit: £21–30
Kilmarnock KA7
01292 611808

## DUMFRIES & GALLOWAY

**Elizabeth Wilson GOsC, BOA**
⊕ ⊕ ⊛ ⊘ ✿
Fees: <£25; Second visit: <£20
Dumfries DG1
01387 267617

**Tim Baker GOsC**
⊕ ⊛
Fees: £26–35; Second visit: £21–30
Dundee DD2
01382 665717

**Neil Falconer GOsC, BOA**
⊕ ⊛ ✿
Fees: £26–35; Second visit: £21–30
Dundee DD5
01382 774200

**Neil Perkes GOsC**
⊕ ✿
Fees: <£25; Second visit: £21–30
Dundee DD5
01382 774200

**I H Flint GOsC, BOA**
⊕ ⊕ ⊛ ⊘
Fees: <£25; Second visit: £21–30
Dumfries DG1
01387 259944

## EAST LOTHIAN

**Thomas McMullen GOsC, BOA**
⊕ ⊕ ⊛ ✿
Fees: £26–35; Second visit: £21–30
Dunbar EH42
01368 864989

## EDINBURGH

**Paul Barratt GOsC**
⊕ ⊕ ⊛ ✿
Fees: <£25; Second visit: £31–40
Edinburgh EH16
0131 667 1234

**Lynn-Marie Bennett GOsC**
⊕ ⊕
Fees: £26–35; Second visit: £21–30
Edinburgh EH1
0131 225 5542

**Alison Bleasby GOsC**
O ⊛ ⊘ ✿
Fees: <£25; Second visit: £21–30
Edinburgh EH10
0131 445 2942

**Heidi Cram GOsC**
⊕ ⊕ ⊕ ⊛ ✿
Fees: £26–35; Second visit: £21–30
Edinburgh EH3,Glasgow G44
0131 225 9949

**Ms Pam Crosbie GOsC, BOA**
⊕ O ⊛ ✿
Fees: <£25; Second visit: £21–30
Edinburgh LEHT
0131 221 1415

**Helen How GOsC**
O ⊛ ✿
Edinburgh EH6
0131 551 1044

**Daniel M Iannarelli GOsC, BOA**
O ⊛ ✿
Fees: £26–35; Second visit: £21–30
Edinburgh EH8
0131 669 7960

**Andrew Patterson GOsC, BOA**
⊕ ⊕ ⊕ ⊛ ✿
Fees: £26–35; Second visit: £21–30
Edinburgh EH54
01506 202526

**Gavin Routledge GOsC, BOA**
⊕ ⊛ ⊘ © ✿
Fees: £26–35; Second visit: £21–30
Edinburgh EH1
0131 221 1415

**W J Stuart-Menteth GOsC**
©
Fees: £26–35; Second visit: £21–30
Edinburgh EH10
0131 447 4080

**Rosalind Stuart-Menteth GOsC**
O ©
Fees: £26–35; Second visit: £21–30
Edinburgh EH10
0131 447 4080

**Katrine Vogt GOsC, BOA**
⊕ ⊕ ⊛ ✿
Fees: £26–35; Second visit: £21–30
Edinburgh EH3
0131 558 3303

**Glynis Fox GOsC, BOA**
⊕ ⊘ ✿
Fees: <£25; Second visit: >£50
Edinburgh EH3
0131 557 2211

**Patrick Harding GOsC, BOA**
⊕ ⊕ ⊛ © ✿
Fees: £26–35; Second visit: £21–30
Edinburgh EH3
0131 558 3303

# Osteopathy

### Jessica Shaw GOsC, BOA
✚ O ⊕ Ⓜ ✚
Fees: <£25; Second visit: £21–30
Edinburgh EH1
0131 221 1415

### Matthew Smith GOsC
✚ ⊘ ✚
Fees: <£25; Second visit: >£50
Edinburgh EH3
0131 557 2211

## FIFE

### Sarah Tongue GOsC
✚ Ⓜ
Fees: £26–35; Second visit: £21–30
Kirkaldy KY16
01334 477000

### Seonaid McLeod GOsC, BOA
✚ Ⓜ ✚
Fees: <£25; Second visit: £31–40
Kirkcaldy KY1
01592 264722

## GLASGOW

### Asif Allauddin GOsC, BOA
✚ O ⊕ ✚
Fees: <£25; Second visit: £21–30
Glasgow G4
0141 552 4420

### Lindsey Campbell GOsC
O ✚
Fees: <£25; Second visit: £21–30
Glasgow G43
0141 571 7911

### Robert D Clarke GOsC, BOA
✚ ⊕ ⊕ Ⓜ ✚
Fees: <£25; Second visit: £21–30
Glasgow G67
01236 781958

### Dennis Cram GOsC, BOA
✚ ⊕ Ⓜ Ⓔ ✚
Fees: £26–35; Second visit: £21–30
Glasgow G4
0141 339 4164

### Alexander Cram GOsC
✚ ⊕ Ⓜ
Fees: £26–35; Second visit: £21–30
Glasgow G4
0141 339 0894

### Elizabeth Cram GOsC, BOA
✚ O ⊕ ✚
Fees: £26–35; Second visit: £21–30
Glasgow G4
0141 339 0894

### Normund Cram GOsC, BOA
✚ O ⊕ Ⓜ ✚
Fees: £26–35; Second visit: £21–30
Glasgow G4
0141 339 0894

### David Drysdale GOsC
✚ O ⊕ ✚
Fees: £26–35; Second visit: £21–30s
Glasgow G12
0141 339 5859

### Hannah Markham GOsC, BOA
✚ ⊕ Ⓜ
Fees: <£25; Second visit: £31–40
Glasgow G12
0141 334 0705

### Gillian E McIntosh GOsC
✚ ⊕ Ⓜ ✚
Fees: <£25; Second visit: £21–30
Glasgow G42
0141 632 1266

### Kirsten Elise Polson GOsC
✚ ⊕ Ⓜ Ⓔ ✚
Fees: <£25; Second visit: <£20
Glasgow G64
0141 762 4162

### Donald Scott GOsC, BOA
✚ O ⊕ ✚
Fees: £26–35; Second visit: £21–30
Glasgow G84
01436 672389

### Hamilton Semple GOsC
✚ ⊕ Ⓜ ✚
Fees: <£25; Second visit: £21–30
Glasgow G2
0141 572 1134

**James Sneddon GOsC, BOA**
Fees: £46–55; Second visit: £41–50
Glasgow G12
0141 339 4340

**Roderick Urquhart GOsC, BOA**
Fees: £26–35; Second visit: £21–30
Glasgow G74
01355 225995

## HIGHLAND

**John Mackenzie GOsC**
Fees: <£25; Second visit: £21–30
Inverness IV40
01599 555369

**Judith Rumbold GOsC, BOA**
Fees: £26–35; Second visit: £21–30
Inverness IV3
01463 713614

**Bryan Mcilwraith GOsC, BOA**
Fees: <£25; Second visit: £21–30
Inverness IV3
01463 222839

**Keith Grieve GOsC, BOA**
Fees: <£25; Second visit: £21–30
Thurso KW14
01847 896363

**Elizabeth Robinson GOsC, BOA**
Fees: <£25; Second visit: £21–30
Inverness IV30
01343 550382

## INVERCLYDE

**John D Cleat GOsC, BOA**
Fees: <£25; Second visit: £21–30
Greenock PA16
01475 888132

## MORAY

**Nigel Robinson GOsC, BOA**
Fees: <£25; Second visit: £21–30
Elgin IV30
01343 550382

## NORTH LANARKSHIRE

**Alexander Malkani GOsC**
Fees: <£25; Second visit: £21–30
Motherwell ML1
01698 267050

**Stuart Wilson GOsC**
Fees: <£25; Second visit: £21–30
Motherwell ML11
01555 665866

## PERTH & KINROSS

**Leonard Armfield GOsC, BOA**
Fees: <£25; Second visit: £21–30
Auchterarder PH3
01764 664600

**Julie Abberton GOsC, BOA**
Fees: £26–35; Second visit: £21–30
Kirkaldy KY13
01577 865665

**Kenneth Blakeley GOsC**
Fees: <£25
Perth PH1
01738 622509

**Boyd C MacKenzie GOsC**
Fees: £26–35; Second visit: £21–30
Perth PH2
01738 622864

## RENFREWSHIRE

**Iona Gray GOsC**
Fees: £26–35; Second visit: £21–30
Paisley PA34
01631 567054

# Osteopathy

**Carole M Mitchell GOsC, BOA**
✛ ⊕ ⓝ ⊘ ✿
**Fees:** <£25; Second visit: £41–50
Paisley PA1
0141 889 8416

## SCOTTISH BORDERS

**Ian Lambert GOsC**
✛ ⊕ ⊕ ⓝ ✿
**Fees:** £26–35; Second visit: £21–30
Peebles EH45
01721 722301

## STIRLING

**Keith Robertson GOsC, BOA**
✛ ⓝ ✿
**Fees:** <£25; Second visit: £31–40
Stirling FK8
01786 479832

# Chiropractic

## ABERDEENSHIRE

**Mark Jackson GCC**
✛ ⓝ ⊘ ✿
**Fees:** £36–45; Second visit: £21–30
Aberdeen AB53
01888 569123

**Les Hall GCC, BCA**
✛ ⓝ ✿
**Fees:** £36–45; Second visit: £21–30
Aberdeen AB15
01224 619240

**Elisabeth Madsen GCC, BCA**
✛ ⓝ ⊘ ⓔ ✿
**Fees:** £46–55; Second visit: £21–30
Aberdeen AB10,Shetland ZE1
01224 211517

## ANGUS

**Mark Cashley GCC**
✛ ⓝ ⓔ ✿
**Fees:** <£25; Second visit: <£20
Dundee DD4
01382 461081

## EDINBURGH

**Sasha Cessford GCC, MCA**
✛ ⓝ ⊘ ⓔ ✿
**Fees:** £36–45; Second visit: £21–30
Edinburgh EH17
0131 666 0314

**Shian Corley GCC, BAAC**
✛ ⊕ ✿
**Fees:** £36–45; Second visit: £31–40
Edinburgh EH1
0131 225 8092

## FIFE

**Alison Benramdane GCC, BCA**
✛ ⊕ ⊕ ⓝ
**Fees:** £26–35; Second visit: £21–30
Kirkcaldy KY1
01592 260791

## GLASGOW

**Allan Dalziel GCC, MCA**
✛ O ⊕ ⓝ ⊘ ✿
**Fees:** £36–45; Second visit: £21–30
Glasgow G76
0141 644 1111

**Carol Latto GCC, BCA**
✛ ⓝ ✿
**Fees:** £26–35; Second visit: £21–30
Glasgow G66
0141 776 1581

**Mette Stopa GCC, BCA**
O ⓝ ⊘ ⓔ ✿
**Fees:** £46–55; Second visit: £21–30
Glasgow G61
0141 570 0090

# Chiropractic

## HIGHLAND

**E Pearce GCC, BCA**
○ ○ ○ ○ ○
**Fees:** £26–35; Second visit: £21–30
Inverness IV3
01463 717084

## PERTH & KINROSS

**Patricia Waite GCC, BCA**
○ ○ ○ ○
**Fees:** £26–35; Second visit: £21–30
Aberfeldy PH15,Aberfeldy PH15
07808 223960

# Western Herbal Medicine

## ABERDEENSHIRE

**J Patterson MNIMH**
○ ○
**Fees:** £26–35; Second visit: <£20
Inverurie AB51
01467 626159

## ANGUS

**H H Cezanne MNIMH,**
○ ○ ○
**Fees:** £46–55; Second visit: £31–40
Dundee DD1
01382 223490

## ARGYLL & BUTE

**J Lambert MNIMH**
○ ○ ○ ○ ○
**Fees:** <£25; Second visit: <£20
Oban PA31
01546 850316

## DUMFRIES & GALLOWAY

**Chloe Bruce MNIMH**
○
**Fees:** <£25
Galloway DG8
01671 830390

## DUMFRIES & GALLOWAY

**Chloe Bruce MNIMH**
○
**Fees:** <£25
Galloway DG8
01671 830390

## EDINBURGH

**C Acott MNIMH**
○ ○ ○ ○ ○
**Fees:** <£25; Second visit: <£20
Edinburgh EH1
0131 225 5542

**D Atkinson MNIMH**
○ ○ ○ ○ ○
**Fees:** <£25; Second visit: <£20
Edinburgh EH1
0131 225 5542

**J M E Austin MNIMH**
○ ○ ○ ○
**Fees:** £26–35; Second visit: <£20
Edinburgh EH2
0131 226 3223

**A L Broughton MNIMH**
○ ○ ○ ○
**Fees:** <£25; Second visit: <£20
Edinburgh EH1
0131 225 5542

**K Brynes MNIMH**
○ ○ ○ ○
**Fees:** <£25; Second visit: <£20
Edinburgh EH1
0131 225 5542

**Z C Capernaros MNIMH**
○ ○ ○
**Fees:** £26–35; Second visit: £21–30
Edinburgh EH1,Bodle Street Green,
Hailsham
0131 556 6110

# Western Herbal Medicine

**DominiqueDavis MNIMH,**
⊕ O ⊕ ⊕ © ✿
**Fees:** <£25; Second visit: <£20
Edinburgh EH1,Hailsham BN27
0131 225 5542

**Sharon Macnish AMH**
⊕ O ⊕ ✿
**Fees:** £26–35; Second visit: £21–30
Edinburgh EH9,Edinburgh EH1
0131 662 0017

**J McGregor MNIMH**
⊕ ⊕ ✿
Edinburgh EH3
0131 315 2130

**Non Owen MNIMH**
⊕ ⊕ ⊕ ✿
**Fees:** <£25; Second visit: <£20
Edinburgh EH30
0131 315 2130

## FIFE

**J Geyer MNIMH**
⊕ ⊕ ⊕ ⊕ © ✿
**Fees:** <£25; Second visit: <£20
Dunfermline KY12,Glasgow G12
0131 315 2130

## GLASGOW

**I Boyd MNIMH**
⊕ ⊕ ✿
**Fees:** £26–35; Second visit: <£20
Glasgow G3
0141 445 4469

**L A Gourlay MNIMH**
O ⊕ ✿
**Fees:** <£25; Second visit: <£20
Glasgow G66
01360 310828

**Jenny Lancaster MNIMH**
⊕ O ⊕ ⊕ ∅ ✿
**Fees:** £26–35; Second visit: <£20
Glasgow G14
07950 161664

**W K Robertson MNIMH**
⊕ ⊕ ⊕ ⊕
**Fees:** £26–35; Second visit: <£20
Glasgow G4
0141 552 4420

**H R Speed MNIMH**
⊕ ⊕ ⊕ © ✿
**Fees:** <£25; Second visit: <£20
Glasgow G12
0141 339 5859

**C A Yarr MNIMH**
⊕ ⊕ ⊕ ✿
**Fees:** £26–35; Second visit: <£20
Glasgow G11
0141 334 0705

## HIGHLAND

**Alison Fraser MNIMH**
⊕ ⊕
**Fees:** <£25; Second visit: <£20
Inverness IV2,Hailsham BN27,Exeter
EX4
01463 238327

## PERTH & KINROSS

**J Hazzard MNIMH**
⊕ ✿
**Fees:** £26–35; Second visit: <£20
Pitlochry PH9
01887 840773

## RENFREWSHIRE

**M Russell MNIMH**
⊕ O ⊕ ⊕ ✿
**Fees:** £26–35; Second visit: £21–30
Bridge of Weir PA11
01505 615516

**M Robertson MNIMH**
⊕ ⊕ ✿
**Fees:** £26–35; Second visit: <£20
Paisley PA1
0141 882 7001

### STIRLING

**D Duncan MNIMH**
O ❀
Fees: <£25; Second visit: <£20
Dunblane FK15,Glasgow G51
01786 825897

**J Sharp MNIMH**
O ❀
Fees: <£25; Second visit: <£20
Stirling FK8
01786 473514

## Chinese Herbal Medicine

### ABERDEENSHIRE

**Kathleen Powderly RCHM**
O ⓦ ⊘ ❀
Fees: £26–35; Second visit: <£20
Aberdeen AB15
01224 326264

### DUMFRIES & GALLOWAY

**Lynda Sharp RCHM**
⊕ ⓖ ⓦ ❀
Fees: £26–35; Second visit: <£20
Dumfries DG1
01387 267617

### EDINBURGH

**James Welsh RCHM**
O ❀
Fees: £26–35; Second visit: £21–30
Edinburgh EH10
0131 466 7005

### FIFE

**Catalina Bowes RCHM**
⊕ ⓦ ❀
Fees: £26–35; Second visit: <£20
Dunfermline KY12
01383 314200

### GLASGOW

**Rhona Fraser RCHM**
⊕ ⓖ ❀
Fees: £26–35; Second visit: £21–30
Glasgow G4
0141 552 4420

**Tom Williams RCHM**
O ❀
Fees: £26–35; Second visit: £21–30
Glasgow G46
0141 638 8801

### HIGHLAND

**Juliette Lowe RCHM**
⊕ O ⓖ ⓦ ❀
Fees: £26–35; Second visit: £21–30
Inverness IV3
01349 884440

# Wales

## Acupuncture

### BRIDGEND

**Michael Williams BMAS**
Fees: £26–35; Second visit: £21–30
Bridgend CF31
01656 752100

### CARDIFF

**Claire Beeson AACP**
Fees: £26–35; Second visit: £21–30
Cardiff CF23
029 2077 3715

**Jacqeeline Brown BAcC, AACP**
Fees: £36–45; Second visit: £31–40
Cardiff CF5
01446 760143

**John V Denning BAcC**
Fees: £26–35; Second visit: £21–30
Cardiff CF10, Aberystwyth SY23,
Lampeter SA48
01974 251307

**Marilyn Irene Godfrey
BAcC, BMAS, AACP**
Fees: £36–45; Second visit: £41–50
Cardiff CF10,Dinas Powys
CF64,Bridgend CF32
029 2040 3010

**Catherine Markey BAcC**
Fees: £36–45; Second visit: £21–30
Cardiff CF11
029 2025 6908

**Kim Rowe AACP**
Fees: £36–45; Second visit: £31–40
Cardiff CF14
029 2048 8121

**Andrew Seary AACP**
Fees: £26–35; Second visit: £21–30
Cardiff CF14
029 20028365

# Acupuncture

## CARMARTHENSHIRE

**Carmel M Richards AACP**
○ ❀ 🔵
Fees: £36–45; Second visit: £21–30
Burry Port SA16
01554 834241

**Ann Francis AACP**
○ 🔵 ⊘ ❀ 🔵
Fees: £36–45; Second visit: £31–40
Kidwelly SA17
01554 890266

**Carey Morgan BAcC**
⊕ ❀ 🔵
Fees: £36–45; Second visit: £21–30
Llandeilo SA19
01558 824235

**Alice Panton BAcC**
⊕ 🔵 ❀ 🔵
Fees: £36–45; Second visit: £21–30
Llandeilo SA19
01558 824235

**Paul De Abreu BAcC**
○ 🔵 ⊘ ❀ 🔵
Fees: £26–35; Second visit: £21–30
Llanelli SA15
01554 756141

**Julian Dundas-Sleath BAcC**
○ ❀ 🔵
Fees: £26–35; Second visit: <£20
Llanelli SA14
01554 757570

## CEREDIGION

**Shion Morgan BAcC**
○ 🔵 ⊘ 🔵
Fees: £26–35; Second visit: £21–30
Aberystwyth SY23
01970 610030

**Alison Mary Kaye BAcC**
⊕ 🔵 🔵
Fees: £26–35; Second visit: <£20
Lampeter SA48
01570 423065

**Helene McMurtrie BAcC**
⊕ ⊘ ❀ 🔵
Fees: £36–45; Second visit: £21–30
New Quay SA45
01545 580686

## GWYNEDD

**Karen Cooper AACP**
⊕ 🔵 🔵
Fees: £26–35; Second visit: £21–30
Caernarfon LL55
01286 674173

**Vicki Creek BAcC**
○ ❀ 🔵
Fees: <£25; Second visit: <£20
Caernarfon LL54
01286 881479

**Anne Marie Williams BAcC**
○
Fees: £26–35; Second visit: £21–30
Llanfairfechan LL33
01248 680745

## ISLE OF ANGLESEY

**Shaun Ekberg BAcC**
⊕ ❀ 🔵
Fees: £46–55; Second visit: £21–30
Bodedern LL65
07747 017911

**Ethnea Scannell BAcC**
⊕ ○ 🔵 ❀ 🔵
Fees: £36–45; Second visit: £21–30
Holyhead LL65
01407 76

## MONMOUTHSHIRE

**Joan Davies AACP**
⊕ 🔵 🔵
Fees: £26–35; Second visit: £31–40
Abergavenny NP7
01873 854711

**Sue Taplin BAcC**
⊕ 🔵 ❀ 🔵
Fees: £36–45; Second visit: £21–30
Abergavenny NP7
01873 850544

# Acupuncture

**Peter Butcher BAcC**
⊕ ⊕ ✿ 📱
Fees: £36–45; Second visit: £21–30
Chepstow NP16, Newport NP20,
Bristol BS9
01291 627722

**Elizabeth Wilson BAcC, AACP**
⊕ ⊕ ⊘ ⊕
Fees: £26–35; Second visit: £21–30
Chepstow NP16
01291 636673

**Colin Biddle BAcC**
⊕ O ⊕
Fees: £26–35; Second visit: £31–40
Monmouth NP25,Bristol BS8
01989 770395

**Lesley Gann BAcC**
⊕ ⊕ ✿ ⊕
Fees: £36–45; Second visit: £21–30
102 Monnow St NP5
01600 772622

## NEATH PORT TALBOT

**Leslie Ross BAcC**
⊕ O ⊕ ⊕ ✿ ⊕
Fees: £36–45; Second visit: £21–30
Port Talbot SA12
01233 733387

## PEMBROKESHIRE

**Niki Oates BAcC**
⊕ ⊕ ⊕
Fees: £36–45; Second visit: £21–30
Narberth SA67,Fishguard
SA65,Carmarthen SA31
01834 860200

**Christian Ashdown BAcC**
⊕ O ⊕ ⊕ ✿ ⊕
Fees: £26–35; Second visit: £21–30
Tenby SA70
01834 871117

## POWYS

**Deborah Smith BAcC**
⊕ ⊕
Fees: £36–45; Second visit: £21–30
Brecon LD3,Kington HR5
01874 623577

**David Smith BAcC**
⊕ © ⊕
Fees: £36–45; Second visit: £21–30
Brecon LD3,Hereford HR1
01874 623577

**Angela Llewellyn BAcC**
⊕ ⊕ © ✿ ⊕
Fees: <£25; Second visit: £21–30
Machynlleth SY20
01650 511350

## SWANSEA

**Duncan Spowart AACP**
O ⊕ ⊕ ⊕
Fees: £26–35; Second visit: £31–40
Swansea SA1
01792 473957

**Simon Webborn BAcC**
⊕ ⊕ ⊕
Fees: <£25; Second visit: £21–30
Swansea SA1
01792 64432

**Limin Zhu BAcC**
⊕ ⊕ ✿ ⊕
Fees: <£25; Second visit: £21–30
Swansea SA1
01792 474488

**David Graham-Woollard AACP**
O ⊘ ⊕
Fees: £26–35; Second visit: £21–30
Swansea SA5
01792 537648

**Andrew Maggs AACP**
⊕ O ⊘ ⊕
Fees: £36–45; Second visit: £31–40
Swansea SA5
01792 774618

## VALE OF GLAMORGAN

**Anne Brown AACP**
O ⊕ ⊘ ✿ ⊕
Fees: £26–35; Second visit: £31–40
Barry CF62
01446 737722

# Acupuncture

### Helen Hopkins AACP
⊕ ⓝ ⬥ ⑩
**Fees:** £36–45; Second visit: £41–50
Cowbridge CF71,Cowbridge CF71
01446 775633

### Kathy Williams AACP
O ⬥ ⑩
**Fees:** £36–45; Second visit: £31–40
Cowbridge CF71
01446 775326

### Fiona John AACP
⊕ ⊕ ⑩
**Fees:** £36–45; Second visit: £31–40
Llantwit Major CF61,Cardiff CF11
01446 794166

### WREXHAM

### L Heaton AACP
⊕ ⓝ ⑩
**Fees:** £26–35; Second visit: £21–30
Wrexham LL13
01978 312407

### Julia James AACP
⊕ ⊘ ⬥ ⑩
**Fees:** £26–35; Second visit: £21–30
Wrexham LL13
01978 312407

# Homeopathy

### BRIDGEND

### Noel Thomas MFHom
O ⓝ ⊘ € ⬥
Maesteg CF34
01656 733262

### CAERPHILLY

### Elaine Watson RSHom
⊕ O ⊕ ⓝ € ⬥
**Fees:** £46–55; Second visit: £31–40
Caerphilly CF83, Cardiff CF10
029 2088 4968

### CARDIFF

### Joseph Beighton RSHom
⊕ O ⊕ ⊕ ⓝ € ⬥
**Fees:** £46–55; Second visit: £20–30
Cardiff CF11,Bridgwater
TA5,Blackwood NP12
029 2022 2221

### Marilyn Godfrey RSHom
⊕ ⊕ ⓝ ⊘ € ⬥
**Fees:** £46–55; Second visit: £41–50
Cardiff CF10,Dinas Powys
CF64,Bridgend CF32
029 2040 3010

### Kathryn Impey RSHom
⊕ O ⊕ ⓝ €
**Fees:** £36–45; Second visit: £20–30
Cardiff CF11
029 2022 8889

### Geraldine Killick RSHom
O € ⬥
**Fees:** £36–45; Second visit: £20–30
Cardiff CF14
029 2075 6130

### Felicity Lee RSHom
⊕ ⊕ ⓝ ⊘ €
**Fees:** £46–55; Second visit: £20–30
Cardiff CF23
029 2048 4555

### Miranda Parsons RSHom
O ⓝ ⬥
**Fees:** £46–55; Second visit: £20–30
Cardiff CF23
029 2076 6225

### CEREDIGION

### Vicky Reed RSHom
⊕ ⊘ €
**Fees:** £46–55; Second visit: £31–40
Aberystwyth SY23
01654 703289

**Hilaire Wood RSHom**
⊕ O ⊕ ⓦ ⓔ ❀
**Fees:** £25–35; Second visit: £20–30
Aberystwyth SY23
01970 880801

## CONWY

**Emlyn Thomas RSHom**
⊕ ⊕ ⓦ ⓔ ❀
**Fees:** £36–45; Second visit: £20–30
Llandudno LL27
01492 642043

## DENBIGHSHIRE

**Anne Johnston RSHom**
⊕ O ⊕ ⊕ ⓦ
**Fees:** £36–45; Second visit: £20–30
Llangollen LL20
01691 718782

**Andrew Kirk RSHom**
⊕ ⊕ ⊕ ⓦ ❀
**Fees:** £36–45; Second visit: £20–30
Ruthin LL15,Chester CH2
01824 707738

## GWENT

**Ian Hamilton RSHom**
O ⓦ ⓔ ❀
**Fees:** £36–45; Second visit: £20–30
Caerleon NP18
01633 423401

## GWYNEDD

**Julie Hodgson RSHom**
⊕ O ⊕ ⊘ ⓔ
**Fees:** £25–35; Second visit: £20–30
Arthog LL39
01341 250065

**Paul Nickson MFHom**
⊕ ⓦ ⊘
**Fees:** £46–55; Second visit: £20–30
Bangor LL57
01248 600212

## MONMOUTHSHIRE

**Jean Child RSHom**
⊕ O ⓦ
**Fees:** £36–45; Second visit: <£20
Caldicot NP26
01291 422037

## NEWPORT

**Gordon Adam RSHom**
⊕ O ⊕ ⓦ ⓔ ❀
**Fees:** £46–55; Second visit: £20–30
Newport NP20,Bristol BS7
01633 843333

## PEMBROKESHIRE

**Judith Williams FFHom, RSHom**
O ⓦ
**Fees:** £36–45; Second visit: <£20
Tenby SA70
01834 844467

## POWYS

**Catherine Evans RSHom**
⊕ ⓦ ⊘
**Fees:** £36–45; Second visit: £20–30
Machynlleth SY20
01650 511626

**Jane Walsh RSHom**
⊕ O ⊕ ⓦ ⓔ
**Fees:** £36–45; Second visit: £20–30
Presteigne LD8
01544 267685

## SWANSEA

**Patricia Bracewell RSHom**
O ⊕ ⓦ ⓔ
**Fees:** £36–45; Second visit: <£20
Abertawe SA6,Swansea SA8
01792 700723

**Siobhan Haynes RSHom**
⊕ ⊕ ⊕ ⓔ ❀
**Fees:** £46–55; Second visit: £20–30
Swansea SA1,Carmarthen
SA31,Swansea SA2
01792 419699

# Homeopathy

**Judith Johnson RSHom**
⊕ ⊕ ⓝ ⓔ ❈
**Fees:** £46–55; Second visit: £20–30
Swansea SA1
01792 874237

## VALE OF GLAMORGAN

**Vivienne Thompson RSHom**
⊕ Ⓞ ⊕ ⓝ ⓔ
**Fees:** >£55; Second visit: £31–40
Cowbridge CF71
01656 890700

**Cathy Thomson RSHom**
Ⓞ ⓝ ⓔ ❈
**Fees:** £46–55; Second visit: £20–30
Penarth CF64
029 2071 1552

# Osteopathy

## BRIDGEND

**Ian Griffiths GOsC, BOA**
⊕ ⓝ ❈
**Fees:** £26–35; Second visit: £21–30
Bridgend CF31
01656 646446

## CAERPHILLY

**Noel Davies GOsC**
⊕
**Fees:** <£25; Second visit: <£20
Blackwood NP12
01495 225655

## CARDIFF

**Angela Cavil GOsC, BOA**
⊕ ⓝ ⊘
**Fees:** £26–35; Second visit: £21–30
Cardiff CF37
01443 485302

**Ian Elias GOsC, BOA**
⊕ ⊕ ⓝ ⊘
**Fees:** £26–35; Second visit: £21–30
Cardiff CF11
029 2023 5220

**Mari Evans GOsC, BOA**
⊕ ⓝ ⓔ ❈
**Fees:** £26–35; Second visit: £21–30
Cardiff CF5
029 2021 4552

**Stephen Mann GOsC, BOA**
⊕ ⓝ ⊘ ❈
**Fees:** £26–35; Second visit: £21–30
Cardiff CF23
07932 043210

**John Mullins GOsC**
⊕ Ⓞ ⊕ ⓝ ❈
**Fees:** <£25; Second visit: £21–30
Cardiff CF24
029 2048 2682

**Erjan Mustafa GOsC, BOA**
⊕ ⓝ ❈
**Fees:** £36–45; Second visit: £31–40
Cardiff CF11
029 2040 9380

**Peter Palmer GOsC, BOA**
⊕ ⊕ ⊕ ⓝ ⊘ ❈
**Fees:** £26–35; Second visit: £21–30
Cardiff CF11
029 2064 0474

**Phil Parry GOsC, BOA**
⊕ ⊕ ⊕ ⓝ ❈
**Fees:** <£25; Second visit: £31–40
Cardiff CF23
029 2076 5522

**Joanne Perkins GOsC, BOA**
⊕ Ⓞ ⓝ ❈
**Fees:** <£25; Second visit: £21–30
Cardiff CF14
029 2069 3258

## CEREDIGION

**Katie Graham-Howell GOsC**
✪ O ⊕ 💬 ❋
Fees: <£25; Second visit: £21–30
Lampeter SA48
01570 421241

## CONWY

**Sarah Foskett GOsC, BOA**
✪ 💬
Fees: <£25; Second visit: £21–30
Llandudno LL49
01766 514680

**Paul Greenhalgh GOsC, BOA**
O 💬 ⓔ ❋
Fees: <£25; Second visit: £21–30
Colwyn Bay LL29
01492 531542

**Sally Ganderton GOsC**
⊕ 💬
Fees: £26–35; Second visit: £21–30
Conwy LL26
01492 640411

**Alison Greenhalgh GOsC, BOA**
O 💬 ❋
Fees: £26–35; Second visit: £21–30
Conwy LL29
01492 531542

**Teresa Harcourt GOsC**
✪ 💬
Fees: <£25; Second visit: £21–30
Llandudno LL31
01492 573500

**Diane Kane GOsC**
✪ ⓔ ❋
Fees: <£25; Second visit: £21–30
Llandudno LL16
01745 813718

**Sharon Tyler GOsC**
✪ O ⊕ 💬 ⊘ ⓔ ❋
Fees: £26–35; Second visit: £21–30
Llandudno LL20
07974 670286

## DENBIGHSHIRE

**Stephen Paul Pitstow GOsC, BOA**
✪ 💬 ⓔ ❋
Fees: <£25; Second visit: <£20
Rhyl LL18
01745 339314

## GWYNEDD

**Coby Langford GOsC**
✪ ⓔ ❋
Fees: £26–35; Second visit: £21–30
Bangor LL57
01248 372037

## MONMOUTHSHIRE

**Alasdair Jacks GOsC, BOA,**
⊕ ⊘
Fees: £36–45; Second visit: £31–40
Chepstow NP16
01291 636100

**Colin Biddle GOsC, BOA**
✪ O 💬
Fees: <£25; Second visit: £21–30
Monmouth NP25
01989 770395

**C Love GOsC**
O 💬
Fees: <£25; Second visit: £21–30
Monmouth NP25
01600 716880

**Andrew Michie GOsC**
✪ O 💬
Fees: £26–35; Second visit: £21–30
Monmouth NP25
01600 716880

## NEWPORT

**Angela Fawcett GOsC, BOA**
✪ ⊕ 💬 ❋
Fees: £26–35; Second visit: £21–30
Newport NP20
01633 843333

# Osteopathy

## Jane Geddes GOsC, BOA
⊕ O ⊕ ⊛ ⊛
**Fees:** <£25; Second visit: £21–30
Newport NP9, Potters Bar EN6,
Dorking RH4
01633 277263

## Julia Griffiths GOsC
⊕ ⊕ ⊛ ⊛
**Fees:** £26–35; Second visit: £21–30
Newport NP16
01291 627374

## Stuart Kramer GOsC
⊕ O ⊛ ⓔ ⊛
**Fees:** £26–35; Second visit: £21–30
Newport NP25
01600 772166

## Charlotte Kramer GOsC
⊕ O ⊛ ⊛ ⓔ ⊛
**Fees:** £26–35; Second visit: £21–30
Newport NP25
01600 772166

## Andrew J Lewis GOsC
⊕ ⊛
**Fees:** <£25; Second visit: £21–30
Newport NP20
01291 424833

## Jonathan Nichols GOsC, BOA
⊕ ⊕ ⊘ ⊛
**Fees:** £26–35; Second visit: £21–30
Newport NP16
01291 627374

### PEMBROKESHIRE

## Richard Blacklaw-Jones GOsC, BOA
⊕ ⊛ ⊛
**Fees:** £36–45; Second visit: £21–30
Haverfordwest SA61
01437 769713

### POWYS

## Genevieve Brown GOsC, BOA
⊕ O ⊕ ⊛ ⊘ ⊛
**Fees:** £26–35; Second visit: £21–30
Builth Wells LD2,Ceredigion SY23
01597 851759

## Simon Guinane GOsC
⊕ ⊛
**Fees:** <£25; Second visit: <£20
Llandrindod Wells LD3
01497 847020

## Jennifer Hodge GOsC, BOA
⊕ O ⊕ ⊛ ⊛
**Fees:** £26–35; Second visit: £21–30
Llandrindod Wells LD8
01544 350241

## Tracey Jones GOsC
⊕ ⊛
**Fees:** <£25; Second visit: <£20
Llandrindod Wells LD3
01497 847020

## David Rodway GOsC, BOA
⊕ ⊕ ⊛ ⊘ ⊛
**Fees:** <£25; Second visit: <£20
Llandrindod Wells LD3
01874 624000

## John Wilden GOsC, BOA
⊕ O ⊕ ⊛ ⊘ ⊛
**Fees:** <£25; Second visit: £21–30
Llanidloes SY18
01686 412230

## Marion Jones GOsC, BOA
⊕ ⊛
**Fees:** £26–35; Second visit: £21–30
Welshpool SY21
01938 556073

### RHONDDA CYNON TAFF

## John Hunt GOsC, BOA
⊕ ⊕ ⊛ ⊛
**Fees:** £26–35; Second visit: £21–30
Pontypridd CF38
01443 204134

## Darius Ridge GOsC
⊕ ⊛ ⊛
**Fees:** <£25; Second visit: <£20
Aberdare CF44
01685 870000

## SWANSEA

**Richard Burden GOsC, BOA**
➕ ⊕ 💊 €
Fees: <£25; Second visit: £21–30
Swansea SA1
01792 654751

**Jill Cantor GOsC, BOA**
➕ O ⊕ 💊 🏵
Fees: £26–35; Second visit: £21–30
Swansea SA43
01239 881308

**Kathy Evans GOsC**
➕ 💊 ⊘ 🏵
Fees: <£25; Second visit: £21–30
Swansea SA3
01792 362150

**David John Rodway GOsC, BOA**
➕ 💊 ⊘ 🏵
Fees: <£25; Second visit: £31–40
Swansea SA2
01792 298767

**Michael Griffiths GOsC, BOA**
➕ 💊 🏵
Fees: <£25; Second visit: £21–30
Swansea SA1
01792 644362

**John Jones GOsC, BOA**
O 💊 🏵
Fees: <£25; Second visit: £21–30
Swansea SA32
01559 384382

**John Palmer GOsC**
➕ ⊘ 🏵
Fees: <£25; Second visit: £21–30
Swansea SA3
01792 362150

## VALE OF GLAMORGAN

**Philippa Slack GOsC**
➕ ⊘ 🏵
Fees: £46–55; Second visit: £31–40
Penarth CF64
029 2070 8350

## WREXHAM

**Paul Dykins GOsC**
➕ 💊 🏵
Fees: <£25; Second visit: £21–30
Wrexham LL12
01978 310197

**Steven Shepherd GOsC, BOA**
➕ O 💊
Fees: £26–35; Second visit: £21–30
Wrexham LL11
01978 262120

# Chiropractic

## CAERPHILLY

**Gary Norman GCC, BCA**
➕ 💊 🏵
Fees: £36–45; Second visit: £21–30
Oakdale CF4
01495 225388

## CARDIFF

**Michael Barber GCC, BCA**
➕ ⊕ 💊 ⊘ 🏵
Fees: £36–45; Second visit: <£20
Cardiff CF71
01446 771114

**Bjorn Hennius GCC, BCA**
➕ 💊 🏵
Fees: £26–35; Second visit: £21–30
Cardiff CF83
029 2088 1882

# Chiropractic

**Annabel Kier GCC, BCA**
⊕ ⊕ ⊘ ✿
Fees: <£25; Second visit: <£20
Cardiff CF71
01446 771114

**Andrew Miles GCC, BCA**
⊕ ⊘ ✿
Fees: £36–45; Second visit: £21–30
Cardiff CF14
029 2055 2299

**Clive Taylor GCC, MCA**
⊕ ⊕ ⊕ ✿
Fees: £26–35; Second visit: £21–30
Cardiff CF23
029 2048 4555

**Shanee Taylor GCC, MCA**
⊕ ⊕ ⊕ ✿
Fees: £26–35; Second visit: £21–30
Cardiff CF23
(029) 20484555

**Rainer Wieser GCC, BCA**
⊕ ⊕ ⊘ ✿
Fees: £36–45; Second visit: £21–30
Cardiff CF14
029 2062 7888

**Barney O'Donnell GCC, MCA**
O ⊕ ✿
Fees: £36–45; Second visit: £21–30
Cardiff CF64
029 2070 0124

## CARMARTHENSHIRE

**Peter Gordon Jarvis GCC, BCA**
⊕ ⊕ ⊕ ⊘ ⊕ ✿
Fees: £26–35; Second visit: £21–30
Carmarthen SA31
01267 231788

## CEREDIGION

**Richard David Purcell GCC, BAAC**
⊕ ⊕ ⊕ ⊕ ✿
Fees: £26–35; Second visit: £21–30
Aberaeron SA46
01545 570000

## DENBIGHSHIRE

**Gail Futcher GCC, MCA**
⊕ ✿
Fees: £26–35; Second visit: £21–30
Corwen LL21
01490 413255

**Janette Keeley GCC, MCA**
⊕ O ⊕ ⊕ ✿
Fees: £26–35; Second visit: £21–30
Ruthin LL15
01824 750463

## GWYNEDD

**S Mack-Smith GCC, BCA**
⊕ ⊕ ⊕ ⊘ ✿
Fees: £36–45; Second visit: <£20
Bangor LL57
01248 370242

## MONMOUTHSHIRE

**Susan Cartlidge GCC, MCA**
⊕ ⊕ ⊕ ⓔ
Fees: £26–35; Second visit: £21–30
Abergavenny NP7,Abergavenny NP7
01873 858391

## NEWPORT

**Ben Bacon GCC, BCA**
⊕ ⊕ ⓔ ✿
Fees: £36–45; Second visit: £21–30
Newport NP20
01633 662022

## PEMBROKESHIRE

**Gillian Roy GCC, MCA**
O ⊕ ⊕ ✿
Fees: £26–35; Second visit: £21–30
Fishguard SA65
01348 840247

## POWYS

**Bethan Riley GCC, MCA**
⊕ ⊘
Fees: £36–45; Second visit: £31–40
Machynlleth SY20,Aberystwyth SY23
01654 702959

# Chiropractic

## SWANSEA

**Andrew Glaister GCC, BCA**
✚ 🅜 ⊘ 🅢
**Fees:** £26–35; Second visit: <£20
Swansea SA67,Carmarthen SA31
01834 860200

**G W Carlisle GCC**
✚ ✚ 🅢
**Fees:** £36–45; Second visit: £21–30
Swansea SA2
01792 281100

## VALE OF GLAMORGAN

**David Byfield GCC, BCA**
✚ 🅜 🅢
**Fees:** <£25; Second visit: <£20
Cowbridge CF71
01446 771114

**S B Lawson GCC, BCA**
✚ 🅜 ⊘ 🅢
**Fees:** £36–45; Second visit: £21–30
Penarth CF64
07813 113050

# Western Herbal Medicine

## CARDIFF

**M Last MNIMH**
✚ 🅐 🅜 🅢
**Fees:** £26–35; Second visit: £21–30
Cardiff CF11
029 2022 2221

**L McCarthy MNIMH**
✚ 🅐 🅜 🅢
**Fees:** £26–35; Second visit: <£20
Cardiff CF10
029 2023 5721

**M Roy MNIMH**
🅞 🅢
**Fees:** £26–35; Second visit: <£20
Cardiff CF24
029 2049 2180

**Rosemary Westlake MNIMH**
✚ 🅞 🅐 🅢
**Fees:** £26–35; Second visit: <£20
Cardiff CF11
0800 018 5090

## CARMARTHENSHIRE

**A-M Goldthorp MNIMH**
🅞 🅔
Trawsmawr SA33
01267 281223

**C Saad MNIMH**
✚ 🅞 🅐 🅜
**Fees:** £26–35; Second visit: £21–30
Ferryside SA17
01267 267653

## CEREDIGION

**A Noon MNIMH**
✚ 🅞 🅐 🅜 🅢
**Fees:** £26–35; Second visit: <£20
Aberystwyth SY23
01970 820713

## CONWY

**Jo Hughes AMH**
🅞 🅜 🅢
**Fees:** £26–35; Second visit: <£20
Llandudno LL30
01492 873506

## DENBIGHSHIRE

**P Waller MNIMH**
✚ 🅞 🅐 🅔 🅢
**Fees:** <£25; Second visit: <£20
Llangollen LL20
01978 869449

# Western Herbal Medicine

## MONMOUTHSHIRE

**M Last MNIMH**
➕ ⓝ ⊘ ❀
Fees: £26–35; Second visit: £21–30
Monmouth NP25
01600 719497

## PEMBROKESHIRE

**Margaret A Moss IRCH**
➕ ⭕ ⊕ ⓝ ❀
Fees: £36–45; Second visit: £21–30
Narberth SA67
01834 861408

## POWYS

**S Millican MNIMH**
➕ ❀
Fees: <£25; Second visit: <£20
Llandysul SA44
01559 384832

**S V Owen MNIMH**
➕ ⊕ ❀
Fees: £26–35; Second visit: <£20
Llandrindod Wells LD1
01982 553398

## RHONDDA CYNON TAFF

**Anthony P Morris IRCH**
⭕ ⓝ ❀
Fees: >£55; Second visit: £41–50
Rhondda CF39
01443 687848

## SWANSEA

**Alexandra Martin AMH**
⭕ ❀
Fees: £26–35; Second visit: <£20
Swansea SA2
01792 299778

## WREXHAM

**T Longhurst MNIMH**
➕ ⊕ ⓝ
Fees: £26–35; Second visit: <£20
Wrexham LL11
01978 364973

# Chinese Herbal Medicine

## CARDIFF

**Pak-Hong Lam RCHM,**
➕ ❀
Fees: <£25
Cardiff CF11
029 2034 3733

**Aileen Oi Leng Yeoh RCHM**
➕ ⊕ ❀
Fees: £36–45; Second visit: <£20
Cardiff CF64
029 2051 2742

## MONMOUTHSHIRE

**Ann Charlton MNIMH, RCHM**
➕ ⭕ ⊕ ❀
Fees: £26–35; Second visit: £21–30
Chepstow NP16
01291 627722

## POWYS

**David Smith RCHM**
➕ ⊕
Fees: £36–45; Second visit: £21–30
Brecon LD3,Hereford HR1
01874 623577

## PEMBROKESHIRE

**Niki Oates RCHM**

✛  ✛  🆖

**Fees:** £36–45; Second visit: <£20
Fishguard SA65,Narberth
SA67,Carmarthen SA31
01348 874384

## SWANSEA

**L A Broom Phd AMH, MNIMH, RCHM**

✛  🔅

Swansea SA3
01792 232144

# Methodology overview

The guide covers complementary therapists who are members of appropriate registration bodies in the fields of acupuncture, homeopathy, osteopathy, chiropractic, and herbal medicine including western herbal medicine, Chinese herbal medicine and Ayurvedic medicine. In the recent House of Lords Select Committee Report on CAM, these therapies were identified by the Lords as being professionally organised, with some scientific evidence of effectiveness and recognised systems of training.

**Establishing scope of research and data collection**

Consumer research was carried out to identify what information people would like to have when they are looking for a complementary therapist. On the basis of this research, questionnaires were constructed in consultation with the Department of Complementary Medicine at the University of Exeter whose specific role was to use their knowledge of orthodox and complementary medicine and their skills of questionnaire design to advise on the content, wording and layout of the questionnaire.

The questionnaires were then circulated to leading institutions and organisations including the Department of Health, the Foundation for Integrated Medicine, NHS Alliance as well as leading institutions and the organisations represented in the guide. In the case of osteopathy and chiropractic, consultation was largely through the leading practitioner bodies.

Questionnaires were then sent to members of the relevant professional organisations. All therapists represented in the guide belong to organisations that maintain a register of members, set educational standards and require members to graduate from an accredited college, run a continuing professional development programme, require members to abide by codes of conduct, ethics and practice, run a complaints system and disciplinary procedure accessible to the public and require members to take out professional indemnity insurance.

The bodies represented in the guide are as follows:

| | |
|---|---|
| **Acupuncture** | British Acupuncture Council |
| | Acupuncture Association of Chartered Physiotherapists |
| | British Medical Acupuncture Society |
| **Homeopathy** | Faculty of Homeopathy |
| | Society of Homeopaths |
| **Osteopathy** | General Osteopathic Council |
| **Chiropractic** | General Chiropractic Council |
| **Herbal Medicine** | National Institute of Medical Herbalists |
| | Association of Master Herbalists |
| | International Register of Consultant Herbalists |
| | Register of Chinese Herbal Medicine |
| | Ayurvedic Medical Association UK |

All herbal bodies represented in the guide are members of the European Herbal Practitioners Association.

It was recognised at the outset that it would be difficult to match previous work by Dr Foster to define 'best practice' in health care, for example, those based on available evidence (eg intervention rates for hospital births) and existing targets in health care (eg door-to-needle time for thrombolysis of 30 minutes). This is because this kind of evidence base is not generally available for complementary medicine, which is still essentially based on tradition and convention. However, in this book we have looked at one important safety issue – whether or not practitioners involve your GP in your care. In looking at this we have chosen to look at practice rather than policy – in other words, how often do practitioners actually communicate with GPs. It is possible therefore that a practitioner may have rarely contacted GPs because the practitioner has never regarded it as necessary. However, we believe that practitioners should, as a matter of course, assuming the patient consents, inform the GP of any therapies provided as this acts as an important safety check. This helps reduce the risk that the practitioner fails to incorrectly diagnose the problems facing the patient. The GP, who will often have a fuller understanding of the patient's background, is a valuable additional check to diagnosis and should always be informed. In practice, relatively few therapists always contact GPs. In this book we have indicated all practitioners who have written to GPs for a significant number of their patients (at least a third) in the last six months.

# Glossary

**AACP: The Acupuncture Association of Chartered Physiotherapists**
Provides training and sets standards for the use of acupuncture by
chartered physiotherapists. It has a strict code of practice, and the
members of the AACP are required to keep up with a stated minimum
number of training hours per year in order to remain on the register.

**Acupuncture points**  Points along the meridians which acupuncturists
claim can be manipulated to aid particular conditions and diseases by
freeing the flow of the body's vital energy.

**Acute condition**  Condition of short duration that starts quickly and
has severe symptoms, eg a cold.

**Adjustment**  Specific directional thrust manoeuvre or application of
force applied to a subluxated vertebra aiming to reduce and/or correct
the vertebral misalignment, thus improving the surrounding affected
tissues and body functions.

**Aggravation of symptoms**  Reaction to taking a homeopathic remedy
where the patient's symptoms from a current or past illness are
temporarily magnified. The aggravation is usually brief and mild and is
followed by a noticeable improvement of the patient's condition.

**Alignment**  The joint surfaces of the body are shaped specifically to
articulate at the correct angle, but the bones can move out of their
proper position; this can lead to problems in the musculo-skeletal
system, including irritation and compression of the nerves.

**Antimicrobial**  Substance that inhibits the growth of microorganisms
including bacteria, viruses and fungi.

**Antioxidant**  Compound that prevents a substance reacting with
oxygen in the air. This is important in food preservation, and is used in
the formulation of paints and plastics. Natural antioxidants, such as
vitamin E and beta-carotene, reduce damage to living cells caused by
toxins.

**Articulation**  Relationships between all types of tissues in the body,
including between bones. According to the founder of osteopathy, Dr

Andrew Taylor-Still, a disturbed articulation (eg after trauma, infection, surgery) will lead to disease in the tissues influenced by this articulation.

**Auricular acupuncture (also known as ear acupuncture)** As the ear has a rich nerve and blood supply, it is believed it may have connections all over the body and can therefore be stimulated on certain acupuncture points to correspond with various parts and organs of the body.

**AMA: The Ayurvedic Medical Association** The professional body for qualified Ayurvedic practitioners in the UK, it holds malpractice insurance and maintains a Code of Ethics.

**Bone density scan** Measures the amount of bone in a particular site, usually the lower part of the spine, the hip, the forearm or the heel. Most scanning machines use narrow beams of X-rays but some use ultrasound instead.

**Bone density** Amount of mineral in bones; low bone density is one of many factors that can increase the risk of fracture.

**BAAB: The British Acupuncture Accreditation Board** Independent body set up to harmonise and regulate the training and qualifications of acupuncture practitioners in the UK. Among its purposes of accreditation, it fosters high educational standards, encourages self-improvement and ensures the competence of its graduates.

**BAAC: The British Association of Applied Chiropractic** The professional body for McTimoney-Corley chiropractors in the UK; it holds malpractice insurance and maintains a Code of Practice.

**BAcC: The British Acupuncture Council** Body that represents and governs professionally qualified acupuncturists, maintaining standards of education, ethics, discipline and Codes of Practice to ensure the safety of the public. It also promotes research and enhances the role that traditional acupuncture can play in the maintenance of the public's health and wellbeing.

**BMA: The British Medical Association** Professional association of doctors that represents their interests and provides services for its members. Its functions include being an independent trade union, a scientific and educational body, a publishing house and a limited company, funded mainly by its members. It does not register, discipline or recommend doctors.

**BCA: British Chiropractic Association** The largest professional association for chiropractors in the UK, it aims to promote, encourage and maintain high standards of conduct, practice, education and training within the profession in this country.

**BMAS: The British Medical Acupuncture Society** Association of medical practitioners interested in or practising acupuncture; it provides services not only to those who use acupuncture in hospitals and general practice, but also for dentists and vets.

**Chartered physiotherapist** Physiotherapist who is a member of a professional regulating body, and has the correct level of education, knowledge and experience needed to treat patients.

**CSP: The Chartered Society of Physiotherapists** Supports and promotes its members and their profession. Nearly every fully trained physiotherapist in the UK is a member of this society and members are bound by a strict professional and ethical code.

**Chronic condition** Persistent or recurring condition, eg eczema; the condition itself may or may not be severe, often starts gradually and changes will be slow.

**Chronic degenerative disorder** Umbrella description for a wide variety of conditions in which there is increased deterioration of the structure and/or function of the body.

**Constitution** General condition of the body, especially with reference to its liability to certain diseases.

**CPD: Continuing Professional Development** Further study relevant to the complementary therapists' profession that most complementary therapy bodies encourage their members to undertake. This is in the form of seminars, research, other training, etc. Most therapists risk expulsion from their professional association if they do not undertake a certain minimum number of hours of CPD.

**Contraindication** Any factor in a patient's condition that makes it unwise to pursue a certain line of treatment. For example, an attack of pneumonia in a patient would be a strong contraindication against the use of a general anaesthetic.

**Decoction** Preparation made by boiling various plants or herbs in water and then straining the fluid in order to drink it.

**'Descending' herbs** Both herbs and food have energetic actions and each substance also exhibits a particular direction of action within the system. Herbalists believe that descending herbs allow the *Qi*, or energy, to circulate downwards through the body by acting as diuretics and laxatives, for example. Ascending herbs would have the opposite effect on the system and include emetics, tonics, detoxifiers and expectorants.

**Detoxification** Process whereby toxic substances are removed or toxic effects neutralised.

**Dilution** The step-by-step process of repeated dilution and shaking by which homeopathic medicines are prepared, which theoretically makes them capable of stimulating the body's own defence system. Homeopaths claim that the effect of homeopathic medicines is strengthened dramatically upon successive dilutions and vigorous shaking between each dilution.

**'Direct' technique** A category of Osteopathic Manipulation Technique (OMT) procedure whereby the osteopath moves 'problem' or 'tight' tissues towards the areas of tightness or restricted movement.

**Doshas** In Ayurvedic thought, all of life, including people, is made up of a combination of three energy-elements which describe your personality and constitution: air (called *vayu* or *vata*), fire (called *pitta*), and water (called *kapha*). Ayurvedic practitioners believe your overall *dosha* will be made up of all three elements but that one element will normally dominate.

**Double-blind, placebo-controlled study** Study in which one group of participants receives the active substance being tested and the other group receives a placebo designed to appear like the real thing. Neither the participants nor the researchers know who is getting the real treatment or the placebo, making it a 'double-blind' experiment; this prevents the researchers from unintentionally biasing their evaluation of the results or influencing the participants' responses.

**Electro-acupuncture** Procedure of selecting and applying special electrical currents to specific acupuncture points situated on the meridian lines, or situated on the outer surface of the ear, in order to correct energy imbalances, release specific neuro-transmitters and promote a return to health.

**EHPA: The European Herbal Practitioners Association**
Represents professional herbal practitioners throughout the EU. It works to protect the rights of practitioners and consumers of herbal medicine within the EU and sets standards of training, practice and quality of herbal medicine.

**GCC: The General Chiropractic Council** Operates a scheme of statutory regulation for chiropractors, similar to the arrangements that cover other health professionals, and is also responsible for setting the standards of chiropractic education, practice and conduct. It is now a criminal offence to describe oneself as any sort of chiropractor without being registered with the GCC.

**GMC: The General Medical Council** The GMC has strong legal powers designed to protect the patient, and is responsible for establishing a register of qualified practitioners, defining their qualifications and appointing examiners. All practising medical doctors in the UK must be registered with the GMC.

**GOsC: The General Osteopathic Council** The GOsC is responsible for regulating, developing and promoting osteopathy in the UK. Since the legislation of May 2000 when the GOsC's statutory register came into force, all osteopaths must register with the Council in order to call themselves osteopaths or to legally practise osteopathy in the UK.

**Healing crisis** Severe symptom, or set of symptoms, that may appear quite suddenly or unexpectedly during the course of natural healing. According to the principles of herbal medicine this is the body's way of rebalancing, and can be temporarily uncomfortable. (Some also refer to this process as detoxifying.)

**Healing reaction** May include resurfacing of symptoms suffered by the patient in previous illnesses and generally appear a few hours or days after starting a homeopathic remedy. Homeopaths regard such reactions as a necessary part of healing and as proof that the chosen homeopathic remedy is the correct one, claiming that improvement soon follows.

**Healing response** TCM proponents believe that acupuncture stimulates the body's internal regulatory system by sending messages to the brain, which releases pain-killing chemicals and encourages the body to generate its own process of natural healing.

**High-velocity** The most common of the 150 chiropractic techniques used is the low-amplitude, high-velocity thrust, involving a tiny calculated movement in the joint at high speed. The purpose of the high-velocity technique is to overcome the conscious patient's protective reflex mechanism that would prevent the separation and movement of the joints.

**Holistic** Chiropractic focuses on what has become known internationally as 'wellness' care, concentrating on maintaining and improving health rather than just treating pain and disease. It describes an approach to patient care in which the physical, mental, and social factors in the patient's condition are taken into account, rather than just the diagnosed disease.

**Holistic medicine** An approach to therapy which focuses on the use of natural substances, and in which all the physical, mental, and social aspects of the patient's life are taken into account in understanding and curing their illness as opposed to merely treating their symptoms.

**'Indirect' technique** A category of Osteopathic Manipulation Technique (OMT) procedure whereby the osteopath pushes the 'tight' tissues away from the area of restricted movement, in the opposite direction to the muscle's resistance, until the tight muscle relaxes.

**Imaging reports** Includes diagnostic procedures such as X-rays, MRI scans, bone density scans, mammograms, CT scans, etc.

**Immuno-suppressing drugs** Reduce the body's resistance to infection and other foreign agents by suppressing the activity of the immune system.

**Infusion** Simplest mode of herbal preparation; simmering water is poured on the active ingredients, then it is infused for a short time before being drunk.

**Laser acupuncture** Using light energy, an infra-red laser is used to exert a photo-chemical action at the cellular level of the tissue. Acupuncturists believe this laser light stimulates any abnormal tissue to activate its normal inter-cellular radiation and thus restart the healing process.

**Low-velocity** Chiropractic technique using light force adjustments, which are swift and dextrous movements to adjust each joint.

**Manipulation** Manual procedure that involves a directed thrust to move a joint past its physiological range of motion.

**MCA: The McTimoney Chiropractic Association**  Professional organisation that supports qualified practitioners of McTimoney chiropractic and supplies a code of professional and ethical conduct, ensuring that the required standards are maintained.

**MCA: The Medicines Control Agency**  The executive agency of the Department of Health which aims to safeguard public health by ensuring that all medicines on the UK market meet appropriate standards of safety, quality and efficacy.

**Meridians**  Practitioners of Traditional Chinese Medicine believe these to be special pathways or channels that *Qi*, the energy force in our bodies, travels along.

**Mobilisation**  Movement applied singularly or repetitively within the range of joint motion, without imparting a thrust or impulse, with the goal of restoring joint mobility.

**Moxabustion**  Process whereby moxa – a dried herb, usually the species mugwort – is burned either directly on the skin, or just above the skin, over acupuncture points. Acupuncturists believe that when lit, moxa burns slowly and provides penetrating heat that can enter the meridians to influence *Qi* and blood flow.

**MRI (magnetic resonance imaging) scan**  Radiology technique that uses magnetism, radio waves and a computer to produce images of body structures. It is particularly useful for examining the central nervous system and musculo-skeletal system and can be used for the noninvasive diagnosis and treatment planning of a wide range of diseases.

**Nerve irritation**  When a nerve is trapped as a result of some structure putting pressure upon the nerve root. If the vertebrae misalign slightly, they may cause the nerves to be irritated or compressed or stretched. Symptoms include pain, numbness, tingling and weakness.

**Nerve root entrapment**  Compression of spinal nerves at the intervertebral foramina, the natural openings between vertebrae through which the nerves run, may result in mechanical disorders of the spine. Entrapment of nerve roots may result in weakness, pain and numbness in the affected area.

**Nervous system**  The vast network of cells specialised to carry information in the form of nerve impulses to and from all parts of the body, in order to bring about bodily activity. The brain and spinal cord together form the central nervous system and the remaining nervous tissue is known as the peripheral nervous system.

**NSAIDs: Non-steroidal anti-inflammatory drugs**  These act both as analgesics to relieve pain and as inhibitors of inflammation. Aspirin is a classic example, but newer compounds such as ibuprofen have been formulated with the aim of producing fewer side-effects, particularly those relating to the gastro-intestinal tract.

**Pancha Karma**  Purgative and detoxifying procedure designed to eliminate toxins that accumulate in the body. In Sanskrit *pancha* means five and *karma* means actions, thus *pancha karma* therapies are five healing modalities unique to Ayurveda. Preliminary procedures include a special diet, massage and steam bath.

**Passive stretching**  Stretching of soft tissues including muscles, etc., induced by someone other than the patients themselves.

**Periosteal acupuncture**  Involves gently tapping areas of the bone near the skin's surface and is useful when a patient does not like needles.

**Phytotherapy (also known as Herbal Medicine)**  The use of plants and plant products for their healing properties to promote better health. Western herbal medicines are prepared from domestically grown plants or collected from the wild.

**Placebo**  Formed from inactive substances, this 'medication' was traditionally given to patients to pacify them without actually benefiting them. Nowadays they are mainly used in controlled studies to determine the efficacy of drugs.

**Protection of title**  Statutorily recognised right of therapists to call themselves by a particular professional title (such as chiropractor). Such protection of title means that any practitioner not registered with a statutory regulated association does not legally have the right to practise that profession.

**Pulse**  A Chinese herbalist takes the pulses from three different areas on each wrist. From the right, they get a reading on the lung, kidney and spleen *yang*, from the left, they get a reading on the heart, liver and kidney *ying*.

**Pulse diagnosis**  Considered the most important part of an Ayurvedic examination, the practitioner performs the diagnosis by placing three fingers on the radial pulse just below the patient's wrist. Each of the three fingers senses one of the three *doshas*; each *dosha* has five sub-*doshas* which have a particular location and function. An imbalance in any one of these can be the precursor of disease.

**Qi** (pronounced Chee) In TCM, Q*i* is believed to be the essence that gives the world and the individual body life. Q*i* moves blood through the body and energises the organs. This energy is derived partly from our genetic make-up, partly from our breathing, and partly from the food we eat. Signs of deficiency are believed to be fatigue, shortness of breath, weak pulse and a pale tongue.

**Randomised controlled trials** A study involving two groups, one treatment group and one control group. The treatment group receives the treatment under investigation, and the control group receives either no treatment or some standard default treatment. Patients are randomly assigned to all groups.

**Referred Pain** Pain felt in a part of the body some distance from its cause; the pain is transmitted along the nerve pathways.

**RCHM: The Register of Chinese Herbal Medicine** Body that regulates the practice of Chinese Herbal Medicine (CHM) in the UK. The Register is a member of the EHPA, the umbrella organisation working towards statutory self-regulation for herbal medicine in Britain.

**Segmental acupuncture** Used to treat internal organs such as the stomach or bladder by inserting needles into areas of the skin or muscle that share the nerve supply that originates from the same level of the spinal cord as the area being treated.

**Seven star hammer** A probe used by acupuncturists to tap over affected areas to stimulate the circulation of Q*i* to relieve many conditions including aches and pains and skin conditions.

**Shen** *Jing, Shen*, and Q*i* describe three concepts of energy in TCM. *Shen* is known as the psyche, mind, or spirit; it is said to be the driving energy behind activities that take place in the mental, spiritual, or creative planes. It is thought that weakened *shen* often manifests itself as anxiety, mild depression, or chronic restlessness.

**Stagnation** When the circulation of Q*i*, blood, or food through the body becomes hampered due to disease, stress or emotional dysfunction.

**Statutory regulation** The primary benefit of effective regulation is that it protects the public. Within a body that has statutory regulation, only practitioners registered with the body and who meet the body's regulations are legally allowed to use that body's title. Unlike voluntary regulation, it has the force of law to ensure its aims are met (see p17).

**Statutory self-regulation** Implies a professional organisation has statutory recognition of its status as the official body to regulate and discipline its own members (see p18).

**Structural damage** Includes the fracture of bones, dislocation or subluxation of spinal joints, and the tearing of joint capsules, discs and other connective tissue, including supporting ligaments, tendons, muscles, nerves and blood vessels.

**Symptomatic pain relief** Relief of pain from one's symptoms.

**TCM** Abbreviation for Traditional Chinese Medicine.

**Tinctures** Herbal tinctures are traditional herbal preparations usually dispensed as alcohol-based liquid medicines.

**'Toggles'** In McTimoney chiropractic, bones are never forced into place, but by adjusting with a very rapid thrust and immediate release, the bone 'toggles' towards its correct position. In a swift thrust known as the 'toggle torque recoil' technique, the practitioner uses one hand as a 'hammer' and the other as a 'nail'. This swift movement is designed to free the joint and ease tension in the surrounding muscles.

**Traction** Application of a pulling force, especially as a means of counteracting the natural tension in the tissues surrounding a broken bone, to produce correct alignment.

**Trigger point acupuncture** A needle is inserted into the overlying skin of a trigger point (painful or tender points in the muscles, tendons, ligaments or on the skin) in order to 'deactivate' it.

***Tui na*** Pronounced 'twee-nah'. This is a form of acupressure that uses many different strokes that are applied to acupressure points, channels and muscle groups. It is believed that the strokes and techniques stimulate an exchange of *Qi* between the practitioner and the patient.

**Voluntary regulation** The primary benefit of effective regulation is that it protects the public. Within a body that has voluntary regulation, the practitioners are voluntarily registered by the body within the body (see p17).

**Voluntary self-regulation** Refers to controls exercised over therapists that are freely chosen by the profession itself and consolidated through the licensing and registration procedures that are legally required of local authorities (see p17).

***Yin(g)/Yang*** In traditional Chinese thought, these are the two elements that form the universe, and are present in every living thing, ideally existing in harmony. *Yin* represents 'dark', 'negative' or 'cold', *yang* represents 'sun light', 'positive' or 'hot'. Traditional Chinese practitioners believe that if one or other of these components is thrown out of balance, it can lead to illness. Herbal medicines are classified according to the *yin* or *yang* component they characterise.

**Yoga** In Ayurveda, yoga means union, and is a traditional system of healing the mind and body. It is believed that yoga cleanses the body of toxins, improving muscle tone and blood circulation.

# Index

homeopathy x, xi, 5, 6, 7, 10, 12, 16, 17,
50, 58-82, 148-9
homeostasis 6
hormonal imbalances 170
hospices 5
hospitals
hot flushes 140
Houghton, P. J. 131n
House of Lords Select Committee on
Science and Technology Sixth Report:
complementary and alternative
medicine (2000) ix, x, 10-11, 14, 16,
17, 20, 21, 53, 492
Hutchful, Tim 118-19
hyperactivity 78, 79
hypercholesterolemia 132
hypertension see high blood pressure
hypnosis 7, 9
hypnotherapy 5, 10, 17

immune system 50, 63, 141, 164, 165,
171
immuno-suppressant drugs 31, 130
Indian head massage 124
indigestion 140, 156
infection 12, 50, 51, 74-5, 141
infertility 30, 34
influenza 50, 51, 62
injuries 60
inoculation programmes 3
insomnia 132, 140, 141
insulin 60, 130
insurance xiii, 17, 22
see also under individual therapies
integrated (integrative) medicine ix, 6-7
intermittent claudication 132

International Register of Consultant
Herbalists 135, 150, 151, 154, 493
Internet 4
iridology 11, 12, 142
irritable bowel syndrome 5, 132, 141

Jackson-Maine, Peter 142-3
Jarrold, Jane 50-51
joint disorders 32, 102, 103-4, 123
Journal of the American Medical Association
2n, 15
Journal of the Royal Society of Medicine 8

Kanpo (Japanese medicine) 127
kapha 170
keyhole surgery 3
kinesiology 11, 172
knee osteoarthritis 14, 84
knee pain 14, 119

labour 7, 61
see also childbirth
lachesis 65
laetrile 5
Lancet, The 15n, 21, 61
laser acupuncture 41
LaStone therapy 12
Lavenant, Maurice 158-9
Law Society 25
Leckridge, Dr Bob 21
lifestyle 4, 6, 64, 88, 103, 125, 128, 142,
144, 157, 160, 170, 171
Linde, K. 131n
Lively, April 148-9
Liverpool: homeopathic hospital 58, 82
Local Health Group 76
London College of Osteopathic Medicine
95
lymphatic system 173

McTimoney, John 103
McTimoney Chiropractic Association
(MCA) 103, 116, 117, 126
McTimoney Chiropractic College 103
McTimoney technique 103, 106, 111,
114, 124
McTimoney-Corley technique 103
magnetic bracelets 14
malaria 59
manipulation 9, 22, 86, 88, 95, 102, 104,
109, 111, 113
marmatherapy 173, 178, 179
Marylebone Health Centre, London 7
massage
Indian head 124
tui na 40
massage therapy 5, 7, 10, 16, 83
mastitis 77
ME 8, 170
measles 141, 156
medical history 23